Common Clinical Presentations

Common Clinical Presentations

Christopher Naugler, BScH, MSc, MD, FCFP, CCFP, FRCPC

Brush
Education Inc.

24 25 26 27 28 5 4 3 2 1

Brush Education is located in amiskwaciwâskahikan, Edmonton, Alberta, within Treaty 6 territory and Métis Nation of Alberta Region 4, and on the traditional and ancestral territories of the Nêhiyawak, Denesuliné, Nakota Sioux, and Saulteaux Peoples.

This book is available in print, PDF, and Global Certified Acessible™ EPUB formats.

Brush Education Inc.
www.brusheducation.ca
contact@brusheducation.ca

Cover design: Dean Pickup; Cover images: © Chingyunsong | Dreamstime.com
Interior design: Carol Dragich, Dragich Design

Library and Archives Canada Cataloguing in Publication

Title: Common clinical presentations / Christopher Naugler, BScH, MSc, MD, FCFP, CCFP, FRCPC.
Names: Naugler, Christopher T. (Christopher Terrance), 1967- author.
Description: Includes bibliographical references and index.
Identifiers: Canadiana (print) 20230526632 | Canadiana (ebook) 20230526675 | ISBN 9781550599428 (softcover) | ISBN 9781550599442 (EPUB) | ISBN 9781550599435 (PDF)
Subjects: LCSH: Physical diagnosis—Handbooks, manuals, etc. | LCSH: Clinical competence—Handbooks, manuals, etc. | LCGFT: Handbooks and manuals.
Classification: LCC RC76 .N38 2024 | DDC 616.07/54—dc23

We acknowledge the support of the Government of Canada
Nous reconnaissons l'appui du gouvernement du Canada | Canada

Acknowledgements

This book is an adaptation of *Strategies for the MCCQE Part II* (Brush Education, 2019). We would like to acknowledge the work of the following contributors to *Strategies*:

Marcia Abbott, BSc, BN, MD, FRCPC, DRCPSC, MIAC

Pavandeep Gill, MD, FRCPC

Alexandra Kirvan, MD, CCFP

Davinder Sidhu, BSc, BPharm, LLB/JD, MD, FRCPC

Amy Thommasen, MD, FRCPC

Researchers: Irene Ma, MSc; Leonard Nguyen, PhD; Vijay S. Kandalam, PhD

Contents

About this resource

This resource is a guide to patient presentations that clinicians and other health care professionals commonly see. If you are a student, it provides essential information for mastering clinical skills. If you are a practicing clinician or health care professional, it is backup information for navigating common patient encounters.

Order of clinical presentations

The clinical presentations are grouped into categories, where appropriate, and organized alphabetically, as shown on the contents page. Categories capture presentations that share a key feature. For example, presentations whose key feature is bleeding are grouped under *bleeding*. Use the contents page to browse categories and locate particular presentations, or look up particular presentations in the index.

Standard sections in each clinical presentation

This resource unpacks 169 common clinical presentations.

The presentations break out key information in standard sections, organized as follows:

Differential diagnosis

This lists common entities in the differential diagnosis for the presentation, and common clinical evidence for each entity. Most presentations include this section, but it is not relevant for all presentations (e.g., burns).

Keys to patient encounter

Key concerns: These are listed first, where helpful, to help focus the patient encounter.

Airway and hemodynamic status: This lists first steps in presentations that have the potential to require emergency management (e.g., hemoptysis). In presentations that are known emergencies (e.g., hypothermia), this is replaced by a section on steps in emergency management.

History: This targets key information about the present illness and past medical history, and other information relevant to the particular presentation (e.g., surgeries, procedures, medications, allergies, family history, and social history).

Physical exam: This targets systems and maneuvers relevant to the particular presentation.

Investigations: These include labs and imaging for general diagnosis, and notes on investigations for specific suspected entities.

Management: This includes notes on steps for diagnosed entities and in cases of uncertain diagnosis.

Patient encounter basics

Overall goal: find evidence, use evidence

Your overall goal is to gather evidence, and use this evidence to focus on what is relevant and useful to the individual case at hand.

Always take these first steps

Always:

- Introduce yourself to the patient.
- Ask the patient for consent to interview and examine them. Be aware that consent may depend on culturally sensitive care, which the patient may not clarify until you ask.
- Offer the patient a chaperone for the encounter.
- Wash your hands.

Use open-ended questions for symptom history

Use open-ended questions, as opposed to yes-no questions, to let the patient tell you about their symptoms. This is more effective than going through a laundry list of possible symptoms. Make eye contact with the patient as they talk and listen carefully. Consider offering a summary of what they tell you, and use this as a basis to ask for clarification or more details.

Focus on diagnostic evidence in physical exams

Approach physical exams with as much focus as possible. Consider what evidence you have in hand from the history. Let this information guide the physical exam, so that you pursue diagnostic manoeuvres relevant to the specific patient.

Focus on relevant investigations

Order investigations that narrow the differential diagnosis, based on evidence from the history and/or the physical exam. Don't order every possible investigation.

Tailor management to the patient

Provide next steps and information that target the situation of the particular patient. This means you need to ask the patient for relevant details about their situation, such as work, recreation, and dietary routines. Think of these details as a way to begin a conversation with the patient about changes to their routines that could help them.

For example, in cases where changes to diet and exercise are relevant:

- Ask what the patient ate yesterday for breakfast, lunch, and supper. Use this to personalize guidelines on dietary changes they need to make.
- Ask what the patient did for exercise last week. Discuss short-term goals with the patient: What could the patient do next week to exercise every day? (For example, when could the patient fit in a 30-minute walk?)

In cases where smoking cessation is relevant:

- Express your concern with the patient's continued smoking. Ask what experience they have had with methods to quit. Provide information about other methods. Ask if there is a method they would like to pursue now, and describe the support you can offer them.

In cases where stress reduction is relevant:

- Ask the patient for an example of a stressful situation they encountered last week. What steps could help relieve that situation?

Respond appropriately to patient needs and challenges

Patients who require culturally sensitive care

Any patient encounter may engage the need for culturally sensitive care. When you ask permission to interview and examine a patient, a refusal from the patient may stem from this.

When a patient withholds consent, engage in a straightforward, respectful conversation about the patient's expectations for care. For example:

- Express confidence in your ability to help the patient.
- Describe specific procedures and investigations you may need to perform in the context of the patient's case.
- Ask the patient how to proceed with their permission (e.g., by providing a same-sex doctor).
- Do your best to meet the patient's expectations while protecting the patient's health and safety.

Patients who are reluctant to talk

Some patients may show reluctance to talk. In these situations:

- Acknowledge the patient's reluctance to talk (e.g., "It seems like you are having some difficulty talking about your health concern.").
- Offer empathy and reassurance (e.g., "Some problems are hard to talk about. It's okay to feel unsettled. I want to help you, not judge you.").
- Express confidence in your ability to help the patient.
- Show your ability to listen respectfully: allow the patient to talk at their own pace.

Abusive patients

Some patients may be angry. In these situations:

- Remain calm.
- Acknowledge the patient's anger.
- Express confidence in your ability to help the patient.
- Ensure your safety and the safety of others. It may be appropriate to assess for homicidal ideation (e.g., "When someone is as upset and angry as you are, they sometimes think about harming others. What thoughts have you had about harming others?"). Seek an emergent admission to a psychiatry ward in the case of homicidal ideation.
- Offer clear next steps. For example, state that you need the patient to answer some questions, so you can better understand their situation.

Noncompliant patients

The health concerns of some patients may stem from noncompliance with prescribed medications.

For example, uncontrolled diabetes can contribute to a variety of presenting problems, such as incontinence, hypertension, and diplopia. Patients may have uncontrolled diabetes because they are not taking their medication, due to forgetfulness or financial constraints.

In any noncompliant patient, seek the reasons for noncompliance.

- In forgetful patients, discuss possible strategies to help with compliance. For example, how could they set up reminders for themselves? How well do they cope with day-to-day tasks in general? What family or friends could they call on for assistance? In patients who are not coping and who do not have social supports, consider community supports such as home care services.
- In patients who cannot afford their medications, express empathy and seek details about the patient's situation. Consider referring the patient to social service agencies, which can help with financial assistance and skills such as budgeting.

ABDOMINAL PRESENTATIONS

Abdominal distention

Differential diagnosis

ASCITES

ASCITES IN GENERAL

Signs and symptoms: normal bowel sounds; "shifting dullness" on percussion of the abdomen

Investigations: abdominal US to detect ascitic fluid

Exudative: low serum-to-ascites albumin gradient (e.g., peritoneal carcinomatosis)

MALIGNANCY

Signs and symptoms: history of abdominal or pelvic malignancy; palpable abdominal mass; enlarged lymph nodes

Investigations: ascites specimen for cytology and culture (the culture rules out bacterial infection)

Transudative ascites: high serum-to-ascites albumin gradient (e.g., portal hypertension)

PORTAL HYPERTENSION

Causes of portal hypertension include CHF, liver disease, and pancreatitis.

CONGESTIVE HEART FAILURE

Signs and symptoms: severe shortness of breath; elevated JVP; edema in the abdomen and legs; pink phlegm; heart murmurs and extra cardiac sounds

History of heart disease or risk factors for heart disease (diabetes, hypertension, hyperlipidemia, and smoking) or hepatic vein thrombosis (Budd-Chiari syndrome)

Investigations: chest x-ray to detect pulmonary edema; NT-proBNP level; echocardiogram imaging to distinguish forms of HF; cardiac stress testing, either with exercise or pharmacological agent

LIVER DISEASE

Signs and symptoms: jaundice; abdominal pain, swelling; palpable, tender liver; swelling in the legs and ankles; systemic symptoms (anorexia, weight loss, weakness, fatigue); itching; easy bruising

History of chronic alcohol abuse; chronic infection with HBV or HCV, or risk factors for these infections (unprotected sex,

IV drug abuse, blood transfusions, tattoos, body piercings, imprisonment, workplace exposure to body fluids); hemochromatosis; autoimmune conditions; α_1-antitrypsin deficiency; primary biliary cirrhosis; CHF

Investigations: tests for liver enzymes (elevated AST, ALT) and liver function (elevated bilirubin; possible abnormal PT/INR); viral serologic tests to detect HBV, HCV; Doppler US; CT scan; MRI; transient elastography; liver biopsy

PANCREATITIS

Signs and symptoms: constant upper abdominal pain that radiates to the back (sitting up and leaning forward may reduce the pain; pain occurs with coughing, vigorous movement, deep breathing); shortness of breath; nausea, vomiting; hypotension; fever; jaundice; abdominal tenderness

History of gallstones or chronic alcoholism (usual); hyperlipidemia; hypercalcemia; change of medication

Investigations: serum amylase and lipase (levels are ≥ 3 times ULN; elevated lipase indicates pancreatic damage); possible elevated calcium; possible elevated cholesterol; possible elevated ALT (this indicates associated liver inflammation); chest x-ray (this may show left-sided or bilateral pleural effusion; atelectasis); abdominal x-ray (this may show calcifications within pancreatic ducts, calcified gallstones, or localized ileus of a segment of small intestine); US

BOWEL DILATATION

Mechanical obstruction (e.g., adhesions, volvulus)

Signs and symptoms (in general): abnormal bowel sounds (increased in early bowel obstruction, decreased in late bowel obstruction); palpable hernia or bowel obstruction

History of abdominal or pelvic surgery; inflammatory bowel disease (ulcerative colitis or Crohn disease); hernia (abdominal, femoral, or inguinal)

Paralytic conditions (e.g., toxic megacolon, neuropathy)

TOXIC MEGACOLON

Signs and symptoms: fever, shock, decreased bowel sounds; history of inflammatory bowel disease, colonic infection (*C. difficile*)

Investigations: elevated WBCs

NEUROPATHY

Examples of diseases with neuropathic effects that can lead to bowel dilation include scleroderma and diabetes.

OTHER

Abdominal mass

Signs and symptoms: abdominal pain, change in bowel habits, constitutional symptoms (fever, weight loss, night sweats), palpable abdominal mass

Investigations: US, CT scan

Irritable bowel syndrome[1]

Irritable bowel syndrome is commonly diagnosed by applying the Rome criteria.

Signs and symptoms (Rome criteria): at least 2 symptoms, present for ≥ 1 day/week for ≥ 3 months

> Symptoms: pain associated with 1) defecation, 2) change of stool frequency, and/or 3) change in stool consistency

Organomegaly (e.g., hepatomegaly)

Signs and symptoms (in general): palpable liver or spleen

Investigations: US

Pelvic mass (e.g., ovarian cancer)

OVARIAN CANCER

Signs and symptoms: postmenopausal female (more common); asymptomatic in early stage (usual); abdominal bloating, discomfort, distention (ascites); ovarian or pelvic mass; urinary urgency, frequency; abnormal vaginal bleeding; fatigue; GI symptoms (nausea, heartburn, diarrhea, constipation, early satiety); shortness of breath

Investigations: transvaginal and abdominal US; CA 125 blood test; pelvic/abdominal CT scan; analysis of ascitic fluid; biopsy

Keys to patient encounter

Key concern

Differentiate ascites from bowel obstruction.

History

HISTORY OF PRESENT ILLNESS

Ask when the abdominal distention started, how constant it is, and what associated symptoms the patient has.

Examples of characteristic symptoms include:

Irritable bowel syndrome: pain with defecation, or with changes in stool frequency or consistency

Liver disease: jaundice, systemic symptoms, and swollen legs

Abdominal or pelvic mass: palpable mass with changes in bowel habits

PAST MEDICAL HISTORY

Ask about heart disease, liver disease, and pancreatitis (these suggest ascites); cancer and bowel surgery (these suggest bowel obstruction); and scleroderma and diabetes (these suggest bowel dilation).

Ask about irritable bowel syndrome (relevant to functional bloating, which is diagnosed in patients who do not meet the criteria for irritable bowel syndrome, but have had a recurrent feeling of bloating or visible distention for at least 3 days per month for at least 3 months).

Ask about psychosocial distress, depression, and anxiety.

Physical exam

Abdominal: Look for masses and ascites.

Cardiovascular: Auscultate the heart for murmurs and extra sounds.

DRE: Look for masses.

Pelvic: Look for masses.

Investigations

CBC

Celiac serology

Liver function (see *Notes on labs and assessments*)

Abdominal x-ray with 3 views of the abdomen

Abdominal US

OTHER INVESTIGATIONS

Order other tests if a specific diagnosis is suspected from the history and physical exam.

Small intestinal bacterial overgrowth: hydrogen breath test following a carbohydrate load; endoscopy and biopsy if warranted

Ascites: paracentesis (cytology for tumor cells; cell count and culture to rule out spontaneous bacterial peritonitis)
Celiac disease: endoscopy and biopsy

Management

Patients with bowel obstruction require emergency referral to a general surgeon. Patients with functional bloating are managed with exercise, diet, simethicone, and possibly other medications for irritable bowel syndrome. TCAs are frequently used to treat functional abdominal pain.

REFERENCE

1. Lacey B, Mearin F, Chang L, et al. Rome IV functional gastrointestinal disorders: disorders of gut-brain interaction. 4th ed. Vol. 2. Raleigh, NC: Rome Foundation; 2017. Chapter 11, Functional bowel disorders; 1393–1407.

ABDOMINAL PRESENTATIONS

Acute abdominal pain

Differential diagnosis

LOCALIZED PAIN

Upper abdominal region

BILIARY TRACT DISEASE

Signs and symptoms: middle-aged woman (more common); epigastric pain, often after eating (the pain is generally constant and often radiates to the right shoulder); right-sided subcostal pain that is worse on deep inhalation; obesity; history of pregnancy

- Cancer or primary biliary cholangitis: fatigue, weight loss
- Obstructive biliary disease: jaundice

Investigations: albumin, PT/INR, bilirubin (total and direct), ALP, AST, ALT, and γ-glutamyl transferase; US or CT scan to detect gallstones; MRCP to detect bile duct obstruction

PANCREATITIS

Signs and symptoms: constant upper abdominal pain that radiates to the back (sitting up and leaning forward may reduce the pain; pain occurs with coughing, vigorous movement, deep breathing); shortness of breath; nausea, vomiting; hypotension; fever; jaundice; abdominal tenderness

History of gallstones or chronic alcoholism (usual); hyperlipidemia; hypercalcemia; change in medication

Investigations: serum amylase and lipase (levels are ≥ 3 times ULN; elevated lipase indicates pancreatic damage); possible elevated calcium; possible elevated cholesterol; possible elevated ALT (this indicates associated liver inflammation); chest x-ray (this may show left-sided or bilateral pleural effusion; atelectasis); abdominal x-ray (this may show calcifications within pancreatic ducts, calcified gallstones, or localized ileus of a segment of small intestine); US

PEPTIC ULCER DISEASE

Signs and symptoms: constant midepigastric pain, often relieved with eating or with antacids; weight loss

Investigations: *H. pylori*; endoscopy to detect ulcer or inflammation of the gastric lining

GASTRITIS

Signs and symptoms: upper abdominal pain; burning, aching pain; pain that is better or worse with eating; feeling of fullness in the upper abdomen with eating; nausea, vomiting

Risk factors: *H. pylori* infection; regular use of NSAIDs (e.g., acetylsalicylic acid, ibuprofen, naproxen); alcohol use; stress; autoimmune disorders (Hashimoto disease, type 1 diabetes)

GASTROESOPHAGEAL REFLUX DISEASE

Signs and symptoms: burning chest pain radiating into the throat (often with a bitter taste in the mouth or regurgitation of food into the mouth; often worse with lying down; often better with standing up or taking antacids; worse with spicy food, coffee, alcohol, fatty foods, peppermint); acid damage to teeth

Risk factors: obesity, pregnancy

ACUTE HEPATITIS

Signs and symptoms: viral-like illness; abdominal pain; jaundice; palpable, tender liver

History of infection with HAV, HBV, HCV or risk factors for these infections (autoimmune conditions, unprotected sex, IV drug abuse, blood transfusions, tattoos, body piercings, workplace exposure to body fluids); toxic ingestion (e.g., acetaminophen); adverse drug reaction (e.g., change of medication)

HCV: often asymptomatic

Investigations: elevated AST, ALT, bilirubin; abnormal PT/INR; positive viral serologic tests (e.g., HAV, HBV, HCV)

CARDIOTHORACIC CONDITION (REFERRED PAIN)

Signs and symptoms: cough, shortness of breath

Heart exam: extra heart sounds or pericardial rub

Lung exam: abnormal breath sounds, absent breath sounds, or lung rales on auscultation; solid sounds on percussion

Risk factors for heart and lung disease: personal or family history of heart and lung disease; hyperlipidemia; diabetes; smoking; occupational exposure to smoke or other lung irritants

Investigations: elevated cardiac enzymes (e.g., troponin), chest x-ray, ECG

MUSCULOSKELETAL CONDITION

Signs and symptoms: palpable abnormalities and point tenderness in abdominal muscles and spine

History of recent trauma, overuse of abdominal muscles, chronic musculoskeletal problems

Lower abdominal pain

APPENDICITIS

Signs and symptoms: child (often); periumbilical pain that migrates over several days to localize in the right lower quadrant; anorexia; fever; localized pain over the McBurney point on abdominal palpation

Investigations: elevated WBCs; US or CT scan to detect distended appendix

MESENTERIC LYMPHADENITIS

Mesenteric lymphadenitis is a common differential diagnosis with appendicitis.

Signs and symptoms: lower abdominal pain; abdominal tenderness (particularly in the right lower quadrant); fever; diarrhea; nausea, vomiting

Investigations: normal appendix on CT scan (this may be useful in distinguishing mesenteric lymphadenitis from appendicitis)

DIVERTICULITIS

Signs and symptoms: constant left lower quadrant abdominal pain; abdominal tenderness; fever; nausea, vomiting; change in bowel habits (constipation and/or diarrhea)

Risk factors: advanced age, obesity, smoking, poor diet, lack of exercise

Investigations: CT scan

INCARCERATED HERNIA

Signs and symptoms: mass or swelling in the abdomen, groin, or upper thigh; rapid-onset acute pain at the site of the mass or swelling; nausea, vomiting; constipation; history of abdominal surgery (this is common in ventral hernias); obesity (this is a risk factor for ventral hernias)

Investigations: US, CT scan

PELVIC INFLAMMATORY DISEASE

Signs and symptoms: lower abdominal and pelvic pain; pain during intercourse; fever; urinary symptoms; vaginal discharge; irregular menstruation; pelvic tenderness and pain associated with 1 or both adnexa

> History of gonorrhea, chlamydia, or risk factors for them (multiple partners, unprotected sex); IUD; childbirth; gynecologic procedure

Investigations: cultures for gonorrhea and chlamydia; US (this has normal findings)

ECTOPIC PREGNANCY

Signs and symptoms: symptoms of pregnancy and/or positive pregnancy test; pelvic pain; vaginal bleeding; painful intercourse; shoulder pain; palpable tubal mass; pelvic tenderness and pain associated with 1 or both adnexa

> Severe symptom: syncope

Risk factors: previous ectopic pregnancy, PID, pregnancy during IUD use

Investigations (pathognomonic): β-HCG above discriminatory zone (> 1500–2000 mIU/mL; 1500–2000 IU/L) **with** transvaginal US findings of a lack of intrauterine gestational sac, complex (mixed solid and cystic) masses in the adnexa, and free fluid in the cul-de-sac

OVARIAN CONDITION (E.G., TORSION OR RUPTURED CYST)

Signs and symptoms: pelvic pain; pain during intercourse; change in bowel habits; nausea, vomiting; fever; worsening or sudden onset of pain (this may indicate ovarian torsion); pelvic tenderness and pain associated with 1 or both adnexa

Investigations: enlarged ovary or ovaries on pelvic US or laparoscopy

URINARY TRACT INFECTION

Signs and symptoms: frequent urination; painful urination; pelvic pain and/or flank pain; fever; tenderness over the bladder

Investigations: urinalysis, urine culture

RENAL COLIC

Signs and symptoms: colicky flank pain; nausea, vomiting; fever; history of kidney stones (common); extreme tenderness at the costovertebral angle on abdominal examination; hematuria

Investigations: KUB x-ray; ureter US, abdominal CT scan

INFLAMMATORY BOWEL DISEASE

Signs and symptoms: younger than 30 (usually); family history of inflammatory bowel disease; fluctuating symptoms with periods of exacerbation and remission; diarrhea (possibly with nocturnal waking); blood in the stool; abdominal pain; weight loss; fever; fatigue; right lower quadrant and periumbilical pain; extraintestinal manifestations (e.g., uveitis, arthritis)

Crohn disease: right lower quadrant mass, uveitis, arthritis

Investigations: elevated CRP (this suggests active inflammation); fecal calprotectin; colonoscopy with biopsy (this is a standard diagnostic procedure); CT scan or MRI (findings: diagnostic structural changes associated with inflammatory bowel disease)

BOWEL OBSTRUCTION

Signs and symptoms: crampy abdominal pain; nausea, vomiting; change in bowel habits (diarrhea or constipation); abdominal distention; palpable mass; increased bowel sounds (this suggests early obstruction; bowel sounds may be decreased in later obstruction); history of colonic diseases (diverticulitis, colon cancer, inflammatory bowel disease)

Risk factors for adhesions: abdominal surgery

Risk factors for paralytic ileus: narcotic medications, chronic neuromuscular disease, diabetes

Investigations: abdominal x-ray to detect distended bowel with air-fluid levels; CT scan to identify etiology of obstruction

DIFFUSE ABDOMINAL PAIN

Generalized peritonitis

BACTERIAL PERITONITIS

Signs and symptoms: fever, abdominal pain, generalized abdominal tenderness, guarding on physical exam, rebound tenderness, ascites

History of abdominal surgery, diverticulitis, appendicitis, recent colonoscopy, inflammatory bowel disease, PUD, pancreatitis, liver disease, PID, peritoneal dialysis, ovarian cyst or mass

Investigations: elevated WBCs; blood and peritoneal cultures

Ruptured abdominal aortic aneurysm

Signs and symptoms: older than 60 (usual); abdominal, back pain; syncope; pulsatile mass; tachycardia; hypotension

Risk factors: history of smoking; family history of AAA; previous aneurysms; hypertension

Investigations: decreased hemoglobin (this may not arise in the context of acute bleeding); US, CT scan, MRI

Ischemic bowel disease

Signs and symptoms: abrupt-onset abdominal pain; abdominal tenderness; nausea, vomiting; fever; blood in the stool; hypotension (this is possible in acute ischemia); localized tenderness (in early presentations) or peritoneal signs (in late presentations) on abdominal exam

> History of pancreatitis, bowel cancer, inflammatory bowel disease, inherited clotting disorders, diseases of blood vessels (peripheral vascular disease, cardiovascular disease, atherosclerosis), diabetes, OC use

Investigations: PT/INR; PTT; elevated lactate (this is possible with ischemic injury); angiography by CT scan or MRI to detect clots; colonoscopy, laparotomy

Gastroenteritis

Signs and symptoms: abrupt-onset diarrhea; crampy abdominal pain; nausea, vomiting; fever; headache; muscle aches; epigastric tenderness on abdominal examination

Risk factors: exposure to persons with similar symptoms or to large groups of people (common: most cases are viral); eating undercooked or contaminated foods, or raw fluids (these are risk factors for bacterial infection)

Irritable bowel syndrome[1]

Irritable bowel syndrome is commonly diagnosed by applying the Rome criteria.

Signs and symptoms (Rome criteria): at least 2 symptoms, present for ≥ 1 day/week for ≥ 3 months

> Symptoms: pain associated with 1) defecation, 2) change of stool frequency, and/or 3) change in stool consistency

Keys to patient encounter

Airway and hemodynamic status

Check the patient's ABCs. Provide emergency management to stabilize the patient as required.

History

PAIN HISTORY

Ask about the location of the pain, when it started, how constant it is, how long it lasts, where it radiates, its quality (e.g., sharp, dull, throbbing), its severity, and what makes it better and worse.

Examples of characteristic pain include:

Pancreatitis: steady upper abdominal pain, worse with coughing, that radiates to the back

PID, ectopic pregnancy, ovarian conditions: pelvic pain made worse with intercourse

Ruptured AAA: diffuse abdominal and back pain

ASSOCIATED SYMPTOMS

Examples of characteristic symptoms include:

Acute hepatitis: viral-like symptoms with jaundice

Hernia: lower abdominal mass or swelling

Inflammatory disease: urinary symptoms, vaginal discharge, irregular menstruation

UTI: frequent and/or painful urination

In particular, ask about:

Constitutional symptoms: fever, weight loss, night sweats, fatigue

Syncope or presyncope: indicators of a possible surgical emergency

Bleeding: vomiting blood or bleeding from the rectum (bright red blood or black, tarry stools)

PAST MEDICAL HISTORY

The relevant previous diagnoses are numerous for this clinical presentation. Check the differential diagnosis.

PAST SURGICAL AND PROCEDURAL HISTORY

Ask about surgeries and procedures, including abdominal surgeries, recent colonoscopy, and gynecological procedures.

MEDICATIONS

Ask about changes in medications.

Check for use of erythromycin and NSAIDs (these can cause gastritis).

SOCIAL HISTORY

Obtain a sexual history, looking for risk factors for infection (multiple sexual partners, unprotected sex).

Ask about substance abuse (IV drugs, alcohol) and occupational exposures.

Physical exam

Vital signs: Look for fever, hypotension, and tachycardia.

Cardiovascular: Assess the heart (relevant to cardiac ischemia) and lungs (pneumonia).

Abdominal:

- Look for masses and tenderness (including rebound tenderness).
- Listen for bowel sounds.
- Look specifically for Murphy sign (this suggests cholecystitis), Carnett sign (relevant to abdominal wall pain), and the psoas sign (appendicitis).

DRE: Look for fecal impaction, palpable masses, and occult blood.

Pelvic: Assess for ectopic pregnancy, vaginitis, and PID.

POINTER

Common and serious presentations of acute abdominal pain by location

LEFT UPPER QUADRANT

Esophagus
Stomach
Pancreas
Spleen
Kidneys
Intestines

RIGHT UPPER QUADRANT

Pulmonary system
Urinary system
Hepatobiliary system

RIGHT LOWER QUADRANT

Appendicitis
Urinary system
Colon
Pelvis

LEFT LOWER QUADRANT

Diverticular disease

Investigations

CBC to assess for infection and anemia

Creatinine

Electrolytes (see *Notes on labs and assessments*)

Liver function (see *Notes on labs and assessments*)

Lipase

Urinalysis
Chlamydia and gonorrhea in patients at risk of STI
β-HCG in women of childbearing age
Abdominal US in patients with right upper quadrant pain
Abdominal CT scan in patients with right and left lower quadrant pain
Transvaginal US in suspected ectopic pregnancy

Management

Management depends on the entity diagnosed: keep in mind the most common presentations, and the most serious presentations, for each anatomic location (see the pointer). Refer the patient to surgery as appropriate.

REFERENCE

1. Lacey B, Mearin F, Chang L, et al. Rome IV functional gastrointestinal disorders: disorders of gut-brain interaction. 4th ed. Vol. 2. Raleigh, NC: Rome Foundation; 2017. Chapter 11, Functional bowel disorders; 1393-1407.

ABDOMINAL PRESENTATIONS

Chronic abdominal pain

Differential diagnosis

CHRONIC ABDOMINAL PAIN IN GENERAL

Definition: abdominal pain lasting > 3 months

UPPER ABDOMINAL PAIN

Gastric cancer

Signs and symptoms: constitutional symptoms (fever, weight loss, night sweats); constant abdominal pain; enlarged lymph nodes; smoking; personal or family history of cancer; epigastric mass on abdominal exam

Investigations: CT scan of abdomen, endoscopy with biopsy

Ulcer and nonulcer dyspepsia

Signs and symptoms: constant midepigastric pain, often relieved with eating or with antacids; weight loss

Investigations: *H. pylori*; endoscopy to detect ulcer or inflammation of the gastric lining

Gastroesophageal reflux disease

Signs and symptoms: burning chest pain radiating into the throat (often with a bitter taste in the mouth or regurgitation of food into the mouth; often worse with lying down; often better with standing up or taking antacids; worse with spicy food, coffee, alcohol, fatty foods, peppermint), acid damage to teeth

Risk factors: obesity, pregnancy

Barrett esophagus

Signs and symptoms: GERD symptoms that don't respond to PPIs; difficulty swallowing food

Investigations: endoscopy with biopsies

Biliary disease

BILIARY TRACT DISEASE

Signs and symptoms: middle-aged woman (more common); epigastric pain, often after eating (the pain is generally constant and often radiates to the right shoulder); right-sided subcostal pain that is worse on deep inhalation; obesity; history of pregnancy

Cancer or primary biliary cholangitis: fatigue, weight loss

Obstructive biliary disease: jaundice

Investigations: albumin, INR, bilirubin (total and direct), alkaline phosphatase, AST, ALT, and γ-glutamyl transferase; US or CT scan to detect gallstones; MRCP to detect bile duct obstruction

Pancreatic disease

PANCREATITIS

Signs and symptoms: constant upper abdominal pain that radiates to the back (sitting up and leaning forward may reduce the pain; pain occurs with coughing, vigorous movement, deep breathing); shortness of breath; nausea, vomiting; hypotension; fever; jaundice; abdominal tenderness

History of gallstones or chronic alcoholism (usual); hyperlipidemia; hypercalcemia; change of medication

Investigations: serum amylase and lipase (levels are ≥ 3 times ULN; elevated lipase indicates pancreatic damage); possible elevated calcium; possible elevated cholesterol; possible elevated ALT (this indicates associated liver inflammation); chest x-ray (this may show left-sided or bilateral pleural effusion; atelectasis); abdominal x-ray (this may show calcifications within pancreatic ducts, calcified gallstones, or localized ileus of a segment of small intestine); US

Hepatic disease

Patients with compensated cirrhosis may be asymptomatic. HCV is often asymptomatic.

Signs and symptoms: jaundice; abdominal pain, swelling; palpable, tender liver; swelling in the legs and ankles; systemic symptoms (anorexia, weight loss, weakness, fatigue); itching; easy bruising

History of chronic alcohol abuse; chronic infection with HBV or HCV, or risk factors for these infections (unprotected sex, IV drug abuse, blood transfusions, tattoos, body piercings, imprisonment, workplace exposure to body fluids); hemochromatosis; autoimmune conditions; α_1-antitrypsin deficiency; primary biliary cirrhosis; CHF

Investigations: tests for liver enzymes (elevated AST, ALT) and liver function (elevated bilirubin; possible abnormal PT/INR); viral serologic tests to detect HBV, HCV; Doppler US; CT scan; MRI; transient elastography; liver biopsy

Cardiothoracic conditions (referred pain)

Signs and symptoms: cough, shortness of breath

Heart exam: extra heart sounds or pericardial rub

Lung exam: abnormal breath sounds, absent breath sounds, or lung rales on auscultation; solid sounds on percussion

Risk factors for heart and lung disease: personal or family history of heart and lung disease; hyperlipidemia; diabetes; smoking; occupational exposure to smoke or other lung irritants

Investigations: elevated cardiac enzymes (e.g., troponin), chest x-ray, ECG

LOWER ABDOMINAL PAIN

Bowel disease

INFLAMMATORY BOWEL DISEASE

Signs and symptoms: younger than 30 (usually); family history of inflammatory bowel disease; fluctuating symptoms with periods of exacerbation and remission; diarrhea (possibly with nocturnal waking); blood in the stool; abdominal pain; weight loss; fever; fatigue; right lower quadrant and periumbilical pain; extraintestinal manifestations (e.g., uveitis, arthritis)

Crohn disease: right lower quadrant mass, uveitis, arthritis

Investigations: elevated CRP (this suggests active inflammation); fecal calprotectin; colonoscopy with biopsy (this is a standard diagnostic procedure); CT scan or MRI (findings: diagnostic structural changes associated with inflammatory bowel disease)

DIVERTICULITIS

Signs and symptoms: constant left lower quadrant abdominal pain; abdominal tenderness; fever; nausea, vomiting; change in bowel habits (constipation and/or diarrhea)

Risk factors: advanced age, obesity, smoking, poor diet, lack of exercise

Investigations: CT scan

IRRITABLE BOWEL SYNDROME[1]

Irritable bowel syndrome is commonly diagnosed by applying the Rome criteria.

Signs and symptoms (Rome criteria): ≥ 2 symptoms, present for ≥ 1 day/week for ≥ 3 months

> Symptoms: pain associated with 1) defecation, 2) change of stool frequency, and/or 3) change in stool consistency

Genitourinary disease

ENDOMETRIOSIS

Signs and symptoms: pelvic pain associated with menstruation (very common); excessive bleeding during menstruation; pain during intercourse; pain during urination or bowel movements; tenderness on pelvic exam; normal findings on abdominal exam (common)

Risk factors: family history of endometriosis; nulliparity; personal history of PID

Investigations: US to detect ovarian cysts (common finding); laparoscopy with biopsy

TUMOR (BENIGN OR MALIGNANT)

Signs and symptoms: weight loss; abdominal pain; blood in the stool; palpable abdominal or pelvic mass

Investigations: elevated CEA, elevated CA 19-9

URINARY TRACT INFECTION

Signs and symptoms: frequent urination; painful urination; pelvic pain and/or flank pain; fever; tenderness over the bladder

Investigations: urinalysis, urine culture

PELVIC INFLAMMATORY DISEASE

Signs and symptoms: lower abdominal and pelvic pain; pain during intercourse; fever; urinary symptoms; vaginal discharge; irregular menstruation; pelvic tenderness and pain associated with 1 or both adnexa

History of gonorrhea, chlamydia, or risk factors for them (multiple partners, unprotected sex); IUD; childbirth; gynecologic procedure

Investigations: cultures for gonorrhea and chlamydia; US (this has normal findings)

Keys to patient encounter

History

PAIN HISTORY

Localize and characterize the pain. Ask where it is, how constant it is, and what makes it better and worse. Make particular note of the location of the pain: this is key evidence in narrowing the diagnosis.

Examples of characteristic pain include:

Radiating pain: pain that radiates to the right shoulder in biliary disease; to the back in pancreatic disease

Constant versus intermittent pain: episodic pain in inflammatory bowel disease, irritable bowel syndrome, or endometriosis

Pain made better by: eating in ulcer and nonulcer dyspepsia; sitting up and leaning forward in pancreatic disease

Pain made worse by: eating in biliary disease, deep breathing in pancreatic disease, and menstruation in endometriosis

ASSOCIATED SYMPTOMS

Establish associated symptoms. Examples of characteristic symptoms include:

Gastric cancer: constitutional symptoms and enlarged lymph nodes

Bowel disease: constipation and/or diarrhea

PID: vaginal discharge and irregular menstruation

GERD: heartburn; regurgitation of food; worse symptoms on lying down

Ask about symptom relationship to dietary factors, especially milk and milk products (lactose intolerance), gluten (celiac disease), and soft drinks and fruit juice (fructose and sorbitol intolerance). Ask about the presence of red flags (see the pointer).

PAST MEDICAL HISTORY

Ask about a history of cancer, HBV, HCV, lung disease, heart disease, hyperlipidemia, and diabetes.

PAST SURGICAL HISTORY

Ask about previous abdominal surgeries.

MEDICATIONS

Determine what prescription medications the patient takes.

POINTER

Red flags in chronic abdominal pain

Fever
Anorexia
Weight loss
Pain that wakes the patient
Blood in the stool or urine
Jaundice
Edema
Abdominal mass
Organomegaly

SOCIAL HISTORY

Ask about illicit drug use; alcohol intake; a history of physical and/or sexual abuse; and recent major psychosocial stressors, such as divorce, job loss, and death of a family member.

Physical exam

Vital signs: Look for fever and tachycardia.

General inspection: Check for peripheral edema, jaundice, and rash.

Cardiovascular: Listen to the heart and lungs, looking for abnormal sounds (relevant to referred cardiothoracic pain).

Abdominal: Look for masses, tenderness, and organomegaly.

DRE: Look for tenderness, masses, and blood.

Pelvic: Look for tenderness and masses.

Investigations

CBC

Liver function (see *Notes on labs and assessments*)

CRP

Lipase

H. pylori with stool antigen or urea breath test

Urinalysis

Abdominal US or CT scan with contrast (consider these)

A

Management

Refer patients with red flags, or patients older than 50 with new abdominal pain, for upper GI endoscopy and colonoscopy.

For patients with functional abdominal pain, consider nonopioid analgesics, H_2 receptor blockers, PPIs, or TCAs. Consider referral for relaxation training, biofeedback, and cognitive behavioral therapy. Encourage a balanced diet, regular exercise, and stress reduction.

POINTER

Barrett esophagus follow-up

Patients with Barrett esophagitis need long-term follow-up because of the risk of progression to esophageal cancer.

REFERENCE

1. Lacey B, Mearin F, Chang L, et al. Rome IV functional gastrointestinal disorders: disorders of gut-brain interaction. 4th ed. Vol. 2. Raleigh, NC: Rome Foundation; 2017. Chapter 11, Functional bowel disorders; 1393–1407.

ABDOMINAL PRESENTATIONS

Hernia (abdominal wall and groin)

Differential diagnosis

INCARCERATED HERNIA IN GENERAL

Any hernia can become incarcerated.

Signs and symptoms: nausea, vomiting, pain, constipation

CONGENITAL HERNIA

Inguinal hernia (infants)

Signs and symptoms: bulge in the internal or external inguinal ring or within the scrotum; bulge that may disappear at rest, and that recurs with crying or straining with a bowel movement

Umbilical hernia (infants and children)

Signs and symptoms: mass that protrudes through the umbilicus, which may be more pronounced with straining; mass that is easily reducible (generally)

ACQUIRED HERNIA

Inguinal hernia

DIRECT

Signs and symptoms: inguinal swelling; swelling that aches and enlarges with straining (usually); palpable bulge above the inguinal canal and **medial** to the internal inguinal ring

INDIRECT

Signs and symptoms: male patient (common); inguinal swelling; swelling that aches and enlarges with straining (usually); palpable bulge above the inguinal canal and **lateral** to the internal inguinal ring

Femoral hernia

Signs and symptoms: female patient (more common); bulge in the upper thigh; palpable bulge below the inguinal ligament

Umbilical hernia

Signs and symptoms: mass that protrudes through the umbilicus, which may be more pronounced with straining

Ventral (incisional) hernia

Signs and symptoms: abdominal bulge that becomes more pronounced on straining; obesity (common)

History of abdominal surgery (common), postoperative wound infection (very common)

Keys to patient encounter

Key concern

Determine if the hernia is incarcerated, because incarcerated hernias require emergent (not elective) repair.

History

HISTORY OF PRESENT ILLNESS

Ask when the patient noticed the mass, and whether it changes with lying down or straining. (A mass that disappears when the patient is supine, and enlarges with straining, is typical for hernia.)

Check in particular for symptoms of:

Incarcerated hernia: sudden severe pain, nausea, vomiting, and constipation

Infection and malignancy: constitutional symptoms (fever, weight loss, fatigue, night sweats)

Ask about recent injuries to the abdomen or groin.

PAST SURGICAL HISTORY

Ask about abdominal surgeries.

Physical exam

Abdominal: Look for redness and tenderness around an umbilical hernia.

Femoral and inguinal: Inspect for bulges while the patient is standing (inguinal hernia).

Valsalva maneuver: Ask the patient to perform the Valsalva maneuver and observe for the accentuation of any hernia masses.

Inguinal ring: Insert a finger into the external inguinal ring and ask the patient to cough, feeling for a bulge. Repeat this on the other side.

GU: Examine the scrotal sack for a mass separate from the testes.

Investigations

Investigations are usually not needed. However, US can help diagnose a scrotal mass in a male patient or an inguinal hernia in a female patient.

Management

Incarcerated hernias are a medical emergency. The patient requires immediate admission, stabilization, and surgical intervention. For other hernias, refer the patient to a general surgeon.

POINTER

Inguinal hernia incidence

Inguinal hernias occur primarily in men (9:1 male:female ratio), and are most common in patients aged 40 to 59.

Some infants have umbilical hernias. These generally close as the children grow. Refer children with umbilical hernias to surgery if the hernia is painful, larger than 1.5 cm in diameter, still present at age 4 years, or incarcerated.

ABDOMINAL PRESENTATIONS

Pediatric abdominal pain

Differential diagnosis

LOWER ABDOMINAL PAIN

Appendicitis

Signs and symptoms: periumbilical pain that migrates over several days to localize in the right lower quadrant; anorexia; fever; localized pain over the McBurney point on palpation

Investigations: elevated WBCs; US or CT scan to detect distended appendix

Constipation

Signs and symptoms: recurrent abdominal pain; straining at hard stools; poor fluid intake; frequent, painful urination (this suggests UTI, which is a possible complication); palpable stool on abdominal exam; impacted stool on rectal exam; anal fissures

Gastroenteritis

Signs and symptoms: abrupt-onset diarrhea; crampy abdominal pain; nausea, vomiting; fever; headache; muscle aches; epigastric tenderness on abdominal examination

Risk factors: exposure to persons with similar symptoms or to large groups of people (most cases are viral); eating undercooked or contaminated foods, or raw fluids (these are risk factors for bacterial infection)

Mesenteric lymphadenitis

Mesenteric lymphadenitis is a common differential diagnosis with appendicitis.

Signs and symptoms: lower abdominal pain; abdominal tenderness (particularly in the right lower quadrant); fever; diarrhea; nausea, vomiting

Investigations: normal appendix on CT scan (this may be useful in distinguishing mesenteric lymphadenitis from appendicitis)

Inflammatory bowel disease

Signs and symptoms: younger than 30 (usually); family history of inflammatory bowel disease; fluctuating symptoms with periods of exacerbation and remission; diarrhea (possibly with nocturnal waking); blood in the stool; abdominal pain; weight loss; fever; fatigue; right lower quadrant and periumbilical pain; extraintestinal manifestations (e.g., uveitis, arthritis)

> Crohn disease: right lower quadrant mass, uveitis, arthritis

Investigations: elevated CRP (this suggests active inflammation); fecal calprotectin; colonoscopy with biopsy (this is a standard diagnostic procedure); CT scan or MRI (findings: diagnostic structural changes associated with inflammatory bowel disease)

Inguinal hernia (incarcerated)

Signs and symptoms: mass or swelling in the groin; rapid-onset acute pain at the site of the mass or swelling; nausea, vomiting; constipation

Investigations: US, CT scan

Urinary tract infection

Signs and symptoms: frequent urination; painful urination; pelvic pain and/or flank pain; fever; tenderness over the bladder

Investigations: urinalysis, urine culture

Gynecological cause in pubertal children

Common causes include dysmenorrhea, PID, ectopic pregnancy, and ovarian torsion.

GENERALIZED PAIN

Peritoneal inflammation

Signs and symptoms: fever, abdominal pain, generalized abdominal tenderness, guarding on physical exam, rebound tenderness, ascites

> History of abdominal surgery, appendicitis, inflammatory bowel disease, PUD, pancreatitis, liver disease, recent colonoscopy

Investigations: elevated WBCs; blood and peritoneal cultures

Bowel

INFANTILE COLIC

Signs and symptoms: age 2 weeks to 4 months (common); crying in the late afternoon or evening; crying > 3 hours per day, > 3 days per week, for ≥ 3 weeks (mnemonic: **rule of 3**)

History of low birth weight, maternal smoking during pregnancy

No evidence of viral or bacterial illness; child abuse; malabsorption; failure to gain weight; frequent or bloody diarrhea; fever

OBSTRUCTION

Signs and symptoms: crampy abdominal pain; nausea, vomiting; change in bowel habits (diarrhea or constipation); abdominal distention; palpable mass; increased bowel sounds (this suggests early obstruction; bowel sounds may be decreased in later obstruction); history of colonic diseases (diverticulitis, colon cancer, inflammatory bowel disease)

Volvulus (surgical emergency): bilious vomiting

Risk factors for adhesions: abdominal surgery

Risk factors for paralytic ileus: narcotic medications, chronic neuromuscular disease, diabetes, CF

Investigations: abdominal x-ray to detect distended bowel with air-fluid levels; CT scan to identify etiology of obstruction

Malabsorption

Signs and symptoms: frequent or bloody diarrhea; failure to gain weight; family history of similar problems; low weight and height for age; reduced muscle and fat (these suggest malnutrition); enlarged liver or spleen (these suggest chronic malabsorption); skin breakdown around the anus (this suggests chronic diarrhea)

Irritable bowel syndrome[1]

Irritable bowel syndrome is commonly diagnosed by applying the Rome criteria.

Signs and symptoms (Rome criteria): at least 2 symptoms, present for ≥ 1 day/week for ≥ 3 months

Symptoms: pain associated with 1) defecation, 2) change of stool frequency, and/or 3) change in stool consistency

FLANK PAIN

Pyelonephritis

Signs and symptoms: frequent urination, painful urination, fever, tenderness over the costovertebral angle

Investigations: elevated WBCs; urinalysis, urine culture, blood culture to identify causative organism

Kidney stones

Signs and symptoms: colicky flank pain; nausea, vomiting; fever; history of kidney stones (common); extreme tenderness at the costovertebral angle on abdominal examination; hematuria

Investigations: KUB x-ray, ureter US, abdominal CT scan

PERIUMBILICAL RECURRENT ABDOMINAL PAIN

Signs and symptoms: age 4 to 16 years (common); recurrent pain centered around the umbilicus

EPIGASTRIC PAIN

Gastroesophageal reflux disease

Signs and symptoms: burning chest pain radiating into the throat (often with a bitter taste in the mouth or regurgitation of food into the mouth; often worse with lying down; often better with standing up or taking antacids; worse with spicy food, coffee, alcohol, fatty foods, peppermint); acid damage to teeth

Risk factors: obesity, pregnancy

Peptic ulcer disease

Signs and symptoms: constant midepigastric pain, often relieved with eating or with antacids; weight loss

Investigations: *H. pylori*; endoscopy to detect ulcer or inflammation of the gastric lining

Biliary tract disease

Signs and symptoms: epigastric pain, often after eating (the pain is generally constant and often radiates to the right shoulder); right-sided subcostal pain that is worse on deep inhalation; obesity; history of pregnancy

Cancer or primary biliary cholangitis: fatigue, weight loss

Obstructive biliary disease: jaundice

Investigations: albumin, INR, bilirubin (total and direct), alkaline phosphatase, AST, ALT, and γ-glutamyl transferase; US or CT scan to detect gallstones; MRCP to detect bile duct obstruction

Keys to patient encounter

Key concerns

Identify patients who need emergency medical or surgical treatment.

Consider that nonorganic causes are the most common causes.

History

PAIN HISTORY

Ask about the location of the pain, when it started, how constant it is, how long it lasts, where it radiates, its quality (e.g., sharp, dull, throbbing), its severity, and what makes it better and worse.

Examples of characteristic pain include:

Appendicitis: pain with periumbilical onset over several days that has localized in the right lower quadrant

Irritable bowel syndrome: recurrent pain associated with defecation, or with changes in stool frequency or consistency

Peptic ulcer: constant midepigastric pain relieved with eating or antacids

ASSOCIATED SYMPTOMS

Examples of characteristic symptoms include:

Gastroenteritis: abrupt-onset diarrhea with fever, vomiting, and muscle aches

Malabsorption: diarrhea and failure to gain weight

UTI: frequent, painful urination

PAST MEDICAL HISTORY

In postmenarcheal girls, ask about menstrual history.

MEDICATIONS

Ask about erythromycin.

FAMILY HISTORY

Ask about sickle cell disease, CF, inflammatory bowel disease, and celiac disease.

SOCIAL HISTORY

In postmenarcheal girls, ask about sexual activity.

Physical exam

Vital signs: Look for fever and hypovolemia.

General inspection:

- Observe the patient for pain behavior (e.g., colic, reluctance to move, guarding).
- Examine the skin for jaundice.

Cardiovascular

Abdominal

GU: Examine the external genitalia looking for penile and scrotal abnormalities in boys, and vaginal discharge in girls.

Pelvic: In sexually active girls, perform a bimanual exam looking for tenderness and adnexal masses.

Investigations

CBC

β-HCG in in postmenarcheal girls

Urinalysis

Abdominal x-ray

US (useful for diagnosing gynecologic causes)

Management

Causes are often age dependent (see the pointer). In children with abdominal guarding, rebound tenderness, or trauma, and in patients whose pain has no obvious etiology, consult a pediatric surgeon.

POINTER

Common causes of abdominal pain in children

YOUNGER THAN 1 YEAR	1 TO 5 YEARS	6 TO 11 YEARS	12 TO 18 YEARS
Gastroenteritis	Gastroenteritis	Gastroenteritis	Appendicitis
Constipation	Appendicitis	Appendicitis	Gastroenteritis
UTI	Constipation	Constipation	Constipation
Intussusception	UTI	Functional pain	Dysmenorrhea
Volvulus	Intussusception	UTI	Mittelschmerz
Incarcerated hernia	Volvulus	Trauma	PID
Hirschsprung disease	Trauma	Pneumonia	Ectopic pregnancy
	Mesenteric lymphadenitis	Mesenteric lymphadenitis	Ovarian/testicular torsion

REFERENCE

1. Lacey B, Mearin F, Chang L, et al. Rome IV functional gastrointestinal disorders: disorders of gut-brain interaction. 4th ed. Vol. 2. Raleigh, NC: Rome Foundation; 2017. Chapter 11, Functional bowel disorders; 1393–1407.

ABUSE, VIOLENCE

Adult abuse, intimate partner abuse

Indicators and risk factors

Signs and symptoms: disclosed abuse (physical, psychological, emotional, sexual, or economic abuse; social isolation); bruising, scars, healed fractures; recurrent symptoms or injuries; resistance by the partner to having the patient interviewed alone (usual)

Note: victims do not always disclose abuse.

Risk factors: pregnancy; threat to leave; partner's history of violence or substance abuse

Keys to patient encounter

Key concerns

Assess the medium- and short-term risk to the patient.

Devise a safe and effective plan for the patient.

History

Note that if the possible abuser is with the patient, the patient may not be honest with answers. Always request to interview the patient alone.

Ask the patient if they are afraid of anyone, and whether they are, or have been, the victim of abuse. Ask specifically about physical, psychological, sexual, and economic abuse, and social isolation. Ask about risk factors for escalating abuse, in particular whether the pattern of abuse has increased in frequency or intensity.

Some patients do not disclose abuse, even in the absence of the perpetrator. In suspected undisclosed abuse, ask about risk factors for abuse: pregnancy; telling the perpetrator about an intention to leave; and substance abuse or a history of violence on the part of the perpetrator.

Establish whether the patient has a plan to protect themselves.

Physical exam

Head and neck: Look for bruises, cuts, and lost teeth.

Musculoskeletal: Look for broken bones.

Dermatological: Look for bruises, cuts, and burns.

Investigations

X-rays for any apparent broken bones

Management

Counsel the patient on making a plan for personal protection. If the patient is facing escalating abuse, alert them that they have a greater risk of permanent injury or death.

Elements of a plan for personal protection include: where to go for help (e.g., a shelter); how to get away; how to get money (e.g., friends, family); how to protect children; and packing a fast-exit suitcase stored with a friend or family member.

Refer the patient to social services if appropriate. Social services can provide assistance with finances, relocation, and protecting and caring for children.

Duty to report

The duty to report risk of harm to an adult varies by jurisdiction (and is absent in some). If in doubt, it is best to discuss the case with a social worker or police.

ABUSE, VIOLENCE

Child abuse

Indicators and risk factors

Signs and symptoms: disclosed abuse (victims do not always disclose abuse); resistance by the parent or caregiver to having the patient interviewed alone (usual)

No evidence of medical conditions that could mimic abuse (e.g., malabsorption; developmental delay due to complications during gestation or delivery; genetic or metabolic disorders)

Risk factors: history of substance abuse by the parents or caregiver; unstable living situation of the parents or caregiver

PHYSICAL ABUSE

This is purposeful action with the intent to physically harm a child. It includes hitting and beating; using an object to hit; kicking; burning; holding under water; tying up; and, in the case of an infant, severe shaking.

Signs and symptoms: inconsistency between an injury and the explanation for the injury and/or the developmental stage of the child; facial contusions; marks on the neck or limbs; burn marks; ligature marks on the wrists and ankles; bite marks; lash marks; bruises or broken bones unexplainable by usual activities; unexplained loss of consciousness in an infant

SEXUAL ABUSE

This is an action done with a child for the sexual arousal and gratification of an adult or significantly older child (greater than a 4-year age difference, chronologically or in mental or physical development).

Signs and symptoms: behavior and knowledge that is inappropriate for the child's age; pregnancy or STI; blood in the child's underwear; trouble walking or sitting, or complaints of genital pain; sexual abuse of other children by the victim

PSYCHOLOGICAL ABUSE

This is injuring a child's self-esteem or emotional well-being. It includes verbal and emotional assault (continually belittling, berating, threatening, intimidating, isolating, or rejecting a child); not providing a child with a safe environment; and withholding or omitting positive contributions to a child's emotional well-being.

Signs and symptoms: problems in school; eating disorders leading to weight loss or poor weight gain; emotional issues (anxiety, low self-esteem); depression; extreme behavior (acting out to seek attention); trouble sleeping

NEGLECT

Neglect involves failure to provide all or some basic physical, emotional, educational, and medical needs. Examples include rejecting a child and not giving love; not feeding a child; not dressing a child in proper clothing; not giving needed medical or dental care; and abandonment by leaving a child at home alone for a long time.

Signs and symptoms: not attending school regularly; poor hygiene, dental care; malnutrition; reports by the child suggesting lack of physical and/or emotional care at home

EXPOSURE TO DOMESTIC VIOLENCE

This involves witnessing an abusive situation within a family, such as violence between parents.

Signs and symptoms: excessive anxiety or crying; fearfulness; difficulty sleeping; depression; social withdrawal; difficulty in school; running away from home; violent tendencies and/or unhealthy tolerance for abuse

Keys to patient encounter

Key concerns

Be aware of presentations that may indicate child abuse.

In suspected abuse, manage with particular attention to safety and prevention.

In disclosed abuse, construct a prevention plan.

History

Generally, parents or adult caregivers accompany children to medical appointments. Ask why the adult is concerned about the child.

If the concern involves an injury, ask the adult and the child to describe how the injury happened.

If the adult is concerned about abuse of the child, ask what the adult knows or why the adult suspects abuse. Seek information from the child, but be aware that victims of abuse often do not disclose abuse.

In suspected abuse, ask to interview the child alone.

Physical exam

Head and neck: Look for bruises, cuts, and lost teeth.
Musculoskeletal: Look for broken bones.
Dermatological: Look for bruises, cuts, and burns.
GU: Look for signs of STI and trauma.

Investigations

X-rays for any apparent broken bones
Gonorrhea if indicated

Management

In cases of disclosed or suspected abuse, where the adult accompanying the child is not the perpetrator, outline a safety plan that the adult could help the child prepare, including safe places where the child could go (e.g., safe friends and relatives); leaving the room if they are witnessing abuse; how to call 911; and knowing their full name and address.

Advise the adult about counseling and mental health services that are available for the child, the family, and caregivers.

Duty to report

Abuse of a minor, or danger of abuse, must be reported to the appropriate authorities. Depending on your region, this may be social services, a child protection agency, or the police.

ABUSE, VIOLENCE

Elder abuse

Indicators and risk factors

Signs and symptoms: disclosed abuse (physical, sexual, psychological, economic, financial or material abuse; neglect); resistance by a caregiver to having the patient interviewed alone (usual); fear of the patient toward a caregiver; isolation; depression;

unexplained changes in financial situation; bruising, scars, healed fractures; poor hygiene; sudden weight loss, malnutrition

Note: victims do not always disclose abuse.

Risk factors:

Victim: female; advanced age (especially older than 80); vulnerability due to a chronic disorder, functional impairment, or cognitive impairment

Perpetrator: substance abuse, psychiatric disorder, history of violence, cohabitation with the elderly person, dependence on the elderly person for support

Keys to patient encounter

Key concerns

Given a state of distress or unexplained findings in an elderly patient, inquire about potential elder abuse.

Identify the immediate level of risk.

History

Note that if the possible abuser is with the patient, the patient may not be honest with answers. Always request to interview the patient alone. Ask the patient if they are afraid of anyone, if anyone hurts them, how they get their food, and who controls their money. Ask about their living arrangements and social contacts, and if anyone controls who they speak to.

Physical exam

Head and neck: Look for bruises, cuts, and lost teeth.

Musculoskeletal: Look for broken bones.

Dermatological: Look for bruises, cuts, and burns.

GU: Look for signs of STI and trauma.

Investigations

X-rays for any apparent broken bones (consider x-rays to look for healed fractures)

Management

In suspected abuse, ensure the immediate safety of the patient and refer the patient to adult protection services.

Duty to report

The duty to report risk of harm to an adult varies by jurisdiction (and is absent in some). If in doubt, it is best to discuss the case with a social worker or police.

ACID-BASE ABNORMALITIES

Acid-base abnormalities

Differential diagnosis

METABOLIC ACIDOSIS

METABOLIC ACIDOSIS IN GENERAL

Investigations: decreased pH; decreased $PaCO_2$; decreased HCO_3^-

High anion gap

Definition: > 12–16 mEq/L (12–16 mmol/L)

Calculation: Anion Gap = (Sodium) – (Chloride + Bicarbonate)

INCREASED ACID PRODUCTION

EXOGENOUS (E.G., METHANOL)

Signs and symptoms (in general): vision changes, abdominal pain, confusion, fever, jaundice, tachycardia, altered level of consciousness, dilated pupils

History of ingesting methanol, acetaminophen, isoniazid, iron, ethanol, ethylene glycol, propylene glycol, salicylate

Investigations: toxin screen to detect particular toxins; elevated urine or serum ketones (possible); elevated lactate (possible); elevated osmolar gap (possible); creatinine

ENDOGENOUS (E.G., KETOACIDOSIS)

KETOACIDOSIS

Common causes of ketoacidosis include type 1 diabetes, alcohol abuse, and starvation.

Symptoms: polydipsia; polyuria; nausea, vomiting; weakness; lethargy; dehydration (tachycardia, hypotension); deep respirations;

fruity odor on the breath (ketone breath); altered mental status; hypertension and bradycardia (these indicate cerebral edema)

History of new-onset type 1 diabetes, signs of infection (e.g., fever), reduced insulin intake, atherosclerotic disease, change in diet, alcohol use, drug use, pregnancy

Investigations: serum glucose (elevated in diabetes; normal–low in alcohol abuse, starvation); acidosis (HCO_3^- < 18 mEq/L [18 mmol/L]; blood pH < 7.3); serum ketones (present); electrolytes (anion gap > 10); CBC with differential; blood gas; urine dipstick to detect ketones; urinalysis; renal and liver function tests; urine culture; blood culture; ECG; chest x-ray

DECREASED RENAL ACID EXCRETION (KIDNEY INJURY)

KIDNEY INJURY

Signs and symptoms: history of kidney disease, chronic renal failure, and/or current renal dialysis; bilateral lower limb swelling; shortness of breath; paroxysmal nocturnal dyspnea; orthopnea

Risk factors: diabetes, diabetic complications, and/or inadequate monitoring; hypertension; smoking

Investigations: renal function tests (reduced calcium; elevated phosphate; elevated creatinine); reduced vitamin D

Normal anion gap

GASTROINTESTINAL BICARBONATE LOSS (E.G., DIARRHEA)

RENAL BICARBONATE LOSS (E.G., RENAL TUBULAR ACIDOSIS, INTERSTITIAL NEPHRITIS)

RENAL TUBULAR ACIDOSIS (PROXIMAL)

Causes include Fanconi syndrome; multiple myeloma; amyloidosis; use of medications such as acetazolamide; renal transplant; autoimmune disease; and low aldosterone.

Investigations: blood tests (reduced HCO_3^-; reduced phosphate; reduced glucose; reduced vitamin D; hyper- or hypokalemia)

INTERSTITIAL NEPHRITIS

Signs and symptoms: fever; rash; arthralgia; use of diuretics, antibiotics, analgesics (usual); history of autoimmune disorders

Investigations: urine eosinophils (their presence is suggestive); urinalysis (normal findings for RBCs, proteinuria, and red cell casts); blood tests (normal creatinine; normal complement level); renal biopsy (definitive)

METABOLIC ALKALOSIS

METABOLIC ALKALOSIS IN GENERAL

Investigations: elevated pH; elevated $PaCO_2$; elevated HCO_3^-

Expanded effective arterial blood volume (e.g., mineralocorticoid excess)

Causes include primary hyperaldosteronism (Conn syndrome), secondary hyperaldosteronism (e.g., renovascular disease, renin-secreting tumor), and hypertension.

Investigations: elevated urine chloride levels

Contracted effective arterial blood volume

GASTROINTESTINAL LOSS (E.G., VOMITING)

RENAL LOSS (E.G., DIURETICS)

Exogenous ingestion

Causes include bicarbonate use (e.g., sodium bicarbonate antacid, IV infusion).

RESPIRATORY ACIDOSIS

RESPIRATORY ACIDOSIS IN GENERAL

Investigations: decreased pH; elevated $PaCO_2$; elevated HCO_3^-

Neuromuscular causes (e.g., medications, illicit drugs)

A common cause is use of sedatives (e.g., opioids, barbiturates, benzodiazepines).

Pulmonary causes of decreased alveolar ventilation (e.g., chronic obstructive pulmonary disease)

CHRONIC OBSTRUCTIVE PULMONARY DISEASE

Signs and symptoms: older than 40 (usual: symptoms do not appear until significant lung damage has occurred); progressive symptoms; wheezing; chest tightness; chronic productive cough; clubbing of fingers; cyanosis around the lips and in the extremities; decreased oxygen saturation; impaired pulmonary function on testing with spirometry

Risk factors: smoking; occupational exposure; intrinsic lung disease

Investigations: chest x-ray; CT scan; ABG

Kyphoscoliosis

Signs and symptoms: poor posture; uneven limb length; abnormal gait; shortness of breath or difficulty breathing

Investigations: x-ray, CT scan of the spine and chest

Hypoventilation (e.g., due to obesity)

Signs and symptoms (in general): excess body weight; snoring; shallow breathing; daytime fatigue; sleep disturbances

RESPIRATORY ALKALOSIS

RESPIRATORY ALKALOSIS IN GENERAL

Investigations: elevated pH; decreased $PaCO_2$; decreased HCO_3^-

Hypoxemia

Causes include living in high altitudes, lung disease (e.g., COPD), and heart disease (e.g., CHD, AVM).

Signs and symptoms: cyanosis

Metabolic disorder (e.g., hepatic failure)

HEPATIC FAILURE

Signs and symptoms: history of liver disease; jaundice; abdominal pain, swelling; palpable, tender liver; swelling in the legs and ankles; systemic symptoms (anorexia, weight loss, weakness, fatigue); itching; easy bruising

> History of chronic alcohol abuse; chronic infection from HBV or HCV (HCV is often asymptomatic); hemochromatosis; autoimmune conditions; α_1-antitrypsin deficiency; primary biliary cirrhosis; CHF
>
> HBV and HCV risk factors: unprotected sex, IV drug abuse, blood transfusions, tattoos, body piercings, imprisonment, workplace exposure to body fluids

Investigations: tests for liver enzymes (elevated AST, ALT) and liver function (elevated bilirubin; possible abnormal PT/INR); viral serologic tests to detect HBV, HCV

Cardiopulmonary disorder (e.g., pneumonia, embolism)

PNEUMONIA

Signs and symptoms: shortness of breath; cough; purulent sputum; chest pain on coughing or deep breaths; fatigue; tachypnea; tachycardia; decreased oxygen saturation; lung crackles on auscultation; lung dullness on percussion

> Children: fever
>
> Elderly: confusion, low body temperature

Risk factors: very old, very young, smoking, immune compromise (e.g., due to chronic illness), hospitalization

Investigations: chest x-ray to detect consolidation

PULMONARY EMBOLISM

Signs and symptoms: sharp chest pain; shortness of breath; cough (possibly with blood); hypoxia; possible unilateral swelling of the lower limbs (this indicates DVT); elevated pulse and respiratory rate; arrhythmias; lung rales on auscultation; lower-lung dullness on percussion; motor or sensory deficits

Risk factors: HF; cancer; surgery; prolonged immobility (e.g., long plane trips); smoking; estrogen replacement therapy; OCs; current pregnancy; previous DVT, embolism, or stroke; family history of embolism

Investigations: elevated d-dimer level; area of reduced pulmonary perfusion on V/Q scan; CT angiography to detect blocked vessel

Central nervous system disorder (e.g., subarachnoid hemorrhage)

SUBARACHNOID HEMORRHAGE

Signs and symptoms: sudden-onset severe symptoms; symptoms that include: severe headache (this is the most common symptom; it is sometimes called a "thunderclap" headache); neck or shoulder pain; meningismus with nuchal rigidity; photophobia; pain with eye movements; nausea, vomiting; seizures; confusion; fever; syncope (prolonged or atypical); neurological abnormalities

History of congenital berry aneurysm; bleeding from an AVM; bleeding disorders or use of blood thinners

Investigations: CT scan, MRI; cerebral angiogram; transcranial US

Drugs (e.g., salicylate)

SALICYLATE POISONING

Signs and symptoms: history of using skin products that contain salicylates, such as OTC acne remedies; abdominal pain; tinnitus; nausea, vomiting (blood in the vomit); hyperthermia; mental status changes (agitation and seizures; or lethargy, CNS depression, and coma)

Other (e.g., fever, pain, pregnancy)

Keys to patient encounter

Key concern

Manage high anion gap metabolic acidosis.

History

Ask about recent vomiting and/or diarrhea; a medical history of type 1 diabetes and renal failure (in particular); medications; and drugs of abuse.

Physical exam

Vital signs: Look for fever and tachypnea.

General inspection: Look for jaundice (skin and sclera) and decreased level of consciousness.

Investigations

ABG

"Chem 7" blood panel: BUN; CO_2 or HCO_3^-; creatinine; glucose; chloride; potassium; and sodium

EVALUATING ACID-BASE STATUS

STEP 1

Look at the pH to determine if the patient has acidemia (decreased pH) or alkalemia (elevated pH). The important principle here is that, while there will be metabolic or respiratory compensation for the primary disorder, the acidemia or alkalemia will never be overcorrected.

STEP 2

Use the following table to classify the primary acid-base abnormality.

TYPE OF DISORDER	PH	$PACO_2$	HCO_3^-
Metabolic acidosis	Decreased	Decreased	Decreased
Metabolic alkalosis	Increased	Increased	Increased
Respiratory acidosis	Decreased	Increased	Increased
Respiratory alkalosis	Increased	Decreased	Decreased

STEP 3

Evaluate for compensation for the primary disturbance:

- **Metabolic acidosis:** For every decrease of HCO_3^- by 10, $PaCO_2$ is expected to decrease by 12.
- **Metabolic alkalosis:** For every increase in HCO_3^- by 10, $PaCO_2$ is expected to increase by 6.
- **Acute respiratory acidosis:** For every increase in $PaCO_2$ by 10, HCO_3^- is expected to increase by 1.
- **Chronic respiratory acidosis:** For every increase in $PaCO_2$ by 10, HCO_3^- is expected to increase by 4.

- **Acute respiratory alkalosis:** For every decrease in $PaCO_2$ by 10, HCO_3^- is expected to decrease by 2.
- **Chronic respiratory alkalosis:** For every decrease in $PaCO_2$ by 10, HCO_3^- is expected to decrease by 5.

STEP 4

If the patient has acidemia, determine if there is an anion gap:

$$\text{Anion Gap} = (\text{Sodium}) - (\text{Chloride} + \text{Bicarbonate})$$

See the pointer for causes of high anion gap metabolic acidosis.

STEP 5

In cases of high anion gap metabolic acidosis, check for a secondary acid-base disturbance (in addition to compensation) by calculating the ratio of the increase in anion gap (AG) to the decrease in HCO_3^- as follows:

$$(\text{Calculated AG} - \text{Expected AG}) \div (24 - \text{Measured } HCO_3^-)$$

This is called the delta:delta ratio. A delta:delta ratio less than 0.4 usually indicates a pure normal anion gap metabolic acidosis; a ratio of 0.4 to 0.8 indicates a mixed normal and high anion gap metabolic acidosis; a ratio of 0.8 to 2.0 indicates a pure high anion gap metabolic acidosis; and a ratio greater than 2 indicates a mixed high anion gap metabolic acidosis and metabolic alkalosis.

Management

Management depends on the specific entity identified. All patients should be admitted to hospital and observed. Consider referral to an internist.

POINTER

Causes of high anion gap metabolic acidosis

Several memory aids exist to help recall the causes of increased anion gap metabolic acidosis (the most common clinical presentation in acid-base abnormalities). The classic mnemonic is **MUDPILES**:

M — Methanol
U — Uremia
D — Diabetic ketoacidosis
P — Paracetamol, propylene glycol, paraldehyde
I — Infection, iron, isoniazid
L — Lactic acidosis
E — Ethylene glycol
S — Salicylates

ALLERGY AND IMMUNOLOGICAL PRESENTATIONS

Allergic reactions and atopy

Differential diagnosis

ANAPHYLAXIS

Signs and symptoms: personal or family history of anaphylaxis; hives; itchiness; peripheral edema; tongue or throat swelling; wheezing; stridor; shortness of breath; tachycardia; cardiovascular collapse; hypotension

URTICARIA OR ANGIOEDEMA

From drugs

Signs and symptoms: drug allergies, change in medication

From food

Signs and symptoms: food allergies, exposure to a known food allergen

Investigations: skin prick testing or serum specific IgE testing

From parasites

Signs and symptoms: history of travel, camping

Investigations: stool analysis to detect ova and parasites

From physical stressors (e.g., cold, exercise)

CRYOGLOBULINEMIA

Signs and symptoms: history of urticaria on exposure to cold; joint pain; positive ice test (applying ice to the skin provokes urticaria); constitutional symptoms (fatigue, weight loss)

> History of autoimmune disease (e.g., arthritis, vasculitis); infection with HBV or HCV, or risk factors for these infections (autoimmune conditions, unprotected sex, IV drug abuse, blood transfusions, workplace exposure to body fluids, tattoos, body piercings)

Investigations: specific laboratory testing for cryoglobulinemia

HYPOTHYROIDISM

Signs and symptoms: history of hypothyroidism or symptoms of hypothyroidism (decreased reflexes, dry skin, weight gain, impaired cognition)

Investigations: elevated thyrotropin (TSH)

EXERCISE-INDUCED URTICARIA

Signs and symptoms: hives during or following exercise

Congenital

URTICARIA PIGMENTOSA

Signs and symptoms: lesions that blister when rubbed; lesions exacerbated by NSAIDs, narcotics, alcohol

Investigations: elevated serum tryptase, elevated urine histamine, lesion biopsy

ATOPIC DERMATITIS

Signs and symptoms: rash that is aggravated by soap, water, dry environments, exposure to allergens; highly pruritic rash; personal or family history of atopic dermatitis, asthma, allergies; wheezing (this suggests coexisting asthma; nasal polyps)

Children (rash location): face, scalp, hands, feet

Adults (rash location): the popliteal fossa, antecubital fossa

RESPIRATORY ALLERGY (E.G., DUST MITES, POLLEN)

Signs and symptoms: wheezing; rhinitis; cough; seasonal symptoms; personal or family history of allergies; allergic "shiners"; eczema; red, watery sclera; nasal polyps; rash

Keys to patient encounter

Key concern

Pay particular attention to findings suggestive of anaphylaxis.

Airway and hemodynamic status

Anaphylaxis is possible in this clinical presentation, so start by checking for key signs and symptoms of anaphylaxis: hypotension, tachycardia, shortness of breath, itchiness, and swelling.

Note that a patient presenting with allergic symptoms can develop anaphylaxis minutes or hours after the triggering event. Stay alert to changes in the condition of any patient who presents with urticaria or angioedema.

Provide emergency care to any patient with unstable vital signs, including administration of epinephrine and transfer to an ED.

History

HISTORY OF PRESENT ILLNESS

Ask about diagnosed allergies and exposure to known triggers.

Ask about previous episodes, including suspected exposures and the timing of the episodes. Note that symptoms within 2 hours of exposure suggest an IgE-mediated process.

Ask about the patient's symptoms, and listen especially for vomiting, diarrhea, GI pain, itching, wheezing, and coughing (these may indicate anaphylaxis). Note symptoms consistent with particular entities (e.g., hives following exercise in exercise-induced urticaria; itchy rash with wheezing in atopic dermatitis; seasonal cough and rhinitis in respiratory allergy).

MEDICATIONS

Ask about new medications, especially penicillin and ACE inhibitors.

Physical exam

Examine the skin for urticaria, angioedema, and rash.

Investigations

In the case of anaphylaxis, no immediate testing is indicated. Pursue investigations for nonemergent allergies as indicated (see the pointer).

POINTER

Recommended allergy evaluations

FOOD ALLERGY

Allergy testing is not indicated for mild atopic dermatitis or isolated respiratory symptoms. Serum IgE testing and skin-prick testing can confirm suspected allergens, but are not indicated for food intolerances that are not IgE mediated.

INHALANT ALLERGY

Serum IgE tests or skin-prick testing are the preferred methods of testing for inhalant allergens (e.g., pollen, fungus, dust mites).

LATEX

This is tested by serum IgE.

DRUGS

Use skin-prick testing for penicillin reaction. Use serum antigen-specific IgE testing for other drugs.

VENOM

Use skin-prick testing or serum antigen-specific IgE testing.

Management

In suspected atopic dermatitis, counsel the patient to avoid too-frequent bathing and exposure to known allergens. Patients should use mild soaps and moisturize their skin frequently (e.g., twice a day).

In patients undergoing anaphylaxis, provide supportive therapy and administer epinephrine, antihistamines, or steroids. Obtain IV access and ensure the patient is in a monitored setting.

Discuss avoidance of triggers and appropriate medication (e.g., antihistamines, steroids). Consider prescribing injectable epinephrine (EpiPen), and counsel the patient about its use.

ALLERGY AND IMMUNOLOGICAL PRESENTATIONS

Urticaria, angioedema

Differential diagnosis

URTICARIA, ANGIOEDEMA IN GENERAL

Signs and symptoms: symptoms that can be chronic with frequent, unpredictable recurrence

Urticaria (this affects the upper dermis): hives (red or white welts), usually on the face, trunk, arms, legs; itching

Angioedema (this affects the dermis, subcutaneous tissue, mucosa, submucosa): swelling with pain or burning that can affect the eyes, cheeks, lips, hands, feet, genitals, inside the throat

IDIOPATHIC

ASSOCIATED WITH IDENTIFIABLE CAUSES

Allergic reaction (e.g., drugs, insects, food)

DRUGS

Anaphylaxis is possible and requires emergent intervention.

Common reactions:

Antibiotics (e.g., penicillins, cephalosporins): IgE-mediated (acute) urticaria that occurs within minutes to 2 hours of exposure (**but** vancomycin allergy causes diffuse erythema or flushing with urticaria: the reaction is due to direct mast cell activation; it is not IgE mediated)

Muscle relaxants (e.g., atracurium, vecuronium, succinylcholine, curare): symptoms associated with direct mast cell activation (IgE-mediated anaphylaxis is also possible)

INSECTS

Anaphylaxis is possible and requires emergent intervention.

Common reactions:

Urticarial lesions: bees, wasps, hornets, fire ants

Papular urticarial lesions on the lower extremities (resolve over weeks): bedbugs, fleas, mites

FOOD

Anaphylaxis is possible and requires emergent intervention.

Common reactions:

IgE-mediated reactions in children (on ingestion): milk, eggs, peanuts, tree nuts, soy, wheat

IgE-mediated reactions in adults (on ingestion): shellfish, fish, tree nuts, peanuts

Direct mast cell activated reactions in young children (on contact or ingestion): tomatoes, strawberries

Direct physical contact with food allergens (e.g., kitchen or food-processing workers): urticaria; IgE-mediated allergic reactions

Direct mast cell release (e.g., opiates, radio-contrast agents)

OPIATES

Examples include dextromethorphan in cough syrup, morphine, and codeine.

Common reaction: acute urticaria with flushing, sweating, asthma, hypotension, sneezing

RADIO-CONTRAST AGENTS

Examples include benzoic acid molecules: ionic monomers, ionic dimer, nonionic monomer, nonionic dimer.

Common reaction: urticaria with angioedema, flushing, bronchospasm, wheezing, laryngeal edema, stridor that occurs within 5 minutes to 1 hour on IV injection of radio-contrast agent

Complement-mediated condition (e.g., serum sickness, infection)

SERUM SICKNESS

This is a less common cause of urticaria. It involves reaction to exogenous proteins, medications, or infectious agents. Examples include antiseizure medications, antibiotics (cefaclor, penicillin, amoxicillin, trimethoprim-sulfamethoxazole), and vaccines (rabies; diphtheria; botulinum; spider or snake venom).

Signs and symptoms: symptoms that present 1 to 3 weeks after exposure (symptoms resolve within a few weeks of exposure cessation); urticarial rash; fever; malaise; polyarthralgia; pruritic rash (not on mucous membranes)

INFECTION

BACTERIAL AND VIRAL INFECTIONS

Causes include UTIs, URTIs, GI infections, and pharyngitis.

Signs and symptoms: acute urticaria (especially in children); history of recent illness with fever, sore throat, cough, rhinorrhea, headache, diarrhea, vomiting

PARASITIC INFECTION

Infections include ascariasis, strongyloidiasis, schistosomiasis, and trichinosis.

Signs and symptoms: acute urticaria with eosinophilia; history of ingesting contaminated raw or undercooked fish or meat; travel to endemic areas

> *Anisakis simplex*: urticaria, angioedema, abdominal pain, and/or anaphylaxis 2 to 24 hours after ingestion

Investigations: stool examination to detect ova and parasites

Physical (e.g., dermatographism, cold)

DERMATOGRAPHISM

This is the most common type of physical urticaria.

Signs and symptoms: rapid-onset (within several minutes) urticaria following physical irritation of the skin (e.g., pressure, scratching, rubbing); welts whose orientation follows the pattern of irritation (e.g., scratching produces linear welts)

COLD

This is a chronic condition that affects young adults and that resolves in 5 to 6 years. Patients with cold urticaria risk anaphylaxis and drowning if they swim in cold water.

Signs and symptoms: urticaria with or without angioedema that forms after cold exposure (e.g., contact with cold air, objects, liquids)

Keys to patient encounter

Key concern

Determine whether the condition is acute and/or life-threatening, and requires immediate treatment.

Airway and hemodynamic status

Anaphylaxis is possible in this clinical presentation, so start by checking for key signs and symptoms of anaphylaxis: hypotension, tachycardia, shortness of breath, itchiness, and swelling.

Note that a patient presenting with allergic symptoms can develop anaphylaxis minutes or hours after the triggering event. Stay alert to changes in the condition of any patient who presents with urticaria or angioedema.

Provide emergency care to any patient with unstable vital signs, including administration of epinephrine and transfer to an ED.

History

HISTORY OF PRESENT ILLNESS

Ask when the patient's symptoms began, how long the symptoms persist, and what the patient knows or suspects about triggers. Ask about recent illness (e.g., UTI, URTI, sore throat).

Listen for evidence of chronic versus acute symptoms, and association of symptoms with systemic disease (serum sickness, infection).

SOCIAL HISTORY

Ask about recent travel, and ingestion of raw or undercooked meat or fish.

Physical exam

Examine the skin for rashes and urticaria.

Investigations

Consider serum IgG tests for specific antigens if the offending agent is unknown.

Management

In patients undergoing anaphylaxis, provide supportive therapy and administer epinephrine, antihistamines, or steroids. Obtain IV access and ensure the patient is in a monitored setting.

Discuss avoidance of triggers and appropriate medication (e.g., antihistamines, steroids). Consider prescribing injectable epinephrine (EpiPen), and counsel the patient about its use.

ALTERED LEVEL OF CONSCIOUSNESS

Coma

Differential diagnosis

COMA IN GENERAL

Definition: severe impairment of consciousness or alertness, and decreased responsiveness to external stimuli; lack of arousal to any stimulation

FOCAL DISEASE (E.G., TUMOR, STROKE)

Brain tumor

Types of brain tumor include meningioma, astrocytoma, oligodendroglioma, glioblastoma, and Schwannoma.

Signs and symptoms: acute-onset headaches; older than 50; change in chronic headache pattern; increasing intensity and frequency of headaches; headaches that disturb sleep; unilateral headache pain, always on the same side; position-evoked crescendo headache; impaired vision; light-headedness

> Other symptoms: focal seizures, confusion, memory loss, personality change

Investigations: imaging for intracranial masses (MRI with contrast enhancement is best for tumors and abscesses); biopsy

Acute stroke

Coma can ensue from extensive cerebrovascular accident.

Signs and symptoms: speech difficulty and hemiparesis (most common symptoms); weakness or paralysis in the extremities or face; arm or leg numbness; confusion; headache; nonorthostatic dizziness; fever

DIFFUSE DISEASE

Vascular disorder (e.g., hypertensive encephalopathy)

HYPERTENSIVE ENCEPHALOPATHY

This occurs during a hypertensive crisis and requires immediate intervention to reduce BP.

Signs and symptoms: history of hypertension (usual), or use of medications (e.g., epinephrine, Ritalin) or drugs (e.g., cocaine, methamphetamine) that can cause hypertension; headache; confusion; blurred vision; seizure; nausea, vomiting; symptoms of end-organ damage (cardiovascular symptoms, hematuria, renal failure)

Infection (e.g., meningitis, encephalitis)

MENINGITIS

Signs and symptoms: fever, headache, Kernig sign (flexing the patient's hip 90 degrees, then extending the knee, causes pain), Brudzinski neck sign (flexing the patient's neck causes flexion of the hips and knees)

Neonates: poor feeding, lethargy, irritability, apnea, listlessness, apathy, hypothermia, seizures, jaundice, bulging fontanelle, pallor, shock, hypotonia, hypoglycemia

Infants and children: nuchal rigidity, opisthotonos, convulsions, photophobia, alterations of the sensorium, irritability, lethargy, anorexia, nausea, vomiting, coma

Investigations: positive culture in CSF; meningeal inflammation (increased pleocytosis, low glucose in CSF); CSF absolute neutrophil count ≥ 1000/μL (1×10^9/L); CSF protein level ≥ 80 mg/dL (0.8 g/L); peripheral blood absolute neutrophil count ≥ 10 000/μL (10×10^9/L); CT scan, MRI

ENCEPHALITIS

Viral infection is the most common cause: HSV-1, HSV-2; EBV; VZV; Enterovirus (e.g., Coxsackievirus); and insect-borne viruses (e.g., West Nile disease, Lyme disease).

Signs and symptoms: seizures, altered mental status (e.g., decreased level of consciousness, lethargy, personality change, behavior change), fever, headache, nausea, vomiting

Infants and neonates: poor feeding, irritability, lethargy

Children and adolescents: irritability, movement disorder, ataxia, stupor, coma, hemiparesis, cranial nerve defect, status epilepticus (severe symptom)

Adults: motor or sensory deficits; speech or movement impairment; flaccid paralysis

Investigations: blood tests (CBC, differential, platelets, electrolytes, glucose, BUN, creatinine, aminotransferases, coagulation); MRI (to detect brain edema; inflammation of the cerebral cortex, gray-white matter junction, thalamus, basal ganglia); CSF tests (perform LP after results of MRI; order CSF protein, glucose, cell count, differential, Gram stain, bacterial culture); EEG (usually abnormal) to differentiate from nonconvulsive seizure activity

Trauma

Investigations: CT scan to detect hematomas, contusions, skull fractures; MRI to detect subtler findings

Metabolic condition (e.g., uremia, hypercalcemia, hypoglycemia)

UREMIA

Signs and symptoms: history of CKD or kidney injury; itchiness

Investigations: blood tests (creatinine, eGFR, potassium, phosphate, calcium, sodium)

HYPERCALCEMIA

Signs and symptoms: constipation, polyuria, polydipsia, dehydration, anorexia, nausea, muscle weakness, altered sensory status

History of sarcoidosis, malignancy, hyperparathyroidism, immobilization

Investigations: blood test (hypercalcemia is total calcium ≥ 10.52 mg/dL [2.63 mmol/L] or ionized calcium ≥ 5.6 mg/dL [1.4 mmol/L]); albumin; parathyroid hormone

HYPOGLYCEMIA

The most common cause is diabetes treatment.

Signs and symptoms: palpitations, pallor, sweating, nightmares, fatigue, hunger

Severe: confusion, disorientation, blurred vision, seizures, coma

Investigations: low plasma glucose (symptoms typically develop at concentrations ≤ 54 mg/dL [3.0 mmol/L])

Substance use and overdose

Examples of common overdose substances include acetylsalicylic acid, acetaminophen, anticholinergics (e.g., TCAs), sympathomimetics (e.g., amphetamines, cocaine), depressants (e.g., alcohol, opiates, sedatives, hypnotics), hallucinogens (e.g., amphetamines), and serotonergic medications (e.g., SSRIs).

Signs and symptoms: personal or family history of substance abuse; excessive worry; loss of interest in friends and usual activities; adverse experience (e.g., abuse, death of a friend or family member); physical evidence (track marks on the arms, nasal septum perforation); tachycardia; tremor and/or sweating

Acetaminophen poisoning: nausea, vomiting; lethargy; pallor; liver enlargement and tenderness

Salicylate poisoning: abdominal pain, tinnitus, nausea, vomiting (blood in the vomit), hyperthermia, mental status changes (e.g., agitation and seizures; or lethargy, CNS depression, and coma)

Investigations: toxicology screen for suspected substance

SEIZURES

Signs and symptoms: history of seizures (e.g., epilepsy)

Investigations: brain and head imaging to detect injury or abnormal brain anatomy; EEG

Keys to patient encounter

History

The patient will be unable to give a history, so seek collateral information from accompanying caregivers and obtain any available medical records.

Ask about the circumstances surrounding the coma: where the patient was found, and what relevant evidence was found with them (e.g., drug paraphernalia).

Ask about medical conditions, medications, trauma, and drug use.

Physical exam

Vital signs: Look particularly for fever (this suggests infection or stroke).

GCS: Document the degree of the patient's unresponsiveness (see the pointer).

General inspection: Examine the patient's arms for evidence of IV drug use.

Neurological

Investigations

Point-of-care glucose (hypoglycemia is a relatively common and reversible cause of coma)

CBC

Urine drug screen

Electrolytes (see *Notes on labs and assessments*)

Calcium

Creatinine

Glucose

Liver enzymes

Thyrotropin (TSH)

CT scan of the head

POINTER

Glasgow Coma Scale

The GSC scores the way a patient's eyes and limbs respond to stimulus, and the patient's facility with speech.

Patients with a normal level of consciousness can open their eyes spontaneously, move appropriately in response to verbal commands, and speak cogently.

Patients whose level of consciousness is compromised may only respond to pain stimulus, and may have garbled speech or only make sounds.

Patients who are unconscious do not respond to any stimulus and do not speak.

Versions of the GCS are available online.

Management

Consider a trial of naloxone for possible opioid overdose.

Admit the patient to ICU and consult a critical-care physician.

ALTERED LEVEL OF CONSCIOUSNESS

Delirium

Differential diagnosis

DELIRIUM IN GENERAL

In addition to the disorders listed in this differential diagnosis, common causes of delirium include sensory deprivation (e.g., a patient in hospital might not have their glasses or hearing aids), urinary retention, fecaloma, and constipation.

Signs and symptoms: sudden-onset (hours to days), fluctuating symptoms that resolve on treatment of the underlying cause; changes in level of consciousness (hypoactivity, hyperactivity, or alternating states); impaired focus (e.g., confusion, disorientation); visual hallucinations

MEDICATIONS (E.G., SEDATIVE, ANTICHOLINERGIC)

Examples of sedatives include benzodiazepines (e.g., alprazolam, clorazepate, diazepam).

Examples of medications with anticholinergic properties include antihistamines, antidepressants (e.g., amitriptyline), cardiovascular medications (e.g., digoxin), antidiarrheals, GI antispasmodics, and antiulcer medications.

The risk of delirium increases with the use of multiple medications, especially psychiatric drugs and sedatives in combination.

METABOLIC CONDITION (E.G., FLUID AND ELECTROLYTE DISTURBANCE)

Metabolic disorders can lead to hormone regulation dysfunction, which can trigger malfunction in brain activity.

Investigations: blood and urine tests to measure electrolyte and hormone levels

HYPOXIA (E.G., ANEMIA, HYPOPERFUSION)

Signs and symptoms (in general): shortness of breath; headache; confusion; history of anemia, heart disease, lung disease, PE

Investigations: CBC, ABG, chest x-ray, echocardiogram

INFECTION

Examples of infections that can cause delirium include UTI, pneumonia, meningitis, and encephalitis.

Investigations: blood tests to analyze immune function; blood and urine cultures; chest x-ray to detect pneumonia; LP (CSF analysis) to detect pathogens

ENDOCRINE CONDITION (E.G., HYPOTHYROIDISM)

Hypothyroidism

Signs and symptoms: history of hypothyroidism or symptoms of hypothyroidism (cold intolerance, decreased reflexes, dry skin, weight gain, impaired cognition)

Investigations: elevated thyrotropin (TSH)

NEUROLOGICAL CONDITION (E.G., STROKE, DEMENTIA)

Acute stroke

Signs and symptoms: speech difficulty and hemiparesis (most common symptoms); weakness or paralysis in the extremities or face; arm or leg numbness; confusion; headache; nonorthostatic dizziness; fever

Dementia

Signs and symptoms: gradual impairment of ≥ 1 cognitive area (complex attention; executive function; learning and memory; language; perceptual-motor skills; social interaction); deficits that interfere with day-to-day life (e.g., ability to pay bills); **no** evidence that the cognitive impairment occurs only with delirium; **no** evidence of depression

POSTSURGICAL CONDITION

Postsurgical delirium is common, especially in the elderly.

Causes may include pain, pain medications, anesthesia, infection, or DVT.

Investigations: EEG to detect brain disturbances associated with pain

WITHDRAWAL (E.G., ALCOHOL, BENZODIAZEPINE)

Alcohol withdrawal

Signs and symptoms:

> Mild withdrawal (symptoms start within 24 hours of cessation): tremulousness, insomnia, anxiety, hyperreflexia, sweating, GI upset, mild autonomic hyperactivity
>
> Moderate withdrawal (symptoms start within 24 to 48 hours of cessation): tremors, insomnia, excessive adrenergic symptoms, intense anxiety
>
> Severe withdrawal (symptoms start > 48 hours after cessation): disorientation, agitation, hallucinations, tremulousness, tachycardia, tachypnea, hyperthermia, sweating

Benzodiazepine withdrawal

Signs and symptoms (symptoms start within 6 to 48 hours of cessation): insomnia, irritability, sweating, dizziness, headache, anxiety, panic attacks, impaired cognition, hallucinations, seizures, nausea

TRAUMA

Investigations: EEG; brain CT scan or MRI

Keys patient encounter

History

The patient will be unable to give a coherent history, so seek collateral information from accompanying caregivers.

DELIRIUM HISTORY

Ask when the delirium began. Listen for triggering events such as change in medication, surgery, substance withdrawal, or trauma.

ASSOCIATED SYMPTOMS

Ask in particular about fever (this suggests infection) and speech difficulty (this suggests stroke).

PAST MEDICAL HISTORY

Ask about a history of hypothyroidism, dementia, and conditions related to hypoxia (e.g., anemia, heart disease, lung disease).

MEDICATIONS

Ask about sedatives, anticholinergic drugs, benzodiazepines, and polypharmacy.

POINTER

Mini-Mental State Exams

MMSEs generally assess:

- orientation to time and place
- recall (e.g., remembering a short list of words)
- calculation (e.g., spelling a word backwards)
- language comprehension (e.g., naming objects; following a written command, a verbal command, and a complex instruction; repeating back a spoken phrase)

SOCIAL HISTORY

Determine the patient's age, and ask about a history of alcohol or drug abuse.

Physical exam

Vital signs: Look for fever (this suggests infection).

Mental status: Administer an MMSE (see the pointer).

Investigations

CBC

Creatinine

Thyrotropin (TSH)

ABG

Blood and urine cultures in suspected infection

CSF culture if symptoms warrant

CT scan of the head (consider this)

Management

Treat any underlying conditions and discontinue any potentially causative medications. Admit the patient to hospital for observation and to ensure their safety. Consider referral to a geriatrician.

POINTER

Proxy decision-making

An important aspect of management in this clinical presentation is to clarify proxy decision-making. Does the patient have an advance directive, or have they named a person to make decisions on their behalf? If the patient has not taken these steps, they may have made "transmitted decisions"—decisions about their care of which they have informed others. In the absence of an advance directive, named proxy decision-makers, or transmitted decisions, individuals who know the patient well may make "hypothetical judgments."

ALTERED LEVEL OF CONSCIOUSNESS

Major or mild neurocognitive disorder (dementia)

Differential diagnosis

MAJOR OR MILD NEUROCOGNITIVE DISORDER IN GENERAL

Signs and symptoms: gradual impairment of ≥ 1 cognitive area (complex attention; executive function; learning and memory; language; perceptual-motor skills; social interaction); **no** evidence that the cognitive impairment occurs only with delirium; **no** evidence of depression

Mild cognitive impairment: deficits that **do not** significantly interfere with day-to-day life

Major cognitive impairment (dementia): deficits that interfere with day-to-day life (e.g., ability to pay bills)

ALZHEIMER DISEASE

Alzheimer disease is generally diagnosed clinically: the goal of imaging studies, when pursued, is to rule out other causes.

Signs and symptoms: older age (rare onset before age 60; prevalence doubles every 5 years after age 65); insidious onset of impairment (key characteristic); memory impairment (most common initial symptom); executive dysfunction and visuospatial impairment (often relatively early symptoms); language deficits and behavioral changes (often later symptoms)

VASCULAR DEMENTIA (E.G., MULTIINFARCT, LACUNAR INFARCT)

Multiinfarct dementia

Deficits manifest after multiple infarcts over time, or suddenly after a stroke.

Signs and symptoms: age 60 to 70 (more common); male (more common); memory loss; confusion (e.g., getting lost in familiar places); difficulty with short-term memory, performing routine tasks (e.g., paying bills), remembering words; misplacing items; personality and mood changes (depression, poor judgment, social withdrawal); sleep disruption; hallucinations, delusions

Risk factors: previous strokes; vascular factors (HF, hypertension, atherosclerosis, AF), smoking, alcohol use, obesity, poor diet, sedentary lifestyle

Investigations: MRI or CT scan

Lacunar infarct

Signs and symptoms: unilateral weakness (face, arm, leg); "dysarthria-clumsy hand syndrome" (facial weakness, difficulty speaking, difficulty swallowing, and slight weakness and clumsiness of 1 hand); ataxic hemiparesis (ipsilateral weakness with limb ataxia); **no** monoplegia, stupor, coma, loss of consciousness, or seizures

> Pure motor hemiparesis (most common): **no** sensory deficit
>
> Pure sensory stroke: **no** motor deficit
>
> Sensorimotor stroke: **no** aphasia, agnosia, neglect, apraxia, hemianopia

Risk factors: systemic hypertension; diabetes; smoking; older age; high LDL

Investigations: MRI or CT scan

BRAIN TRAUMA (E.G., POSTCONCUSSIVE CONDITION, ANOXIA)

BRAIN TRAUMA IN GENERAL

This is injury to brain tissue that likely results in functional impairment.

Investigations: EEG depending on symptom severity; CT scan or MRI if swelling or bleeding is suspected

Concussion

This is a less severe type of brain injury.

Signs and symptoms: history of concussion; headache; impaired alertness; loss of consciousness; memory loss; confusion; drowsiness

Anoxia

Examples of causes include severe asthma attack, heart attack, carbon monoxide poisoning, and near drowning.

DRUGS (E.G., ALCOHOL, SUBSTANCE ABUSE)

TOXINS (E.G., HEAVY METALS, ORGANIC TOXINS)

Sources of heavy metal exposure include lead (lead paint, lead in water pipes), mercury (eating fish contaminated with mercury), and arsenic (pesticides).

Sources of organic toxin exposure include organophosphate pesticides.

Signs and symptoms: sudden weight loss or gain; changes in skin and hair condition; anemia (fatigue, pallor, dizziness, shortness of breath, tachycardia); abdominal pain; diarrhea

Investigations: blood and urine testing to detect markers of heavy metal or toxin poisoning (e.g., liver function, blood chemistry, urinalysis)

NEURODEGENERATIVE DISORDERS (E.G., PARKINSON DISEASE, LEWY BODY DEMENTIA, HUNTINGTON DISEASE)

Parkinson disease

Signs and symptoms (mnemonic **TRAP**): **t**remor at rest; **r**igidity of the lower limbs; **a**kinesia, bradykinesia; **p**ostural instability

> Other symptoms: cognitive impairment; dementia; shuffling gait with stooped posture and loss of arm swing; micrographia; hypophonia; masklike facies; "pill rolling"; lack of blinking; orthostatic hypotension
>
> History of use of antipsychotics, antiemetics; toxin ingestion (e.g., carbon monoxide, cyanide); head trauma; vascular disease; other neurodegenerative disease (e.g., Lewy body dementia, Huntington disease); brain tumor; hydrocephalus; metabolic conditions (e.g., hypoparathyroidism, Wilson disease, chronic liver failure); infections that spread to the brain (HIV/AIDS, syphilis, prion disease, toxoplasmosis, encephalitis lethargica, progressive multifocal leukoencephalopathy)

Lewy body dementia

Signs and symptoms: visual hallucinations, movement disorder (slowed movement, rigid muscles, tremor, shuffling walk), dizziness, constipation, sleep difficulties

Risk factors: family history of Lewy body dementia or Parkinson disease; male; older than 60

Huntington disease

Signs and symptoms: family history of Huntington disease; abnormal eye movements; tics (uncontrolled movement in the fingers, feet, face, trunk); myoclonus; chorea (progressive chorea in late-onset Huntington disease; older than 50); psychiatric symptoms (depression; apathy; anxiety; obsessions, compulsions; irritability; psychosis; paranoid and acoustic hallucinations; hypersexuality); cognitive symptoms (impaired executive function; loss of mental flexibility, concentration, judgment, memory, awareness); motor symptoms (bradykinesia, dystonia, muscle weakness); profuse sweating from autonomic disturbance

Investigations: DNA analysis (PCR or Southern blot); neuroimaging (MRI, CT scan, SPECT, PET scan) for progression monitoring

NORMAL PRESSURE HYDROCEPHALUS

Signs and symptoms (classic triad):

Gait disturbance (most common and earliest symptom): dizziness; balance and walking difficulty (e.g., tripping, wide stance, short shuffling steps)

Cognitive impairment: organization and concentration difficulty; daytime sleepiness; psychomotor slowing; loss of precise fine movement; short-term memory problems; apathy; reduced speech; dementia

Urinary symptoms: frequent urination, especially at night; urgency; permanent incontinence

Investigations: MRI to detect ventricular enlargement with no macroscopic CSF obstruction; normal or mildly elevated LP opening pressure

INTRACRANIAL MASS (E.G., TUMOR, SUBDURAL MASS, BRAIN ABSCESS)

Brain tumor

Types of brain tumor include meningioma, astrocytoma, oligodendroglioma, glioblastoma, and Schwannoma.

Signs and symptoms: acute-onset headaches; older than 50; change in chronic headache pattern; increasing intensity and frequency of headaches; headaches that disturb sleep; unilateral headache pain, always on the same side; position-evoked crescendo headache; impaired vision; light-headedness

Other symptoms: focal seizures, confusion, memory loss, personality change

Investigations: imaging for intracranial masses (MRI with contrast enhancement is best for tumors and abscesses); biopsy

Subdural hematoma

Signs and symptoms: history of head trauma or use of anticoagulants; local neurological findings (cranial nerve abnormalities; mono- or hemiparesis or hemiplegia); global neurologic findings (confusion, coma); pupil abnormalities; retinal hemorrhage

Investigations: imaging for intracranial masses (CT scan with contrast enhancement is best for hematomas)

Brain abscess

This is caused by bacteria (most common), fungi, or parasites.

Signs and symptoms: headache (most common); fever; focal neurologic deficits (vision or hearing loss; tingling; weakness; behavior or cognitive change); seizures; nausea, vomiting; recent or current infections, or recent trauma or surgery; signs of infection on the skin, or in the sinuses, oral cavity, eye fundus, ears, or other locations (e.g., lung)

Investigations: blood cultures; culture of brain lesion; imaging for intracranial masses (MRI with contrast enhancement is best for tumors and abscesses)

INFECTION (E.G., HIV, NEUROSYPHILIS)

HIV

HIV develops into AIDS when the CD4 cell count is < 200 cells/μL (0.2×10^9/L) (reference range of CD4: 500–2000 cells/μL [$0.5–2.0 \times 10^9$/L]).

Signs and symptoms: flu-like symptoms in the first, acute phase; leukopenia in the second, latent, asymptomatic stage (200–499 CD4 cells/μL [$0.2–0.499 \times 10^9$/L]); lymphadenopathy

> Neurocognitive symptoms: behavioral changes; difficulty in making decisions; difficulties with attention, concentration, memory; tremors; loss of coordination
>
> AIDS: recurrent, severe opportunistic infections or malignancies

Risk factors: unprotected sex; IV drug use

Investigations: positive HIV-1 p24 antigen in the blood followed by HIV antibody testing (positive ELISA result); PCR to determine HIV RNA level or viral load

Neurosyphilis

Symptoms can present within weeks or years of infection. Some patients are asymptomatic.

Signs and symptoms: headache; stiff neck; nausea, vomiting; loss of vision or hearing; general paresis (changes in personality, mood)

Risk factors: unprotected sex, HIV

Investigations: positive test for syphilis

ENDOCRINE, METABOLIC, OR NUTRITIONAL DISORDER (E.G., HYPOTHYROIDISM, VITAMIN B_{12} DEFICIENCY)

Hypothyroidism

Signs and symptoms: history of hypothyroidism or symptoms of hypothyroidism (cold intolerance, decreased reflexes, dry skin, weight gain, impaired cognition)

Investigations: elevated thyrotropin (TSH)

Vitamin B_{12} deficiency

Signs and symptoms: neuropsychiatric symptoms including memory or cognitive impairment, dementia, depression; anemia (fatigue, pallor, dizziness, shortness of breath, tachycardia), peripheral neuropathy

Investigations: low serum vitamin B_{12} (or cobalamin); CBC with peripheral smear (low hemoglobin, macrocytosis)

Keys to patient encounter

Key concerns

Identify deterioration in cognitive function.

Look for reversible risk factors.

Differentiate early Alzheimer disease from other causes.

History

COGNITIVE SYMPTOMS

Obtain collateral information on the patient's symptoms (e.g., from an accompanying caregiver), if possible. Ask how long the patient has had cognitive problems and how quickly the problems have developed. Note that insidious onset is a hallmark of Alzheimer disease.

ASSOCIATED SYMPTOMS

Ask about other symptoms the patient has had.

Examples of characteristic symptoms include:

Lacunar infarct: weakness

Toxic exposure and neurosyphilis: GI symptoms

Neurodegenerative disorders: movement abnormalities

Screen for symptoms of depression: depressed mood, loss of interest in usual activities, psychomotor changes (agitated or slowed, as observed by others), significant weight change, sleep disturbance, fatigue, indecisiveness, and recurrent thoughts of death or suicide.

PAST MEDICAL HISTORY

Ask about a history of stroke, vascular disorders, hypertension, diabetes, dyslipidemia, heart disease, HIV, and head trauma or concussions.

SOCIAL HISTORY

Ask about drug and alcohol abuse.

Physical exam

Mental status: Administer an MMSE (see the pointer).

Neurological

Investigations

Thyrotropin (TSH)

Vitamin B_{12}

Brain imaging (MRI or CT scan) to diagnose any masses or infarcts

VDRL or other syphilis test

Management

Management depends on the specific diagnosis. Consider referral to a neurologist, psychiatrist, or geriatrician.

POINTER

Mini-Mental State Exams

MMSEs generally assess:

- orientation to time and place
- recall (e.g., remembering a short list of words)
- calculation (e.g., spelling a word backwards)
- language comprehension (e.g., naming objects; following a written command, a verbal command, and a complex instruction; repeating back a spoken phrase)

ALTERED LEVEL OF CONSCIOUSNESS

Seizures

Differential diagnosis

PRIMARY NEUROLOGICAL DISORDERS (E.G., IDIOPATHIC EPILEPSY, HEAD TRAUMA, ENCEPHALITIS)

Idiopathic epilepsy

This presents with generalized seizures or partial (focal) seizures. Cognition is normal. In children, it often resolves on its own at a later age.

Risk factors: family history of epilepsy

IDIOPATHIC GENERALIZED EPILEPSY

Signs and symptoms:

Childhood absence epilepsy: age 4 to 10 years; absence seizures (brief losses of awareness with staring, eye blinking, lip smacking); episodes of loss of consciousness without loss of body tone that are brief (4 to 20 seconds) and frequent (up to 10 times a day) (hyperventilation provokes episodes); EEG showing generalized spike wave activity at 2.5–5 Hz

Juvenile absence epilepsy: onset at age 10 to 12 years; absence seizures; generalized tonic-clonic seizures (possible; these are not seen in childhood absence epilepsy)

Juvenile myoclonic epilepsy (this disorder does not completely resolve in adulthood, so it requires lifelong therapy): myoclonic jerks, generalized tonic-clonic seizures, and absence seizures (absence seizures begin several years before the onset of other seizure types); seizures that are provoked by sleep deprivation or waking; EEG showing spike wave at 4–6 Hz

IDIOPATHIC FOCAL EPILEPSY

Signs and symptoms:

Benign epilepsy of childhood with centrotemporal spikes: onset at age 3 to 13 years (peak incidence age 7 to 9 years); seizures with facial numbness or twitching, guttural vocalizations, hypersalivation, drooling, dysphasia, speech arrest (**no** loss of consciousness); nighttime seizures or on waking; EEG showing centrotemporal sharp waves

Panayiotopoulos syndrome: onset before age 5 years; seizures with vomiting, sudden loss of muscle tone, unresponsiveness, pale skin, incontinence, coughing, hypersalivation; nighttime seizures (duration > 5 minutes); interictal EEG showing occipital spikes and epileptiform activity from other or multiple areas

Benign occipital epilepsy of childhood: onset at age 8 to 9 years; seizures with blindness, visual hallucinations, hemiclonic activity, automatisms, migraines, versive movements; daytime seizures (duration < 5 minutes); interictal EEG showing epileptiform activity that is mostly occipital and long bursts of spike-wave activity on closing the eyes

Seizures or epilepsy due to head trauma

Head trauma includes bullet wounds, severe sports-related injuries, and other severe physical trauma to the head.

Early posttraumatic seizures (these develop within days of trauma) are usually focal.

Late posttraumatic seizures (these develop within weeks of trauma) are associated with a high risk of later epilepsy (posttraumatic epilepsy).

Prompt treatment of active seizures (with IV phenytoin and sodium valproate) is needed to prevent further damage.

Investigations: MRI

Seizures or epilepsy due to encephalitis

Seizures are common in encephalitis.

Viral infection is the most common cause: HSV-1, HSV-2; EBV; VZV; Enterovirus (e.g., Coxsackievirus); and insect-borne viruses (e.g., West Nile disease, Lyme disease).

Signs and symptoms: altered mental status (e.g., decreased level of consciousness, lethargy, personality change, behavior change), fever, headache, nausea, vomiting

Infants and neonates: poor feeding, irritability, lethargy

Children and adolescents: irritability; movement disorder; ataxia; stupor; coma; hemiparesis; cranial nerve defect; status epilepticus (severe)

Adults: motor or sensory deficits; speech or movement impairment; flaccid paralysis

Investigations: blood tests (CBC, differential, platelets; electrolytes; glucose; BUN; creatinine; aminotransferases; coagulation); MRI to detect brain edema, inflammation of the cerebral cortex, gray-white matter junction, thalamus, basal ganglia; CSF tests (perform LP after results of MRI; order CSF protein, glucose, cell count, differential, Gram stain, bacterial culture); EEG (usually abnormal) to differentiate from nonconvulsive seizure activity

SYSTEMIC DISORDER (E.G., HYPOGLYCEMIA, ELECTROLYTE DISORDERS)

Hypoglycemia

Hypoglycemic seizures are common in diabetic patients who take excessive insulin or oral hypoglycemics.

Signs and symptoms: palpitations, pallor, sweating, nightmares, fatigue, hunger

Severe: confusion, disorientation, blurred vision, seizures, coma

Electrolyte disorders

Status epilepticus in older adults is associated with electrolyte imbalance.

Signs and symptoms:

Hyponatremia (this is a medical emergency): serum sodium < 135 mEq/L (135 mmol/L) (severe: < 115 mEq/L [115 mmol/L]); in adults, generalized seizures; in children, acute symptomatic nonfebrile seizures; nonspecific findings on EEG

Hypocalcemia: total calcium < 8.5 mg/dL (2.15 mmol/L); mental status changes and generalized tonic-clonic or focal motor seizures, with or without muscular tetany (acute hypocalcemia); positive Chvostek sign; Trousseau sign; EEG showing background rhythm with evolution from alpha to theta, diffuse increase in slow wave activity in theta and delta range

Hypomagnesemia: serum magnesium < 1.8 mg/dL (0.70 mmol/L) (severe: < 1.25 mg/dL [0.50 mmol/L]); generalized tonic-clonic seizures (severe hypomagnesemia); neuromuscular irritability; cardiac arrhythmia; higher risk of hypomagnesemia in HIV-positive patients

Hypophosphatemia (symptoms usually arise only in cases of chronic and severe serum phosphate depletion: < 2.5 mg/dL [0.81 mmol/L]): paresthesias; generalized seizures; impaired muscle contractility; history of chronic alcoholism, refeeding syndrome, Fanconi syndrome

OTHER (E.G., FEBRILE SEIZURE, WITHDRAWAL)

Febrile seizure

Signs and symptoms: young child (age 3 months to 6 years; peak incidence age 12 to 18 months); fever > 38°C; symptoms of cold, influenza, ear infection (febrile seizure is usually the first sign of illness); **no** intracranial infection, CNS inflammation, acute systemic metabolic abnormality; **no** previous afebrile seizures

Simple febrile seizure (most common): generalized tonic-clonic phase (loss of consciousness, followed by both arms and legs shaking uncontrollably); generalized convulsions lasting ≤ 15 minutes; quick return to baseline after convulsions (**no** confusion, agitation, drowsiness); **no** recurrence within 24 hours

Complex febrile seizure: younger child with abnormal development; focal convulsions (1 limb or 1 side of the body shakes); convulsions lasting > 15 minutes

Risk factors for recurrence: first febrile seizure at younger than 18 months; family history of febrile seizure; high fever; viral infection

Withdrawal seizures (alcohol)

Signs and symptoms: chronic alcoholism (onset at age 40 to 50); tonic-clonic seizures; single seizure or a brief period of multiple seizures that occur 12 to 48 hours after the last alcoholic drink

Keys to patient encounter

Key concerns

Differentiate seizure from other transient nonseizure conditions (e.g., syncope, pseudoseizure).

Consider seizure in the context of episodic neurological symptoms (e.g., inattention, psychosis).

Provide emergent treatment of a patient presenting with seizure.

Provide immediate management of secondary causes of seizure.

History

HISTORY PRESENT ILLNESS

A main goal of the history is to differentiate true seizure from nonseizure conditions and to determine secondary causes of seizure. Ask whether the patient has lacked sleep or experienced unusual stress. Ask what happened immediately before the event (e.g., getting up from a sitting or lying position), whether there was a warning (aura) before the event, and whether the patient was exposed to flashing lights or computer screens before the event. Ask about recent illness.

For children and infants, ask whether the child has had a fever, and whether the event was observed by others. Ask about abnormal body movements during the seizure, the time of day it happened, whether the child lost control of bowel or bladder function, and whether the child bit their tongue or cheeks. Ask whether the child was aware of what was happening and could speak normally. Ask how the child felt after the event (e.g., tired or confused; headache; muscle aches). Ask whether the child has previously experienced anything similar.

PAST MEDICAL HISTORY

Ask about coexisting medical conditions (e.g., diabetes, malignancy) and a history of head trauma.

If the patient is diabetic, ask about insulin routines, looking for possible noncompliance with medication.

Ask about possible pregnancy and any known complications (preeclampsia/eclampsia).

MEDICATIONS

Ask about current medications to assess for electrolyte disturbances. Ask about chemotherapy and other immunosuppressing drugs.

SOCIAL HISTORY

Ask about alcohol use, including the frequency and amount of use, and the date of the last drink.

FAMILY HISTORY

Ask about a family history of epilepsy.

Physical exam

Vital signs: In a child, look for fever.

Neurological: Conduct a full neurological examination, looking in particular for focal neurologic signs.

Investigations

Glucose and electrolytes to rule out hypoglycemia

β-HGC to rule out eclampsia

LP in immunocompromised patients to rule out CNS infection

CT scan or MRI of the head to rule out intracranial pathology

EEG to investigate the seizure type

Management

Management depends on the cause of the event. Nonseizure events (e.g., syncope, pseudoseizure) may require referral to a cardiologist or psychiatrist respectively. For true seizures, neuroimaging and laboratory testing may indicate an etiology requiring specific management (e.g., neurosurgery referral, management of a metabolic condition). In unprovoked seizures (seizures with no identifiable secondary cause), new-onset epilepsy is the most common cause.

Alcohol withdrawal seizures require hospital admission and urgent management. Seizures associated with eclampsia require hospital admission and emergency obstetrical consultation.

> **POINTER**
>
> **Monitoring antiseizure medication complications**
>
> Patients taking antiseizure medications often experience weight gain and develop high lipids. These are complications that require monitoring.

In febrile seizure in children, provide the parents with information and reassurance.

In suspected primary neurological disorder, refer the patient to a neurologist.

Manage any coexisting medical conditions.

ANORECTAL PAIN

Anorectal pain

Differential diagnosis

ANORECTAL DISEASE

Inflammatory bowel disease

Signs and symptoms: younger than 30 (usually); family history of inflammatory bowel disease; fluctuating symptoms with periods of exacerbation and remission; diarrhea (possibly with nocturnal waking); blood in the stool; abdominal pain; weight loss; fever; fatigue; right lower quadrant and periumbilical pain; extraintestinal manifestations (e.g., uveitis, arthritis)

Crohn disease: right lower quadrant mass, uveitis, arthritis

Investigations: elevated CRP (this suggests active inflammation); fecal calprotectin; colonoscopy with biopsy (this is a standard diagnostic procedure); CT scan or MRI (findings: diagnostic structural changes associated with inflammatory bowel disease)

Fissures, fistulas

Signs and symptoms: pain with bowel movements; small amounts of bright red blood following bowel movements; anal fissures or fistulas on physical exam

Hemorrhoids

Signs and symptoms: anal pain (if hemorrhoids are thrombosed); anal bleeding (bright red blood), often following a bowel movement; hemorrhoids on physical exam

DERMATOLOGIC DISEASE

Psoriasis

Signs and symptoms (general): nail pitting; current or prior erythematous scaly rashes; family history of psoriasis or similar skin conditions; history of other autoimmune diseases

Anal psoriasis: pain during bowel movements; anal bleeding; excessive anal dryness and itching

Contact dermatitis or atopic dermatitis

Signs and symptoms: redness, itchiness, dry cracked skin, blisters, swelling, burning

MALIGNANCY

Signs and symptoms: weight loss, abdominal pain, blood in the stool, constipation, change in stool caliber, personal or family history of colorectal cancer, palpable mass (anal or rectal)

Investigations: colonoscopy; CEA

INFECTION

Sexually transmitted infections

Signs and symptoms: lower abdominal and pelvic pain; pain during intercourse; fever; urinary symptoms (often); vaginal or urethral discharge (anal discharge in anal sex); irregular menstruation

Risk factors: unprotected sex, multiple sexual partners

Investigations: positive cultures for gonorrhea and/or chlamydia

Bacterial, fungal, or parasitic infections

BACTERIAL INFECTIONS

Food-borne bacterial infections are a more common source of anorectal pain than fungal or parasitic infections.

Signs and symptoms (in general): nausea, vomiting, abdominal pain, diarrhea, fever

Risk factors: ingesting raw meat, poultry, seafood, or eggs, or unpasteurized milk, or contaminated water; travel (e.g., travel to developing countries, camping); close exposure to birds or reptiles; antibiotic use (which can lead to *C. difficile* infection)

FUNGAL AND PARASITIC INFECTIONS

These are less likely to cause anorectal pain, except in severe infection.

Risk factors for severe infection: AIDS; other factors causing immunosuppression (e.g., chemotherapy)

TRAUMA

Examples of causes include occupational trauma, intimate partner violence, and sexual assault. If the trauma comes from a high-force injury, associated pelvic fracture is possible.

Investigations: proctoscopy, sigmoidoscopy

COCCYGEAL PAIN

Signs and symptoms: female patient (more common); pain that is worse with standing from a sitting position; history of prolonged sitting on hard surfaces; history of trauma (falling on the coccyx); obesity

Keys to patient encounter

Key concern

Identify anorectal pain caused by underlying disease.

History

PAIN HISTORY

Ask when the pain started, what the pain is like, and how constant it is.

Examples of characteristic pain include:

Chronic pain in a chronic disorder such as anorectal disease

Pain other than anal pain such as abdominal pain in inflammatory bowel disease, crampy pain in bacterial infection, pain from pelvic fracture in trauma

Episodic pain triggered by bowel movements in anal fissures, fistulas, or hemorrhoids

Episodic pain triggered by standing after sitting in coccygeal pain

Constant pain in trauma

ASSOCIATED SYMPTOMS

Ask, in particular, about constipation.

Examples of characteristic symptoms include:

Anal fissures, fistulas, and hemorrhoids: small amounts of bright red blood following bowel movements

Malignancy: blood in the stool and constitutional symptoms

Bacterial infection: nausea and diarrhea

STI: vaginal and/or anal discharge

PAST MEDICAL HISTORY

Ask about risk factors for underlying disease (see the pointer). Ask about trauma, including sexual trauma.

MEDICATIONS

Ask about medications known to cause constipation: antidepressants, antipsychotics, levodopa, antihistamines, antacids, and iron supplements. Ask about recent antibiotic use (relevant to *C. difficile* infection).

Physical exam

Vital signs: Look for fever and hypotension.

Abdominal: Look for masses.

Anal: Inspect the anus for masses, bleeding, hemorrhoids, and anal fissures.

DRE: Look for masses.

POINTER

Risk factors for underlying disease in anorectal pain

- Family history of inflammatory bowel disease
- Family history of psoriasis
- Family history of colorectal cancer
- Unprotected sex, multiple sexual partners (STI)
- AIDS or other immunosuppressive factors (infection)

Investigations

CBC to look for anemia and infection

Other specific investigations as indicated in the differential diagnosis

Management

If the patient has a benign cause of anorectal pain (e.g., hemorrhoids or anal fissures), advise conservative treatment: increased fiber, increased exercise, stool softeners, analgesics, and sitz baths. In the absence of an obvious benign cause, refer the patient for proctoscopy or colonoscopy to rule out malignancy and inflammatory bowel disease.

BLEEDING

Bleeding, bruising

Differential diagnosis

LOCALIZED BLEEDING (E.G., EPISTAXIS, LACERATION)

HEMOSTASIS DISORDERS

Platelet or blood vessel disorders (e.g., von Willebrand disease, collagen disorder, medication-induced disorder)

VON WILLEBRAND DISEASE

Signs and symptoms: family history of von Willebrand disease

Investigations: decreased von Willebrand factor on vWF antigen test; decreased ristocetin cofactor activity assay (this indicates a functional problem with von Willebrand factor)

COLLAGEN DISORDER

Signs and symptoms: history of collagen vascular disease (e.g., Ehlers-Danlos syndrome); hypermobile joints; hyperelastic skin; skin that tears easily

Investigations: genetic test for collagen vascular disease

MEDICATION-INDUCED DISORDER

Signs and symptoms: recent use of anticancer drugs, antibiotics (especially sulfonamide, penicillin, cephalosporin, rifampin, and vancomycin), heparin, digoxin, thiazide diuretics, H_2 antagonists, phenytoin, valproic acid, carbamazepine, oral anticoagulants, antiplatelet agents

Coagulation disorders (e.g., factor VIII deficiency, vitamin K deficiency, fibrinolysis)

FACTOR VIII DEFICIENCY

Signs and symptoms: family history of hemophilia, hemarthrosis

Investigations: decreased factor VIII or factor IX

VITAMIN K DEFICIENCY

Signs and symptoms: use of warfarin; diet restricting vitamin K intake (rare); conditions that cause fat malabsorption (celiac disease, Crohn disease, chronic pancreatitis, CF, small bowel surgery)

Investigations: elevated INR

FIBRINOLYSIS

Signs and symptoms (disseminated intravascular coagulopathy): history of recent, severe infection, especially sepsis; recent heat stroke; current pregnancy or recent delivery; organ transplant or recent blood transfusion; pancreatitis; malignancy; hepatic failure

Investigations: peripheral blood smear to detect RBC fragments (diagnostic); decreased platelets on CBC; elevated d-dimer level; elevated INR; elevated PTT; decreased plasma fibrinogen

Keys to patient encounter

Key concern

Recognize that some presentations are self-limiting.

Airway and hemodynamic status

If the patient is actively bleeding, check their ABCs. Provide emergency management, if indicated (e.g., apply pressure and gauze to the site of bleeding; apply a tourniquet to a limb to control life-threatening bleeding; apply nasal packing for epistaxis).

History

HISTORY OF PRESENT ILLNESS

Ask how easily the patient bleeds. For example, does the patient find it difficult to stop bleeding after minor injuries or dental work? Ask about bleeding that has required surgical intervention, blood transfusion, or replacement therapy.

PAST MEDICAL HISTORY

Ask about hemostasis disorders; and conditions associated with vitamin K deficiency, including celiac disease, Crohn disease, chronic pancreatitis, CF, and small bowel surgery.

MEDICATIONS

Ask about medications associated with bleeding and bruising (see the information in the differential diagnosis).

FAMILY HISTORY

Ask about a family history of bleeding problems. In women, ask about a history of menorrhagia, or hysterectomy for postpartum bleeding.

Physical exam

Vital signs

Dermatological: Examine the skin and mucous membranes for petechiae and bruising.

Joints: Look for hemarthroses.

Abdominal: Look for hepatosplenomegaly.

Investigations

CBC and peripheral blood smear to look for anemia and thrombocytopenia

PT/INR and PTT to look for clotting factor deficiencies

Coagulopathy screen (or hemostasis screen), which would generally include:

- circulating anticoagulant (inhibitory screen)

- factor assays (factors II, V, VII, VIII, IX, X, XI, XII, XIII)
- inhibitor screen or assay
- 50:50 mixing study
- von Willebrand factor workup (von Willebrand factor antigen, von Willebrand factor activity)

Platelet function studies to look for platelet disorders (consider this)

Management

Consider referring the patient to a hematologist for assistance with management, especially in ongoing suspicion of a bleeding disorder despite a nondiagnostic workup.

BLEEDING

Blood in sputum (hemoptysis)

Differential diagnosis

AIRWAY DISEASE

Inflammatory (e.g., bronchiectasis, bronchitis)

BRONCHIECTASIS

Signs and symptoms: long-standing symptoms, productive cough, shortness of breath, chest pain, fever, general physical wasting

Investigations: CT scan to detect abnormal bronchial tree dilatation

BRONCHITIS

Signs and symptoms: productive cough, shortness of breath, fever, minimal hemoptysis, abnormal lung sounds (wheezing, crackles, rhonchi)

Chronic bronchitis: symptoms of acute bronchitis lasting > 3 months, with exacerbations (this identifies chronic bronchitis); history of asthma, COPD; general physical wasting

Neoplasm (e.g., bronchogenic carcinoma)

BRONCHOGENIC CARCINOMA

Signs and symptoms: constitutional symptoms (fever, weight loss, night sweats, fatigue); abnormal lung sounds on auscultation; areas of dullness on percussion of the chest; enlarged lymph nodes

Risk factors: smoking, asbestos exposure

Investigations: chest x-ray and CT scan; biopsy

Other (e.g., foreign body, trauma)

FOREIGN BODY

Signs and symptoms: history of inhaling a foreign body; wheezing (possible: this suggests a partially obstructed bronchus)

Investigations: chest x-ray or CT scan

TRAUMA

Signs and symptoms: absence of lung sounds (this suggests pneumothorax); tender spine, ribs, spleen; history of a medical procedure (e.g., bronchoscopy)

PULMONARY PARENCHYMAL DISEASE

Infectious disease (e.g., tuberculosis, necrotizing pneumonia)

TUBERCULOSIS

Signs and symptoms: constitutional symptoms (fever, weight loss, night sweats, fatigue), chest pain

Risk factors: contact with TB-infected individuals; use of IV street drugs; factors causing immunosuppression (HIV infection, cancer, immunosuppressant medications, autoimmune disease, and malnutrition); hypoxia

Investigations: positive tuberculin skin test (purified protein derivative) in suspected latent TB; sputum mycobacterial culture, PCR of sputum in suspected active TB; chest x-ray

NECROTIZING PNEUMONIA

Signs and symptoms: rapid onset and progression of symptoms; rapidly worsening shortness of breath; fever; hypoxia; recent history of pneumonia

Investigations: CBC to detect leukopenia (leukopenia may rapidly worsen); chest x-ray to detect lung consolidation

Inflammatory or immune disease (e.g., vasculitis)

VASCULITIS

Signs and symptoms: personal or family history of vasculitis; cutaneous vasculitis (polyarteritis nodosa: palpable purpura, petechiae, ulcers); abnormal lung sounds; neuropathy (numbness, weakness); hematuria in pulmonary-renal syndrome (e.g., Goodpasture syndrome)

Investigations: elevated serum ANCA; CT scan to detect diffuse alveolar infiltrates; anti-GBM; biopsy

Other (e.g., coagulopathy)

COAGULOPATHY

Signs and symptoms: use of anticoagulants; history of liver disease (this can lead to deficits in clotting factor production); bruising and petechiae on the skin and in the mouth

Investigations: elevated PT/INR; serum liver enzyme tests to detect liver disease

CARDIAC OR VASCULAR DISEASE

Pulmonary embolus with infarction

Signs and symptoms: sharp chest pain; shortness of breath; cough (possibly with blood); hypoxia; possible unilateral swelling of the lower limbs (this indicates DVT); elevated pulse and respiratory rate; arrhythmias; lung rales on auscultation; lower-lung dullness on percussion; motor or sensory deficits

Risk factors: HF; cancer; surgery; prolonged immobility (e.g., long plane trips); smoking; estrogen replacement therapy; OCs; current pregnancy; previous DVT, embolism, or stroke; family history of embolism

Investigations: elevated d-dimer level; area of reduced pulmonary perfusion on V/Q scan; CT angiography to detect blocked vessel

Elevated pulmonary capillary pressure (e.g., mitral stenosis, left ventricular failure)

Signs and symptoms (in general): chest pain; shortness of breath; history of heart disease (especially acute MI or ischemia); hypoxia; lung rales; heart murmur (this suggests mitral valve stenosis)

Investigations: chest x-ray to detect pulmonary edema; ECG; echocardiogram

Pulmonary arteriovenous malformation

Signs and symptoms: often asymptomatic until bleeding begins; shortness of breath on exertion; localized abnormal lung sounds (this suggests the location of the pulmonary AVM); orthodeoxia (characteristic: this is oxygen desaturation with upright position)

Long-standing hypoxia: digital clubbing, cyanosis

Investigations: elevated hemoglobin (this indicates long-standing hypoxia); imaging to detect pulmonary AVM

POINTER

Common causes of hemoptysis

CHILDREN

Lower respiratory tract infection
Foreign body aspiration

ADULTS

Note that in up to a third of cases no cause can be identified.

Bronchitis
Bronchogenic carcinoma
Pneumonia

Keys to patient encounter

Key concern

Determine if the patient requires urgent intervention and stabilization, or if the patient requires further investigation to rule out serious underlying disease.

Airway and hemodynamic status

Check the patient's ABCs. Look in particular for hypotension and tachycardia. Begin resuscitation, as required: administer bolus(es) of isotonic crystalloid solution to maintain systolic BP at > 100 mmHg.

In cases of massive hemoptysis, mortality is secondary to asphyxiation (and not exsanguination). It is thus essential to protect the airway with intubation (if necessary). If the source of hemoptysis is known (e.g., right-sided bronchiectasis), have the patient lie on the side of the source (e.g., right lateral decubitus position).

History

HISTORY OF PRESENT ILLNESS

Ask how much blood the patient is coughing up and how often.

Listen for evidence of massive hemoptysis (> 200 mL per day), which is a medical emergency. Note that bleeding can start and stop unpredictably: patients may not be bleeding when you see them.

Ask about the nature of the blood (e.g., bright red, blood-tinged sputum, "coffee grounds").

ASSOCIATED SYMPTOMS

Ask about associated symptoms. Examples of characteristic symptoms include:

Bronchogenic carcinoma: constitutional symptoms and enlarged lymph nodes

TB: chest pain

PAST MEDICAL HISTORY

Ask about TB, vasculitis, liver disease, heart disease, cancer, PE, and HIV and other conditions that cause immune-system suppression.

Ask about recent medical procedures, such as bronchoscopy (relevant to trauma).

MEDICATIONS

Ask about anticoagulants, acetylsalicylic acid, and NSAIDs; and about estrogen replacement therapy and OCs (relevant to PE).

SOCIAL HISTORY

Ask about occupational exposures to asbestos (e.g., from work in asbestos mining, construction, firefighting, industrial work, shipyard work).

Ask about a history of smoking, including exposure to second-hand smoke.

Physical exam

Vital signs: Look for fever, tachycardia, tachypnea, dyspnea, and hypoxia.

Head, neck:

- Look for enlarged lymph nodes in the neck, supraclavicular region, and axillae (relevant to infection, malignancy, HIV).
- Check for jugulovenous distention.

B

- Examine for facial tenderness and mucopurulent nasal discharge (infection).
- Examine the mucus membranes for petechia (low platelets or other bleeding disorder).

Cardiovascular:

- Auscultate the heart for abnormal sounds.
- Look for edema (edema in the legs and unilateral leg pain may indicate pulmonary thromboembolic disease).
- Examine the hands and feet for clubbing (this may indicate lung cancer or chronic lung disease).

Respiratory:

- Examine the lungs for dullness to percussion (this may indicate pneumonia; dullness in the lower lung fields may indicate CHF).
- Auscultate the lungs for pleural friction rub and rales (unilateral rales may indicate pneumonia; bilateral rales and/or decreased lung sounds may indicate CHF).

Abdominal: Look for masses (relevant to malignancy) or an enlarged liver (CHF).

Investigations

CBC to assess for anemia

Electrolytes (see *Notes on labs and assessments*)

Creatinine

PT/INR

Chest X-ray or CT scan

V/Q scan on suspicion of PE

Management

Admit patients reporting massive hemoptysis to hospital. For anemic patients, order blood transfusion. The transfusion threshold may vary depending on comorbidities and can be as low as 7 g/dL (70 g/L) in patients without cardiac disease. Consider platelet transfusions to keep the platelet count above 50, and vitamin K or FFP to keep the PT/INR at or below 1.5. Consult a general surgeon, gastroenterologist, or respirologist, as appropriate, for bronchoscopy or endoscopy. Bronchoscopy or endoscopy will facilitate diagnosis, biopsy, and possible treatment (e.g., banding of varices). Refer patients who may need surgery to a thoracic or general surgeon.

BLEEDING

Blood in urine (hematuria)

Differential diagnosis

RENAL CONDITION

Glomerular disease (e.g., systemic lupus erythematosus, hemolytic uremic syndrome, vasculitis)

GLOMERULAR DISEASE IN GENERAL

Investigations: abnormal findings on urine microscopy (dysmorphic RBCs, proteinuria, and red cell casts); elevated creatinine; decreased serum complement level

SYSTEMIC LUPUS ERYTHEMATOSUS

Signs and symptoms: personal or family history of SLE; malar rash; arthritis; cytopenias

Investigations: elevated ANA titer; elevated dsDNA level

HEMOLYTIC UREMIC SYNDROME

This commonly follows infection from Shiga-toxin-producing *E. coli.*

Signs and symptoms: GI symptoms (abdominal pain, bloody diarrhea); anemia (fatigue, weakness, pallor); neurologic symptoms (irritability, confusion, seizures); peripheral edema (this is a sign of renal failure); thrombocytopenia

Investigations: low platelet count; elevated PT/INR; schistocytes on blood smear; microangiopathic hemolytic anemia

VASCULITIS

Signs and symptoms: personal or family history of vasculitis; cutaneous vasculitis (polyarteritis nodosa: palpable purpura, petechiae, ulcers); abnormal lung sounds; neuropathy (numbness, weakness); hematuria in pulmonary-renal syndrome (e.g., Goodpasture syndrome)

Investigations: elevated serum ANCA; CT scan to detect diffuse alveolar infiltrates; anti-GBM; biopsy

Nonglomerular disease (e.g., acute interstitial nephritis, renal tumor, exercise)

NONGLOMERULAR DISEASE IN GENERAL

Signs and symptoms: possible history of autoimmune disorders

Investigations: normal findings on urine microscopy, normal creatinine, normal serum complement level

ACUTE INTERSTITIAL NEPHRITIS

This is the usual cause of nonglomerular disease.

Signs and symptoms: fever; rash; joint pain; use of diuretics, antibiotics, analgesics (usual); history of autoimmune disorders

Investigations: urine eosinophils (their presence is suggestive); urinalysis (normal findings for RBCs, proteinuria, and red cell casts); blood tests (normal creatinine, normal complement level); renal biopsy (definitive)

RENAL TUMOR

Signs and symptoms: flank pain, constitutional symptoms (weight loss, night sweats), hypertension (this can indicate certain renal tumors), palpable renal mass

Investigations: CT scan, US

EXERCISE

This is hematuria that occurs after strenuous exercise and resolves with rest.

POSTRENAL CONDITION (E.G., STONES, BLADDER TUMOR, BENIGN PROSTATIC HYPERPLASIA, CYSTITIS)

Kidney stones

Signs and symptoms: flank pain, history of kidney stones

Investigations: IV urography, US, CT scan

Bladder tumor or benign prostatic hyperplasia

Signs and symptoms: change in urinary habits (reduced urination in prostate conditions; blood in the urine; reduced and/or frequent urination in bladder conditions); bladder mass or enlarged prostate on palpation

Investigations: urine cytology; CT scan or cytoscopy to detect bladder mass

Cystitis

Signs and symptoms: increased frequency of urination; painful urination; pelvic and/or flank pain; fever; tenderness over the bladder

Investigations: urinalysis, urine culture

HEMATOLOGIC CONDITION (E.G., COAGULOPATHY, SICKLE CELL HEMOGLOBINOPATHY)

Coagulopathy

Signs and symptoms: use of anticoagulant medication; history of liver disease (this can lead to deficits in clotting factor production); bruising and petechiae on the skin and in the mouth

Investigations: elevated PT/INR; serum liver enzyme tests to detect liver disease

Sickle cell disease

Signs and symptoms: family history of sickle cell disease; painful swelling of the hands and feet

Investigations: CBC to detect anemia, sickle cells; positive sickle cell screen; abnormalities on peripheral blood smear; abnormalities on hemoglobin electrophoresis

Keys to patient encounter

Key concern

Differentiate glomerular from nonglomerular causes using urinalysis.

History

HISTORY OF PRESENT ILLNESS

Establish symptoms associated with the hematuria. Examples of characteristic symptoms include:

Hemolytic uremic syndrome: GI and neurologic symptoms

Urologic malignancy or infection: constitutional symptoms

Cystitis or UTI: frequent and painful urination

If pain is present, ask how constant it is (intermittent colicky pain suggests stones).

PAST MEDICAL HISTORY

Ask about kidney or bladder disease, and kidney stones; a history of pelvic irradiation; and risk factors for malignancy (see the pointer).

MEDICATIONS

Ask whether the patient takes NSAIDs and/or anticoagulants.

POINTER

Urologic malignancy

RISK FACTORS

Male
Older than 35
History of smoking
Exposure to benzenes or aromatic amines (through, for example, work in chemical manufacturing)

INCIDENCE

Malignancy is present in up to 5% of patients with microscopic hematuria and up to 40% of patients with gross hematuria.

Physical exam

Vital signs: Look for hypertension.

Abdominal

Prostate: Look for abnormalities (relevant to BPH, prostatitis, and prostate cancer).

Pelvic: Look for atrophic vaginitis, masses, and uterine bleeding.

Investigations

Significant hematuria is defined as 3 or more RBCs per HPF.

Urine microscopy and culture to assess for:

- pyuria and/or bacteriuria
- casts and/or dysmorphic red cells (these suggest a glomerular cause)
- intact RBCs and the absence of casts (this suggests a nonglomerular cause)

CT urography in cases of microscopic hematuria

Renal and pelvic US instead of CT scan for pregnant patients or in patients with poor renal function

Management

Many patients will not have an identifiable cause. These patients should have annual urinalysis with a repeat workup performed within 3 to 5 years.

Refer patients with risk factors for malignancy to a urologist for cystoscopy. Urine cytology has lower sensitivity, but may also be useful in patients with risk factors for malignancy.

Refer patients with hypertension, elevated serum creatinine, dysmorphic RBCs, cellular casts, or proteinuria to a nephrologist.

Refer patients who have masses for biopsy.

BLEEDING

Lower gastrointestinal bleeding

Differential diagnosis

COLORECTAL CANCER OR POLYPS

Signs and symptoms: weight loss, abdominal pain, blood in the stool, constipation, change in stool caliber, personal or family history of colorectal cancer, palpable mass (anal or rectal)

Investigations: CEA, colonoscopy

DIVERTICULOSIS

Signs and symptoms: often asymptomatic, history of diverticular disease, painless rectal bleeding

ANGIODYSPLASIA

Signs and symptoms: older age (usual), rectal bleeding

ANORECTAL DISEASE

Fissures, hemorrhoids

Signs and symptoms: small amounts of bright red blood following bowel movements; pain, irritation; constipation

Fistulas, abscesses

These are often related to inflammatory bowel disease.

Signs and symptoms: history of inflammatory bowel disease (e.g., Crohn disease, ulcerative colitis), diarrhea, blood in the stool, abdominal pain, weight loss, fever, fatigue

ENTEROCOLITIS

Signs and symptoms: abdominal pain, cramping, tenderness; diarrhea; nausea, vomiting; rectal bleeding

Investigations: colonoscopy

BRISK BLEEDING FROM THE UPPER GASTROINTESTINAL TRACT

Signs and symptoms: blood in the stool; epigastric pain; difficulty or pain with swallowing; acid reflux; food becoming impacted in the esophagus, especially foods that are solid or difficult to chew

History of trauma to the chest or abdomen; liver disease (esophageal varices and/or impaired production of clotting factors)

Investigations: endoscopy or barium swallow

RECTAL TRAUMA

If the trauma comes from a high-force injury, associated pelvic fracture is possible.

Risk factors: substance abuse, intimate partner violence, homelessness, occupational hazards

Investigations: proctoscopy, sigmoidoscopy

Keys to patient encounter

Key concerns

Determine the hemodynamic status of the patient and the need for immediate specialized care.

Identify patients at high risk of colorectal cancer for colonoscopy.

Airway and hemodynamic status

Check the patient's ABCs. Look in particular for hypotension and tachycardia. Begin resuscitation, as required: administer bolus(es) of isotonic crystalloid solution to maintain systolic BP at > 100 mmHg.

History

HISTORY OF PRESENT ILLNESS

Ask about the nature of the blood: bright red blood, versus clots, versus dark tarry stools (melena).

Ask about associated symptoms and vomiting in particular: vomiting with blood suggests an upper GI source; vomiting without blood may indicate an intestinal blockage.

Examples of other characteristic symptoms include:

Abdominal pain: colorectal cancer, inflammatory bowel disease, enterocolitis

Constitutional symptoms: malignancy, liver disease

PAST MEDICAL HISTORY

Ask about colorectal cancer, diverticular disease, hemorrhoids, inflammatory bowel disease, and liver disease, including chronic liver disease (portal hypertension with varices).

MEDICATIONS

Ask about acetylsalicylic acid and NSAIDs.

PAST PROCEDURAL HISTORY

Ask about a recent colonoscopy with polypectomy (relevant to a postpolypectomy bleed), and abdominal or pelvic radiation (radiation colitis).

SOCIAL HISTORY

Ask about a history of alcoholism.

Physical exam

Vital signs: Obtain the patient's BP in supine and standing positions to look for orthostatic changes.

General inspection: Look for signs of liver disease (gynecomastia in men, palmar erythema, Dupuytren contractures, leukonychia).

Abdominal: Look for tenderness, masses, and signs of liver disease (hepatomegaly, splenomegaly, caput medusa, spider nevi).

Nasogastric lavage: Use this in patients without hematemesis to rule out an upper GI tract source of blood.

B

DRE: Look for masses and frank blood.

POINTER

Common causes of lower gastrointestinal bleeding

The most common cause is diverticulosis, followed by hemorrhoids, ischemic colitis, postpolypectomy bleed, inflammatory bowel disease, cancer or polyps, and vascular ectasia.

INVESTIGATIONS

CBC to assess for anemia

Liver function tests (see *Notes on labs and assessments*)

PT/INR

Creatinine

Electrolytes (see *Notes on labs and assessments*)

Urgent colonoscopy

- This is the main method of establishing a diagnosis, and treatment (e.g., banding) may be administered at the same time.
- Consider a tagged RBC scan (technetium-99m-labeled RBCs) or mesenteric angiography to localize a source of bleeding if urgent colonoscopy is not possible or does not yield a diagnosis.

MANAGEMENT

For anemic patients, order blood transfusion. The transfusion threshold may vary depending on comorbidities and can be as low as 7 g/dL (70 g/L) in patients without cardiac disease. Consider platelet transfusions to keep the platelet count above 50, and vitamin K or FFP to keep the PT/INR at or below 1.5. Consult a general surgeon or gastroenterologist for colonoscopy, and a general surgeon for consideration of surgical correction of a bleeding source.

BLEEDING

Upper gastrointestinal bleeding

Differential diagnosis

ULCERATIVE OR EROSIVE PROCESSES

Peptic ulcer disease

Signs and symptoms: constant midepigastric pain, often relieved with eating or with antacids; weight loss

Investigations: *H. pylori*; endoscopy to detect ulcer or inflammation of the gastric lining

Esophagitis

Signs and symptoms: difficulty swallowing or pain with swallowing; food becoming impacted in the esophagus, especially foods that are solid or difficult to chew; acid reflux; oral *Candida* infection; oral ulcers; epigastric tenderness (this could arise from associated PUD or reflux)

> History of food allergies or environmental allergies (e.g., pollen); factors causing immunosuppression, such as HIV, cancer, immunosuppressant medications, autoimmune disease, malnutrition (immunosuppression creates a higher risk for bacterial, viral, and fungal infections of the esophagus); use of antiinflammatories and bisphosphonates (these present a particular risk if they are not swallowed properly and remain in the esophagus)

Investigations: upper GI series (barium swallow) or endoscopy

Gastritis

Signs and symptoms: constant epigastric pain that may be relieved by antacids; constitutional symptoms (fever, night sweats, weight loss, fatigue); epigastric tenderness; history of using gastric irritants (antiinflammatories, smoking, alcohol)

Investigations: *H. pylori*

PORTAL HYPERTENSION

Signs and symptoms: enlarged or tender liver; enlarged spleen; abdominal masses; ascites

> History of cirrhosis (common) (risk factors: alcohol abuse, hepatitis); portal vein thrombosis (less common) (risk

factors: chronic liver disease, prothrombin *G20210A* mutation)

Investigations: endoscopy to detect esophageal varices

TRAUMA (E.G., MALLORY-WEISS TEAR)

Signs and symptoms: coughing; severe or prolonged hiccups; recurrent vomiting or retching; abdominal pain; history of trauma to the chest or abdomen

Investigations: endoscopy

TUMORS

Signs and symptoms: epigastric pain; difficulty swallowing or pain with swallowing; food becoming impacted in the esophagus, especially foods that are solid or difficult to chew; acid reflux; constitutional symptoms (fever, night sweats, weight loss, and fatigue); smoking; alcohol use; personal or family history of malignancy; palpable abdominal mass

Investigations: CT scan, MRI; endoscopy with biopsy

Keys to patient encounter

Key concern

Determine the hemodynamic status of the patient and resuscitate if necessary.

Airway and hemodynamic status

Check the patient's ABCs. Look in particular for hypotension and tachycardia. Begin resuscitation as required: administer red cell transfusions and bolus(es) of isotonic crystalloid solution to maintain systolic BP at > 100 mmHg.

History

HISTORY OF PRESENT ILLNESS

Ask when the bleeding started, and about the quantity and the nature of the blood.

Ask about associated symptoms. Examples of characteristic symptoms include:

Peptic ulcer disease: blood with a "coffee grounds" appearance and constant midepigastric pain

Trauma: recent-onset bleeding with bright red blood, and abdominal pain or chest pain

Mallory-Weiss tear: coughing, vomiting, or hiccups

Tumor: epigastric pain, difficulty swallowing, and constitutional symptoms

Ask about bleeding from the rectum (tarry stools or bright red blood).

PAST MEDICAL HISTORY

Ask about PUD, liver disease (relevant to portal hypertension), HIV and allergies (esophagitis), and cancer (tumor).

PAST SURGICAL HISTORY

Ask about abdominal surgery.

MEDICATIONS

Ask about clopidogrel, warfarin, NSAIDs, acetylsalicylic acid, SSRIs, and corticosteroids.

SOCIAL HISTORY

Ask about smoking, alcohol abuse, and use of illicit drugs.

Physical exam

Vital signs: Obtain the patient's BP in supine and standing positions to look for orthostatic changes.

Abdominal: Look for signs of liver disease (hepatomegaly, splenomegaly, caput medusa, spider nevi), abdominal tenderness, masses, and surgical scars.

DRE: Look for melena or bright red blood (the presence of melena is consistent with upper GI bleeding; bright red blood indicates lower GI bleeding).

Investigations

CBC

PT/INR

PTT

Creatinine

BUN

Liver function (see *Notes on labs and assessments*)

H. pylori via a stool antigen or urea breath test

Blood typing and cross-matching

Emergency endoscopy to (possibly) identify a source of bleeding, and also allow treatment of any discovered lesions with epinephrine injection, thermocoagulation, application of clips, or banding

POINTER

Cirrhosis follow-up

Patients with cirrhosis should have regular upper-endoscopy screening to identify the presence or development of esophageal varices. The recommended frequency of screening depends on findings of the initial screening.

B

Management

For patients with coagulopathy, give transfusions with FFP. For patients with low platelet counts, give platelet transfusions.

If bleeding remains uncontrolled after medical or endoscopic treatment, refer the patient to a surgeon. Discontinue any NSAIDs. Treat *H. pylori* infection, if present. Assess the patient's risk of rebleeding (this risk increases with older age, the presence of shock, and with increasing comorbidities).

BLOOD PRESSURE PRESENTATIONS

Hypertension

Differential diagnosis

HYPERTENSION IN GENERAL

Definition: ≥ 135/85 mmHg for nondiabetic individuals; ≥ 130/80 mmHg for diabetic individuals

PRIMARY

Signs and symptoms: often asymptomatic, headache

Risk factors: family history of hypertension; lack of exercise; high-sodium diet; obesity

SECONDARY

Renal parenchymal disease (e.g., kidney injury, polycystic kidney disease)

KIDNEY INJURY

Signs and symptoms: history of kidney disease, chronic renal failure, and/or current renal dialysis; bilateral lower limb swelling; shortness of breath; paroxysmal nocturnal dyspnea; orthopnea

Risk factors: diabetes, diabetic complications, and/or inadequate monitoring; hypertension; smoking

Investigations: renal function tests (elevated creatinine, reduced calcium, elevated phosphate), reduced vitamin D

POLYCYSTIC KIDNEY DISEASE

This is the most common inherited cause of kidney disease. It may not be detected in patients younger than 30.

Signs and symptoms: family history of polycystic kidney disease; hypertension with pain (abdomen, flank, lower back); hematuria; UTIs

Investigations: renal US; genetic testing; serum creatinine and GFR to assess disease; urine tests (hematuria, micro or gross; culture to detect UTI or cyst infection)

Metabolic or endocrine conditions (e.g., adrenal adenoma or hyperplasia, thyroid conditions)

FUNCTIONAL ADRENAL ADENOMA OR HYPERPLASIA

Adrenal adenoma is usually asymptomatic. Secretion of cortisol (Cushing syndrome), aldosterone (hyperaldosteronism), or catecholamines (pheochromocytoma) might result in hypertension.

Signs and symptoms: round face, pronounced abdominal weight, hump on the upper back, thin arms and legs, stretch marks, acne (these are signs of Cushing syndrome); hypokalemia (signs of hyperaldosteronism); episodes of palpitations, diaphoresis, anxiety (signs of pheochromocytoma)

Investigations: 24-hour urine free cortisol or 1 mg dexamethasone suppression test (Cushing syndrome); plasma aldosterone:renin ratio (hyperaldosteronism); 24-hour urine collection for catecholamines and metanephrines (pheochromocytoma); CT scan to detect adrenal mass

HYPERTHYROIDISM

In the context of hypertension, hyperthyroidism typically exhibits high diastolic BP.

Signs and symptoms: history of hyperthyroidism or symptoms of hyperthyroidism (changes in menstrual patterns, enlarged thyroid, tachycardia, palpitations, diarrhea, muscle weakness, tremor, hyperactive reflexes, weight loss, sweating, thinning hair)

Investigations: elevated thyrotropin (TSH)

HYPOTHYROIDISM

Signs and symptoms: history of hypothyroidism or symptoms of hypothyroidism (decreased reflexes, dry skin, weight gain, impaired cognition)

Investigations: elevated thyrotropin (TSH)

Vascular conditions (e.g., unilateral renal artery stenosis, coarctation of the aorta)

UNILATERAL RENAL ARTERY STENOSIS

Signs and symptoms: personal or family history of renal disorders; renal artery bruits; signs and symptoms of diabetes (personal or family history of diabetes; history of diabetic complications and/or inadequate monitoring; polydipsia, polyuria, weight loss)

Investigations: elevated creatinine; urinalysis (to detect proteinuria, eosinophils, and WBCs or white cell casts); fasting glucose or HbA_{1c} to detect diabetes

COARCTATION OF THE AORTA

Signs and symptoms: weaker pulse in the legs than in the arms; heart murmur

Investigations: CT scan of the chest and/or abdomen

Catecholamine excess (e.g., pheochromocytoma, drug-induced conditions)

CATECHOLAMINE EXCESS IN GENERAL

Signs and symptoms: cardiac rate and rhythm abnormalities (possible)

Investigations: elevated catecholamine level on 24-hour urine collection; CT scan to detect adrenal mass

PHEOCHROMOCYTOMA

Signs and symptoms: tachycardia; pallor; headaches; shortness of breath; symptoms that occur in brief spells (up to 20 minutes) with no symptoms between (these spells may be mistaken for panic attacks)

DRUG-INDUCED CATECHOLAMINE EXCESS

Associated drugs include NSAIDs; anabolic steroids; erythropoietin; cocaine and other stimulants; and thyroxine replacements.

Obstructive sleep apnea

Signs and symptoms: excessive or loud snoring; disturbed sleep (e.g., not feeling rested in the morning); obesity (common); allergic rhinitis (sneezing, runny nose, eye irritation); morning headache; palpable masses in the oral cavity or neck

Investigations: sleep study (polysomnography); hypertrophic adenoid tissue on lateral neck x-ray

Keys to patient encounter

Key concerns

Identify patients with urgent or emergent hypertension.

Assess patients for cardiac risk and end organ damage.

Although most hypertensive adults have primary (essential) hypertension, it is important to rule out secondary causes.

History

HISTORY OF PRESENT ILLNESS

Ask about symptoms of high BP: headaches, shortness of breath, nosebleeds, chest pain, numbness or weakness, vision changes, and back pain. Ask about snoring (relevant to obstructive sleep apnea).

RISK FACTORS

Ask about cardiac risk factors: family history of heart disease, and a personal history of dyslipidemia and smoking. Ask about other risk factors for hypertension: lack of exercise, high-sodium diet, alcohol abuse, and recent emotional stressors.

PAST MEDICAL HISTORY

Ask about kidney disease, adrenal tumor, and thyroid disease.

MEDICATIONS AND DRUGS

Ask about OCs, decongestants, caffeine, cocaine, and amphetamines.

FAMILY HISTORY

Ask about hypertension, focusing on age of onset, and about kidney disease, adrenal tumor, and thyroid disease.

Physical exam

Vital signs: Take 2 BP measurements 2 minutes apart on each arm (see the pointer for interpreting BP readings).

Weight and height: Calculate the patient's BMI (see *Notes on labs and assessments*).

Head and neck:

- Examine the thyroid.
- Check for bruits.

Funduscopy: Look for papilledema.

Cardiovascular:

- Auscultate the heart.
- Check the lower extremities for edema.

Respiratory

Abdominal: Check for bruits.

Neurological

POINTER

Interpreting blood pressure readings

Normal BP: < 120/80 mmHg

Elevated BP: systolic 120–129 mmHg, diastolic < 80 mmHg

Stage 1 hypertension: systolic 130–139 mmHg or diastolic 80–89 mmHg

Stage 2 hypertension: systolic ≥ 140 mmHg or diastolic ≥ 90 mmHg

Investigations

INVESTIGATIONS FOR SECONDARY CAUSES

Creatinine

Electrolytes (see *Notes on labs and assessments*)

Thyrotropin (TSH)

Urinalysis

Urinary catecholamines

B

INVESTIGATIONS FOR CARDIOVASCULAR RISKS

Lipids (see *Notes on labs and assessments*)

Fasting glucose or HbA_{1c} to screen for diabetes

INVESTIGATIONS FOR END ORGAN DAMAGE

Urine test for microalbuminuria

ECG

Echocardiogram (consider this)

Management

Identify any existing hypertensive emergency. This is defined as systolic BP > 180 mmHg and/or diastolic BP > 120 mmHg, with end organ dysfunction (aortic dissection, acute coronary syndrome, stroke, encephalopathy, acute renal failure, pulmonary edema, eclampsia). Treat hypertensive emergencies with IV medications; the choice of medication depends on the context (e.g., nitroglycerin in pulmonary edema or acute coronary syndrome; labetalol in aortic dissection).

Counsel all patients on lifestyle modifications, including reduced sodium intake, regular exercise, maintaining a healthy weight, and limiting alcohol intake. Counsel the patient to follow a diet rich in fruits, vegetables, whole grains, poultry, fish and low-fat dairy. Treat any secondary causes and manage additional cardiovascular risk factors (e.g., smoking cessation).

Most patients will also require antihypertensive medication. First-line therapy is often a thiazide diuretic (e.g., hydrochlorothiazide). Thiazide diuretics or CCBs are often more effective in patients of African descent and older individuals than other antihypertensives. ACE inhibitors or angiotensin II receptor blockers are other first-line medications, and may be a better choice in patients with diabetes or chronic liver disease.

BLOOD PRESSURE PRESENTATIONS

Hypertension disorders of pregnancy

Differential diagnosis

HYPERTENSION DISORDERS OF PREGNANCY IN GENERAL

Signs and symptoms:

Preeclampsia: BP > 140/90 mmHg, and proteinuria or other symptoms

Eclampsia: preeclampsia and neurological symptoms

CHRONIC HYPERTENSION WITH OR WITHOUT PREECLAMPSIA OR ECLAMPSIA

Signs and symptoms: preexisting hypertension; headaches; changes in vision; decreased urine output; seizures (this is a sign of eclampsia)

Investigations: CBC (to detect thrombocytopenia, hemolytic anemia); renal function tests; chest x-ray to detect pulmonary edema; urinalysis

GESTATIONAL HYPERTENSION WITH OR WITHOUT PREECLAMPSIA OR ECLAMPSIA

Signs and symptoms: headaches, changes in vision, seizures, **no** history of preexisting hypertension

Investigations: CBC (to detect thrombocytopenia, hemolytic anemia); renal function tests; chest x-ray to detect pulmonary edema; urinalysis

Keys to patient encounter

Key concern

Identify patients with eclampsia and preeclampsia, and take urgent action.

History

Ask if the patient has a history of hypertension, and if previous pregnancies were complicated by hypertension or preeclampsia. Ask about cerebral and visual disturbances.

Physical exam

BP:

- Nonsevere hypertension in pregnancy is defined as systolic BP of 140–159 mmHg and/or diastolic BP of 80–109 mmHg.
- Severe hypertension is defined as systolic BP ≥ 160 mmHg and/or diastolic BP ≥ 110 mmHg.

Respiratory: Examine the lungs for edema.

Abdominal: Look for right upper quadrant pain (relevant to preeclampsia).

Investigations

CBC to look for thrombocytopenia

Liver function to look for thrombocytopenia

24-hour urine collection to look for urine protein (≥ 0.3 g in preeclampsia, and ≥ 5 g in eclampsia)

Fetal US to look for IUGR

Management

Refer the patient to an obstetrician for management and follow-up. Antihypertensive therapy is recommended for patients with systolic BP ≥ 140 mmHg or diastolic BP ≥ 90 mmHg. Start antihypertensive therapy with oral labetalol, methyldopa, long-acting nifedipine, or other beta-blockers (acebutolol, metoprolol, pindolol, and propranolol). ACE inhibitors and angiotensin receptor blockers should not be used in pregnant women.

BLOOD PRESSURE PRESENTATIONS

Hypertension in childhood

B

Differential diagnosis

HYPERTENSION IN CHILDHOOD IN GENERAL

In children, hypertension from a secondary cause is usual.

In adolescents, essential hypertension is more likely, but secondary causes must be ruled out.

NEONATES AND YOUNG INFANTS

Renal artery thrombosis after umbilical artery catheter

Signs and symptoms: history of umbilical artery catheterization (rare); renal artery bruits

Investigations: elevated creatinine; urinalysis (to detect proteinuria; eosinophils; WBCs or white cell casts)

Coarctation of the aorta

Signs and symptoms: pale skin; failure to thrive; presence of symptoms since birth (often); family history of coarctation of the aorta; weaker pulse in the legs than in the arms; heart murmur

Turner syndrome (common associated condition): female; small stature; skeletal abnormalities

Investigations: CT scan of the chest and/or abdomen

Congenital renal disease

Signs and symptoms: failure to thrive, family history of hereditary renal disease

Investigations: elevated creatinine; urinalysis (to detect proteinuria; eosinophils; WBCs or white cell casts); US or CT scan to detect abnormalities in renal size or shape

Renal artery stenosis

Signs and symptoms: failure to thrive, renal artery bruits, family history of hereditary renal disease

Investigations: elevated creatinine; urinalysis (to detect proteinuria; eosinophils; WBCs or white cell casts); US or CT scan to detect abnormalities in renal size or shape

CHILDREN AGED 1 TO 10 YEARS

Renal disease

Signs and symptoms: failure to thrive, family history of hereditary renal disease

Investigations: elevated creatinine; urinalysis (to detect proteinuria; eosinophils; WBCs or white cell casts); US or CT scan to detect abnormalities in renal size or shape

Coarctation of the aorta—see above

CHILDREN OLDER THAN 10 YEARS

Essential hypertension

Signs and symptoms: often asymptomatic, headache

Risk factors: family history of hypertension; lack of exercise; high-sodium diet; obesity

Renal disease

Signs and symptoms: failure to thrive; family history of hereditary renal disease; symptoms and signs of diabetes (personal or family history of diabetes; history of diabetic complications and/or inadequate monitoring; polydipsia, polyuria, and/or weight loss)

> Poststreptococcal glomerulonephritis: history of group A β-hemolytic streptococcus infection

Investigations: elevated creatinine; urinalysis (to detect proteinuria; eosinophils; WBCs or white cell casts); US or CT scan to detect abnormalities in renal size or shape; fasting glucose or HbA_{1c} to detect diabetes

Coarctation of the aorta—see above

Keys to patient encounter

Key concern

Distinguish primary from secondary hypertension.

History

HISTORY OF PRESENT ILLNESS

Ask about symptoms of hypertensive emergency: headache, vomiting, and altered level of consciousness.

Ask about snoring (a symptom of sleep apnea); and symptoms of hyperthyroidism (heat intolerance, tachycardia, and weight loss).

PAST MEDICAL HISTORY
Ask about kidney, heart, and endocrine disease, complications during the patient's birth, and failure to thrive during growth and development.

MEDICATIONS AND DRUGS
Ask whether the patient is taking amphetamines, anabolic steroids, cocaine, phencyclidine, caffeine, and/or OCs.

FAMILY HISTORY
Ask about hypertension and cardiovascular disease.

Ask about maternal smoking during pregnancy (this increases risk of hypertension in the child).

SOCIAL HISTORY
Ask about the patient's diet, looking for evidence of a diet high in fat and sodium (e.g., full of fast food).

Physical exam

BP:

- Confirm that hypertension is present: compare the patient's BP with a table of normal pressures for the age, height, weight, and sex of the patient.
- Measure BP in both arms (it should be equal) and in 1 leg in prone position (it should be slightly higher in the leg). Unequal arm pressures, or a lower BP in the leg, may indicate coarctation of the aorta.
- To diagnose hypertension in a pediatric patient, the patient must present with a high BP reading for at least 3 visits in a row.

Femoral pulses: Decreased pulses may indicate coarctation of the aorta.

General inspection: Look for acne, hirsutism, striae, moon facies, and truncal obesity (relevant to Cushing syndrome).

Weight and height: Calculate the patient's BMI (see *Notes on labs and assessments*).

Funduscopy: Look for papilledema.
Abdominal: Listen for bruits (relevant to renovascular disease).

POINTER

When to start regular blood pressure measurement

Children 3 years of age and older should have their BP measured at every office visit.

Investigations

These investigations are appropriate in children with confirmed hypertension.

CBC
Creatinine
Electrolytes (see *Notes on labs and assessments*)
Renal US
Urinalysis
Urine drug screen if illicit drug use is a possibility (consider this)
Fasting glucose or HbA_{1c}
Lipids
Echocardiogram
Polysomnography in suspected sleep apnea

Management

Counsel the patient on lifestyle modifications: weight reduction if the patient is overweight or obese; regular physical activity; a diet rich in fresh fruit and vegetables, and fiber; avoidance of alcohol and tobacco; and sodium reduction (1.2 g/day in children 4 to 8 years old, 1.5 g/day in children older than 8 years). Most children will require antihypertensive medication.

BLOOD PRESSURE PRESENTATIONS

Hypotension, shock

Differential diagnosis

HYPOTENSION IN GENERAL

Definition: systolic BP < 90 mmHg or diastolic BP < 60 mmHg

CARDIAC OUTPUT DIMINISHED

Hypovolemia

HEMORRHAGE

Causes include recent massive blood loss from trauma or the disruption of a large internal blood vessel.

THIRD SPACE LOSS

Signs and symptoms: history of CHF, chronic liver disease, recent extensive burns, renal disease, overzealous fluid replacement

Investigations: blood tests (albumin, sodium, creatinine, CBC)

Cardiac dysfunction

INTRINSIC

MYOPATHY (E.G., ISCHEMIC CONDITION)

Signs and symptoms: chest pain (usual; this is a symptom of MI, which is generally the cause of cardiogenic shock), sweating, pallor, shortness of breath, abnormal heart sounds

Investigations: elevated troponin; ECG; chest x-ray to detect cardiac enlargement and pulmonary edema

RHYTHM ABNORMALITIES

Signs and symptoms: tachycardia or bradycardia; light-headedness; fainting; shortness of breath

Investigations: ECG

MECHANICAL ABNORMALITIES

Signs and symptoms: heart murmurs (these suggest valvular abnormalities or cardiac shunt)

EXTRINSIC OR OBSTRUCTIVE

PULMONARY EMBOLUS

Signs and symptoms: sharp chest pain; shortness of breath; cough (possibly with blood); hypoxia; possible unilateral swelling of the lower limbs (this indicates DVT); elevated pulse and respiratory rate; arrhythmias; lung rales on auscultation; lower-lung dullness on percussion; motor or sensory deficits

Risk factors: HF; cancer; surgery; prolonged immobility (e.g., long plane trips); smoking; estrogen replacement therapy; OCs; current pregnancy; previous DVT, embolism, or stroke; family history of embolism

Investigations: elevated d-dimer level; area of reduced pulmonary perfusion on V/Q scan; CT angiography to detect blocked vessel

TENSION PNEUMOTHORAX

Signs and symptoms: history of trauma or recurrent spontaneous pneumothorax; absence of breath sounds on auscultation; deviated trachea

PERICARDIAL DISEASE

Signs and symptoms: increased JVP, multiple heart sounds, pulsus paradoxus (decrease of ≥ 10 mmHg in systolic pressure with inspiration); history of conditions that can lead to fluid accumulation in the pericardial space, which compresses the heart and causes hypotension (cardiac surgery, trauma to the chest, MI, pericarditis)

Investigations: echocardiogram to detect pericardial effusion

AORTIC DISSECTION

Signs and symptoms: intense "ripping" chest pain; tachycardia; different pulses in the arms versus the legs; heart murmur

Risk factors: long-standing hypertension; hereditary connective tissue disorders (especially Marfan syndrome); deceleration trauma; AAA; arteritis; pregnancy

Investigations: elevated troponin; CT scan, echocardiogram, or MRI

VENA CAVAL OBSTRUCTION

Signs and symptoms: tachycardia; edema of the lower extremities (this indicates inferior vena cava syndrome)

History of malignancy (especially renal cell carcinoma); liver transplantation or other invasive procedures involving the inferior vena cava; hepatic vein thrombosis (Budd-Chiari syndrome); coagulopathy; OCs; pregnancy

Investigations: elevated hemoglobin (this indicates polycythemia, which is a related condition); abnormal serum liver enzyme tests (this indicates Budd-Chiari syndrome); CT scan with contrast to detect obstruction of the vena cava

DISTRIBUTIVE CONDITIONS

Sepsis

Definition: infection with systemic inflammatory response, dysfunction of ≥ 1 organ system

Signs and symptoms: fever or hypothermia; tachycardia; tachypnea; infection (most common: pneumonia, abdominal infection, kidney infection, bacteremia)

Severe: oliguria; mental status changes; shortness of breath; extreme hypotension, unresponsive to fluid replacement (this indicates septic shock)

Risk factors: very young or very old; compromised immune system; wounds, burns; catheterization, intubation

Investigations: CBC with differential; cultures (blood, CSF, urine) to detect causative organism; ABG to detect acidosis; elevated creatinine; chest x-ray to detect pulmonary edema

Anaphylaxis

Signs and symptoms: personal or family history of anaphylaxis; hives; peripheral edema; swelling; tongue or throat swelling; wheezing; stridor; shortness of breath; tachycardia; cardiovascular collapse; hypotension

Inadequate tissue oxygenation

Signs and symptoms: bradycardia

History of autonomic dysfunction (e.g., multiple system atrophy, Parkinson disease, tabes dorsalis, stroke); use of beta-blockers; spinal cord injury (common: the injury is usually acute); Addison disease or symptoms of Addison disease (muscle weakness, weight loss, skin hyperpigmentation)

Investigations (Addison disease): decreased serum cortisol; elevated serum ACTH

Postprandial hypotension

This occurs in up to one-third of older adults and is caused by blood redistribution to the GI tract after eating.

Signs and symptoms: dizziness, faintness, or falls following meals

Keys to patient encounter

Key concerns

Pay particular attention to the presence or absence of shock.

General life-saving measures are usually indicated, regardless of the underlying cause.

Airway and hemodynamic status

Check the patient's ABCs. Begin resuscitation, as required: give oxygen, insert 2 large bore IV lines, give a 1 liter bolus of crystalloid, and then reassess the patient's vital signs.

History

In emergency situations, perform a history and physical exam at the same time.

HISTORY OF PRESENT ILLNESS

Ask what symptoms the patient has, how long the patient has had them, how constant they are, and what may trigger them. Ask female patients if they are pregnant.

Examples of characteristic symptoms include:

CHF and other chronic conditions: long-standing symptoms, such as light-headedness and fatigue

Cardiomyopathy: chest pain, shortness of breath, and sweating triggered by exertion

Pericarditis: chest pain alleviated by leaning forward

Anaphylaxis: hives and itching triggered by known allergens

Postprandial hypotension: dizziness after eating

PAST MEDICAL HISTORY

Ask about anaphylaxis and known triggers; recent infections and symptoms of infection (fever, cough, pain); recent blood loss (relevant to anemia); recent severe vomiting or diarrhea (relevant to dehydration); Addison disease; and thyroid disease.

MEDICATIONS

Ask about antihypertensives, anticoagulants, and OCs.

FAMILY HISTORY

Ask about cardiac problems.

Physical exam

BP: Measure with the patient supine and standing (if the patient can stand).

General inspection:

- Assess the patient's peripheral perfusion (symptoms of poor perfusion include cold, clammy skin and delayed capillary refill).
- Examine the skin (including the lips) for hives and swelling.
- Look for sources of infection.
- Assess the patient's mental status for confusion.

Cardiovascular: Assess heart rate and rhythm.

Respiratory: Listen to the lungs for rales and wheezing.

Investigations

CBC to assess for anemia and infection

Blood glucose to assess for hypoglycemia and hyperglycemia

Creatinine

Electrolytes (see *Notes on labs and assessments*)

Urinalysis

Blood and urine cultures

ECG

Other specific investigations as indicated in the differential diagnosis (consider these)

IN SUSPECTED CARDIAC DISORDERS

Echocardiogram

Exercise stress test to assess for ischemic heart disease

24-hour Holter monitor

IN SUSPECTED INFECTION

Chest x-ray

Urinalysis

Management

Treat any specific disorders identified. Consult a critical-care physician and admit the patient to ICU for monitoring and treatment.

BREAST PRESENTATIONS

Breast discharge

Differential diagnosis

GALACTORRHEA

Idiopathic

Signs and symptoms: bilateral discharge (usual)

Investigations: elevated prolactin (possible)

Hyperprolactinemia

PHYSIOLOGIC

Signs and symptoms: current pregnancy; recent stress; recent nipple stimulation; history of hypothyroidism or symptoms of hypothyroidism (decreased reflexes, dry skin, weight gain, impaired cognition)

DRUG-INDUCED

Examples of drugs include atypical antipsychotics, SSRIs, or MAOIs; and herbal supplements (fennel, anise, or fenugreek seed).

PITUITARY TUMOR

Signs and symptoms: menstrual abnormalities; infertility; vision changes and/or headaches

Investigations: LH, FSH, ACTH; MRI of the brain

BREAST NEOPLASM

Signs and symptoms: breast pain or swelling; unilateral discharge (often); palpable mass in the breast and/or axilla

Risk factors: personal or family history of breast cancer; smoking; HRT

Investigations: cytology of breast discharge; mammogram

Keys to patient encounter

Key concern

Differentiate galactorrhea from other causes of breast discharge.

History

POINTER

Red flags in breast discharge

Spontaneous
Unilateral
Bloody
Involves a single duct
Associated with a mass

HISTORY OF PRESENT ILLNESS

Ask when the discharge started, how it started, and what color it is. Listen, in particular, for red flags (see the pointer).

Ask whether the patient is pregnant, or has been pregnant recently. In patients who do not think they are pregnant, ask about sexual activity and symptoms of possible current pregnancy (amenorrhea, nausea, breast tenderness).

Ask about symptoms of pituitary tumor (headaches, vision changes, menstrual changes) and hypothyroidism (dry skin, cold intolerance).

MEDICATIONS

Ask about verapamil, cimetidine, metoclopramide, estrogen, OCs, opiates, antipsychotics, MAOIs, neuroleptics, SSRIs, and TCAs. Ask about herbal supplements.

Physical exam

Breast:

- Look for masses, discharge (note the color), asymmetry, and changes to the skin.
- Look for axillary lymph node enlargement.

Investigations

In patients with bilateral milky discharge, order a pregnancy test to rule out pregnancy. If this is negative, order tests for prolactin (relevant to pituitary tumor) and thyrotropin (TSH) (hypothyroidism). If red flags are present, send a sample of the discharge for cytology, and order a mammogram and breast US. Abnormal prolactin should be followed up with an MRI of the pituitary.

Management

Patients with pathologic discharge should be referred to a surgeon for duct excision.

BREAST PRESENTATIONS

Breast masses and enlargement

Differential diagnosis

MALIGNANT BREAST MASSES

Ductal carcinoma in situ

Signs and symptoms: palpable breast mass (this occurs in 10% of patients); nipple discharge (occasionally); microcalcifications on mammogram (this is usually how it is detected)

Lobular carcinoma in situ

This has a higher risk of subsequent invasive breast carcinoma.

Signs and symptoms: **no** specific clinical presentation; **no** palpable lump; incidental breast biopsy finding (this is usually how it is detected); rarely visible on mammogram

Invasive breast cancer

Signs and symptoms: women (most common), older age (the risk increases with age); palpable mass; nipple inversion; skin redness or dimpling; nipple discharge

> History of estrogen replacement therapy in postmenopausal women; excessive alcohol consumption; lack of physical activity; obesity

Risk factors: increasing age; family history of breast cancer and/or *BRCA1* and *BRCA2* mutations

Investigations: mammogram, biopsy

NONMALIGNANT BREAST MASSES

Fibrocystic change

Signs and symptoms: tender, bilateral lumps that fluctuate in size and tenderness with menstrual cycle; possible green or dark brown nipple discharge

Infection

Signs and symptoms: pain; redness; breast tenderness; fever and flu-like symptoms; unilateral symptoms, sometimes confined to a small segment of the breast; redness; tenderness; skin warmth; tender lymph nodes in the ipsilateral axilla

Risk factors: current lactation, nipple piercings, breast implants, TB

Investigations: US

GYNECOMASTIA

Physiological (newborns, adolescents, elderly)

Most male infants have some degree of gynecomastia at birth due to the effect of maternal estrogen. The gynecomastia generally goes away by 2 to 3 weeks of age.

Gynecomastia is common during puberty and in the elderly.

Pathological (e.g., testosterone deficiency or increased estrogen production, medications)

TESTOSTERONE DEFICIENCY

Signs and symptoms: use of antiandrogen medications (e.g., flutamide, finasteride) (these treat prostate enlargement and prostate cancer); use of spironolactone (this treats hypertension and edema); possible hypogonadism; history of liver disease, Klinefelter syndrome, hypothyroidism

Investigations: testosterone, thyrotropin (TSH)

INCREASED ESTROGEN PRODUCTION

Signs and symptoms: use of medications that increase estrogen levels (e.g., estrogen, spironolactone, verapamil, cimetidine); history or symptoms of hypothyroidism (decreased reflexes, dry skin, weight gain, impaired cognition); symptoms of pituitary tumor (headaches, vision changes); testicular abnormalities (hypogonadism, asymmetry, masses)

Investigations: abnormal LH levels; elevated estradiol; abnormal thyrotropin (TSH); MRI scan of the brain to detect pituitary tumor

MEDICATIONS

Medications known to cause gynecomastia include antiandrogen drugs, anabolic steroids, diazepam, TCAs, some antibiotics, spironolactone, cimetidine, digoxin, CCBs, and methadone.

Keys to patient encounter

History

HISTORY OF PRESENT ILLNESS

Ask when the patient discovered the mass and how the mass has changed.

Ask about other symptoms, and whether they correspond to the menstrual cycle.

Examples of characteristic symptoms include:

Invasive breast cancer: nipple inversion, nipple discharge with skin redness, or dimpling

Fibrocystic change: fluctuating bilateral lumps with breast tenderness

Infection: fever with breast pain and redness

RISK FACTORS FOR BREAST CANCER

Ask about general risk factors for breast cancer and specific risk factors for hereditary breast cancer (see the pointer).

POINTER

Risk factors for breast cancer

GENERAL RISK FACTORS	SPECIFIC RISK FACTORS FOR HEREDITARY BREAST CANCER
First-degree relative with breast or ovarian cancer Personal history of atypical ductal hyperplasia or lobular carcinoma in situ Personal history of breast or ovarian cancer Alcohol consumption Current or prior use of hormone therapy or OCs Menarche before age 12 Menopause after age 55 Nulliparity Older than age 35 at first delivery High breast density on mammography Thoracic radiation exposure	Breast cancer diagnosed at age 35 or younger "Triple negative" (ER, PR, HER2 receptors) breast cancer diagnosed at age 60 or younger Male breast cancer 2 primary breast cancers with at least 1 diagnosed at age 50 or younger Ovarian cancer at any age Breast or ovarian cancer and Ashkenazi Jewish heritage Family member with confirmed *BRCA1* or *BRCA2* mutation 1 breast cancer and 1 ovarian cancer in first-degree relatives 2 first-degree relatives with breast cancer diagnosed at age 50 or younger 2 first-degree relatives with ovarian cancer 3 breast cancers in first-degree relatives, with 1 diagnosed at age 50 or younger

MEDICATIONS

Ask about estrogen, OCs, SSRIs, haloperidol, spironolactone, and digoxin.

B

Physical exam

Vital signs: Look for fever.

Breasts:

- Palpate the breast tissue.
- Inspect the breasts for asymmetry, nipple discharge, and skin changes.
- Inspect the axillae, supraclavicular area, and chest wall.

Investigations

Mammography in women aged 30 and older

US in women younger than 30 (more sensitive than mammography in this age group)

US-guided core needle biopsy for all masses

Management

Refer patients with malignant breast masses to a surgeon for excisional biopsy or mastectomy. Refer patients with risk factors for hereditary breast cancer (see the pointer) for *BCRA1* and *BCRA2* gene testing.

BURNS

Burns

Keys to patient encounter

Key concern

Manage major thermal trauma.

Airway and hemodynamic status

Check the patient's ABCs. Begin resuscitation, as required.

RESUSCITATION

Remove the patient's clothing: This ensures the burning process has stopped. Cool the burnt area with cool, running water for 20 minutes.

Establish large-bore IV access: Go through burned skin if necessary.

Assess ABG: Administer oxygen or hyperbaric oxygen to patients with elevated carboxyhemoglobin.

History

In an emergency situation, take a history at the same time as you perform other tasks.

BURN HISTORY

Ask how the burn happened. Note that burns can result from thermal, chemical, electrical, or radiation injuries.

RISK FACTORS FOR INHALATION INJURY

Risk factors include being inside a burning building, being involved in an explosion, and losing consciousness. Ask whether the patient's voice sounds different.

PAST MEDICAL HISTORY

Ask about current and/or chronic medical conditions. Determine the patient's tetanus immunization status.

Physical exam

TBSA burned: Estimate as follows (mnemonic: **rule of 9s**): each arm: 9%; face and/or scalp: 9%; back: 18%; front: 18%; each leg: 18%; perineum: 1%; any area as big as the patient's own hand: 1%.

Inhalation injury: Examine the patient for traces of carbon around the nose and mouth, and in the throat or sputum; burned or singed facial hair and facial swelling; and stridor, hoarseness, black sputum, or respiratory distress.

B

Management

ADMIT OR TRANSFER THE PATIENT TO A BURN UNIT, AS WARRANTED

Patients require treatment in a burn unit if they have:

- burns to 20% or more TBSA (any age)
- burns to 10% or more TBSA (younger than 10 years or older than 50 years)
- full-thickness burns to more than 5% TBSA (any age) (see the pointer on assessing burn depth)
- superficial partial-thickness burns or full-thickness burns to the hands, feet, face, perineum, genitalia, or major joints (any age)
- inhalation injury (any age)

POINTER

Assessing burn depth

Superficial burns: dry, painful, minor blisters; red skin; brisk capillary return

Superficial partial-thickness burns: moist, painful, red, broken blisters; brisk capillary return

Deep partial-thickness burns: moist, painless, white-or-red mottled, sloughed skin; sluggish capillary return

Full-thickness burns: dry, painless, charred skin or white skin; absent capillary return

PROVIDE ONGOING FLUID SUPPORT, AS WARRANTED

Patients who require treatment in a burn unit also require fluid support for the first 24 hours after injury (use Hartmann's solution).

Use the Parkland formula to calculate the patient's 24-hour fluid requirement:

$$4 \text{ cc} \times \% \text{ TBSA burned} \times \text{weight in kg}$$

Give half the calculated amount in the first 8 hours from the time of injury, and half in the subsequent 16 hours.

TREAT PAIN

Provide immediate pain relief (e.g., IV morphine 0.1 mg/kg in titrated boluses).

PREVENT SECONDARY INFECTION

Administer systemic antibiotics and tetanus prophylaxis.

Dress the patient's wounds (apply topical antibiotic ointment on facial burns and topical silver sulfadiazine on other burns).

CARDIAC PRESENTATIONS

Abnormal heart sounds and murmurs

Differential diagnosis

ABNORMAL HEART SOUNDS AND MURMURS IN GENERAL

Systolic murmurs are often innocent, but diastolic murmurs are almost always pathological.

ABNORMAL HEART SOUNDS

S1 (e.g., mitral stenosis, atrial fibrillation)

MITRAL STENOSIS

Signs and symptoms: chest pain; shortness of breath (on exertion or when lying down); fatigue; swollen feet or legs; dizziness or fainting; heavy coughing; severe headache and other stroke symptoms; pulmonary edema; arrhythmia

Risk factors: history of rheumatic fever, untreated *Streptococcus* infections

ATRIAL FIBRILLATION

Signs and symptoms: chest pain, shortness of breath, palpitations, weakness, fatigue, dizziness

Risk factors: older age; personal or family history of heart disease; hypertension; chronic disease (thyroid disease, obstructive sleep apnea, diabetes, kidney disease, lung disease); obesity; alcohol use

S2 (e.g., hypertension, aortic stenosis)

HYPERTENSION

Signs and symptoms: systolic BP ≥140 mmHg and/or diastolic BP ≥ 90 mmHg

History of renal conditions; diabetes; adrenal or thyroid conditions; vascular conditions; catecholamine excess; obstructive sleep apnea; family history of hypertension

Risk factors: lack of exercise, high-sodium diet, obesity

AORTIC STENOSIS

Signs and symptoms: chest pain; feeling faint, fainting with exertion; shortness of breath, especially on exertion; fatigue, especially during and after exertion; palpitations

Risk factors: bicuspid aortic valve; older age; history of rheumatic fever

Investigations: echocardiogram; chest x-ray; cardiac catheterization with contrast dye, CT scan, MRI; ECG to measure electrical impulses from the heart muscle; exercise testing

S3 (e.g., congestive heart failure)

CONGESTIVE HEART FAILURE

Signs and symptoms: history of heart disease (or risk factors for heart disease: diabetes, hypertension, hyperlipidemia, and smoking) or hepatic vein thrombosis (Budd-Chiari syndrome); severe shortness of breath; elevated JVP; edema in the abdomen and legs; pink phlegm; heart murmurs and extra cardiac sounds

Investigations: chest x-ray to detect pulmonary edema; NT-proBNP; echocardiogram to distinguish forms of HF; cardiac stress testing, either with exercise or pharmacological agent

S4 (e.g., hypertension—see above)

Abnormal splitting (e.g., atrial septal defect)

ATRIAL SEPTAL DEFECT

Signs and symptoms: shortness of breath; fatigue; swelling of the feet, legs, or abdomen; palpitations or skipped beats; frequent lung infections; stroke symptoms

Risk factors: history of rubella infection; history of in-utero exposure to tobacco, alcohol, cocaine; maternal history of diabetes, SLE, phenylketonuria, obesity

SYSTOLIC MURMURS

Ejection murmurs (e.g., physiologic, aortic stenosis)

PHYSIOLOGIC (FUNCTIONAL) MURMUR

An example cause is high cardiac output (because of, for example, athletic training, anemia, or pregnancy).

AORTIC STENOSIS—SEE ABOVE

PANSYSTOLIC MURMURS (E.G., MITRAL REGURGITATION)

Mitral regurgitation

Signs and symptoms: shortness of breath; fatigue; palpitations; swollen feet or ankles

Risk factors: personal or family history of valve disease; history of heart attack or heart disease; use of ergotamine, cabergoline; history of endocarditis, rheumatic fever; older age

DIASTOLIC MURMURS

DIASTOLIC MURMURS IN GENERAL

Diastolic heart murmurs are generally low-pitched sounds of softer intensity and longer duration than other heart sounds.

Other sounds or murmurs are generally higher pitched and louder, with a possible click or thrill, and heard in either the systole phase alone or continuously throughout the cardiac cycle.

Early (e.g., aortic regurgitation)

AORTIC REGURGITATION

Signs and symptoms: fatigue; shortness of breath; swollen ankles and feet; chest pain that increases with exercise; light-headedness or fainting; arrhythmia; palpitations

Risk factors: history of endocarditis, rheumatic fever; aortic stenosis; CHD; hypertension; Marfan syndrome; ankylosing spondylitis; older age

Middiastolic (e.g., mitral stenosis—see above)

PERICARDIAL FRICTION RUBS

PERICARDIAL FRICTION RUBS IN GENERAL

This is caused by movement of inflammatory adhesions between pericardial layers, which results in systolic or multiphase high-pitched squeaking.

Acute pericarditis

Signs and symptoms: sudden-onset, stabbing chest pain; pain made worse with inhalation or lying down, made better with sitting up or leaning forward (usual); radiation of pain to the neck, arms, left shoulder, and especially to the trapezius muscle

> History of recent viral illness; infection (e.g., TB); autoimmune disease (e.g., SLE, RA, scleroderma); uremia; MI; aortic dissection; chest wall trauma; thoracic surgery

Diagnosis: ECG; chest x-ray to detect pericardial effusion

Cardiac tamponade

Signs and symptoms: history of invasive heart procedures; chest pain, radiating to the neck and jaw; right upper quadrant abdominal pain (due to hepatic venous congestion); tachycardia; elevated JVP; pulsus paradoxus

Investigations: abnormal ECG; normal chest x-ray

Keys to patient encounter

History

HISTORY OF PRESENT ILLNESS

Ask about chest pain. Classic angina pain is diffuse and retrosternal, radiating to the left arm and jaw. The pain is exacerbated by exertions and relieved by rest. However, not all cardiac pain follows this pattern and atypical chest pain may be particularly common in women. Also ask about the presence of exercise intolerance, palpitations, shortness of breath, peripheral edema, fatigue, and syncope.

Examples of characteristic symptoms include:

Mitral stenosis: chest pain, coughing, severe headache

Aortic stenosis: chest pain, symptoms triggered by exertion (feeling faint, shortness of breath, fatigue)

Acute pericarditis: stabbing chest pain that radiates to the trapezius and is made worse on inhalation

Cardiac tamponade: upper right quadrant abdominal pain, tachycardia

PAST MEDICAL HISTORY

The relevant previous diagnoses are numerous for this clinical presentation. Check the differential diagnosis.

PAST SURGICAL HISTORY

Ask about previous cardiac surgery or procedures, and thoracic surgery.

MEDICATIONS

Ask about ergotamine and cabergoline.

FAMILY HISTORY
Ask about heart disease and hypertension.

SOCIAL HISTORY
Ask about alcohol use and athletic training.

Physical exam

Vital signs

Cardiovascular and pulmonary:

- Look for elevated JVP.
- Examine the extremities for edema.
- Auscultate the heart and lungs for abnormal sounds, as listed in the differential diagnosis. Heart sounds from specific valves are best heard at the following locations:

Aortic valve: second intercostal space at the right sternal border

Pulmonic valve: second intercostal space at the left sternal border

Tricuspid valve: left lower sternal border

Mitral valve: fifth intercostal space at the midclavicular line (cardiac apex)

Investigations

ECG

Echocardiography

Management

Refer the patient to a cardiologist. Consider the need for endocarditis prophylaxis (see the pointer).

POINTER

Recommendation for endocarditis prophylaxis

Routine antibiotic prophylaxis is appropriate for patients with a prosthetic cardiac valve; a history of infective endocarditis; unrepaired or incompletely repaired cyanotic CHD; a recently repaired (within the past 6 months) congenital heart defect; and a limited number of additional indications.

CARDIAC PRESENTATIONS

Cardiac arrest

Differential diagnosis

CORONARY ARTERY DISEASE

Signs: ST elevation on the cardiac monitor or defibrillator

CARDIAC CONDUCTION ABNORMALITIES

Signs: VT or VF on the cardiac monitor or defibrillator

MYOCARDIAL ABNORMALITIES

This is typically identified on autopsy.

NONCARDIAC CAUSES (E.G., PULMONARY EMBOLUS)

Pulmonary embolism

Signs and symptoms: sharp chest pain; shortness of breath; cough (possibly with blood); hypoxia; possible unilateral swelling of the lower limbs (this indicates DVT); elevated pulse and respiratory rate; arrhythmias; lung rales on auscultation; lower-lung dullness on percussion; motor or sensory deficits

Risk factors: HF; cancer; surgery; prolonged immobility (e.g., long plane trips); smoking; estrogen replacement therapy; OCs; current pregnancy; previous DVT, embolism, or stroke; family history of embolism

Investigations: elevated d-dimer level; area of reduced pulmonary perfusion on V/Q scan; CT angiography to detect blocked vessel

Hypoxia

Signs: cyanosis of ≥ 1 extremity; low oxygen saturation on pulse oximetry (but be aware that low oxygen saturation will be present as a consequence of the cardiac arrest itself)

Tension pneumothorax

Signs: absence of breath sounds over 1 or both lungs on auscultation, deviated trachea

Acidosis

Investigations: low pH on ABG test

Hypo- or hyperkalemia

Investigations: abnormal electrolyte concentrations on ABG test, normal ECG findings

Drugs

Common overdose drugs include TCAs, beta-blockers, CCBs, and cocaine.

Hypovolemia

Common causes are severe dehydration or bleeding.

Cardiac tamponade

Common causes are chest trauma and recent MI.

Keys to patient encounter

Key concern

Initiate immediate cardiac life support.

Airway and hemodynamic status

Perform a primary survey for ABCs. Be aware of possible cervical spine injury and maintaining cervical stabilization. If the patient has no pulse, begin chest compressions at a rate of 100 to 120 per minute. If breathing is absent, begin ventilation at a rate of 10 per minute using a bag-valve mask. If bag-mask ventilation is not adequate, insert an advanced airway device: laryngeal mask airway (LMA), Combitube, or endotracheal tube. Confirm placement of the airway device by observation and confirming the presence of lung sounds in 4 lung fields. Attach ECG leads and identify the patient's rhythm. Establish IV or intraosseous (IO) access. Follow the appropriate ACLS protocol for the rhythm identified. Look for reversible causes.

History

Obtain a brief history from accompanying caregivers, witnesses, and first responders. Ask about clinical features relevant to the arrest: what they noticed about the patient before the arrest, what the patient was doing when the arrest happened, and whether the patient has a history of CAD. (Check for a sternotomy scar.) Ask what treatment the patient received before arriving at the hospital.

Consider stopping CPR if ACLS produces no response after 20 minutes of efficient resuscitation (no return of spontaneous circulation, no shockable rhythm, no reversible causes).

Management in cases of death

If the patient is deceased, talk to the family.

First, offer condolences and determine the extent of the family's understanding of the medical condition of their relative.

Determine if the patient is an organ donor. The family may know the answer to this. If not, they may have the patient's wallet, which might contain the patient's driver's license (which often lists organ donor status) or an organ donor card.

If the patient is not a donor, counsel the family about the possibility of organ donation. If the family consents to donation, determine which organ(s) they are consenting to.

If the patient is an organ donor or the family consents to donation, contact the organ transplant team.

CARDIAC PRESENTATIONS

Chest pain

Differential diagnosis

CARDIOVASCULAR CONDITIONS

Ischemic

ACUTE CORONARY SYNDROME

Some patients present with atypical pain (this is more common in women).

Signs and symptoms: squeezing pain that radiates to the left arm or jaw (often); pain that started with exertion or exercise and has not subsided; decreased oxygen saturation

Left heart failure: extra cardiac sounds and lung rales on auscultation

Right heart failure: edema in the feet and legs

Risk factors: personal or family history of cardiac disease; high cholesterol; hypertension; diabetes; smoking; renal failure; anemia; electrolyte abnormalities

Investigations: 12-lead ECG (possible findings: ST-segment elevation, T-wave inversion); CBC to detect anemia; creatinine; electrolytes; elevated troponin (this may take 4 to 6 hours to appear); chest x-ray

STABLE ANGINA PECTORIS

Some patients present with atypical pain.

Signs and symptoms: pain on exertion or exercise that subsides with rest or nitroglycerin medication; squeezing pain that radiates to the left arm or jaw (often); decreased oxygen saturation

Left heart failure: extra cardiac sounds and lung rales on auscultation

Right heart failure: edema in the feet and legs

Risk factors: high cholesterol; smoking; hypertension; diabetes; family history of cardiac disease; anemia; electrolyte abnormalities

Investigations: 12-lead ECG; CBC to detect anemia; electrolytes; chest x-ray (this is normal)

Nonischemic

AORTIC ANEURYSM

Signs and symptoms: pain in the chest or midback, often described as tearing pain; shortness of breath; cough; hoarse voice; difficulty swallowing

Risk factors: hypertension, Marfan syndrome

Investigations: US, MRI, or CT scan

PERICARDITIS

Signs and symptoms: sudden-onset stabbing chest pain; pain made worse with inhalation or lying down, made better with sitting up or leaning forward (usual); radiation of pain to the neck, arms, left shoulder, and especially to the trapezius muscle; pericardial rub on auscultation (usual)

History of recent viral illness; infection (e.g., TB); autoimmune disease (e.g., SLE, RA, scleroderma); uremia; MI; aortic dissection; chest wall trauma; thoracic surgery

Diagnosis: ECG; chest x-ray for pericardial effusion

PULMONARY OR MEDIASTINAL CONDITIONS

Pulmonary embolism or pulmonary infarct

PULMONARY EMBOLISM

Signs and symptoms: sharp chest pain; shortness of breath; cough (possibly with blood); hypoxia; possible unilateral swelling of the lower limbs (this indicates DVT); elevated pulse and respiratory rate; arrhythmias; lung rales on auscultation; lower-lung dullness on percussion; motor or sensory deficits

Risk factors: HF; cancer; surgery; prolonged immobility (e.g., long plane trips); smoking; estrogen replacement therapy; OCs; current pregnancy; previous DVT, embolism, or stroke; family history of embolism

Investigations: elevated d-dimer level; area of reduced pulmonary perfusion on V/Q scan; CT angiography to detect blocked vessel

Pleuritis

Signs and symptoms: chest pain aggravated by breathing; shortness of breath; fever; decreased oxygen saturation; areas of lung consolidation on auscultation (this suggests pneumonia)

Risk factors: viral or bacterial infection; autoimmune disease, especially RA; TB; heart surgery

Investigations: CBC to detect elevated WBCs, chest x-ray

Pneumothorax

Signs and symptoms: sudden-onset shortness of breath with pain; absence of breath sounds over 1 lung on auscultation; deviated trachea (this suggests a tension pneumothorax)

Risk factors: prior pneumothorax; COPD; smoking; emphysema

Investigations: chest x-ray

Malignancy

Signs and symptoms: shortness of breath (often; this symptom is consistent with a space-occupying lesion); constitutional symptoms (fever, weight loss, night sweats, fatigue)

Risk factors: smoking, exposure to asbestos, history of cancer

Investigations: CT scan of the lungs

GASTROINTESTINAL CONDITIONS

Esophageal spasm or esophagitis

ESOPHAGEAL SPASM

Signs and symptoms: squeezing chest pain, difficulty swallowing, regurgitation of food

ESOPHAGITIS

Signs and symptoms: difficulty swallowing or pain with swallowing; food becoming impacted in the esophagus, especially foods that are solid or difficult to chew; acid reflux; oral *Candida* infection; oral ulcers; epigastric tenderness (this could arise from associated PUD or reflux)

> History of food allergies or environmental allergies (e.g., pollen); factors causing immunosuppression, such as HIV, cancer, immunosuppressant medications, autoimmune disease, malnutrition (immunosuppression creates a higher risk for bacterial, viral, and fungal infections of the esophagus); use of antiinflammatories and bisphosphonates (these present a particular risk if they are not swallowed properly and remain in the esophagus)

Investigations: upper GI series (barium swallow) or endoscopy

Peptic ulcer disease

Signs and symptoms: constant midepigastric pain, often relieved with eating or with antacids; weight loss

Investigations: *H. pylori*; endoscopy to detect ulcer or inflammation of the gastric lining

Mallory-Weiss syndrome

Common causes include vomiting, coughing, hiccups, and abdominal trauma (e.g., a fall, car accident).

Signs and symptoms: abdominal pain, vomit with blood

Investigations: endoscopy

Biliary disease or pancreatitis

BILIARY DISEASE

Signs and symptoms: middle-aged woman (more common); epigastric pain, often after eating (the pain is generally constant and often radiates to the right shoulder); right-sided subcostal pain that is worse on deep inhalation; obesity; history of pregnancy

> Cancer or primary biliary cholangitis: fatigue, weight loss
>
> Obstructive biliary disease: jaundice

Investigations: elevated ALP, bilirubin (this indicates biliary obstruction); elevated aminotransferases (AST, ALT) (this indicates liver injury); US or CT scan to detect gallstones; MRCP to detect bile duct obstruction

PANCREATITIS

Signs and symptoms: constant upper abdominal pain that radiates to the back (sitting up and leaning forward may reduce the pain; pain occurs with coughing, vigorous movement, deep breathing); shortness of breath; nausea, vomiting; hypotension; fever; jaundice; abdominal tenderness

History of gallstones or chronic alcoholism (usual); hyperlipidemia; hypercalcemia; change of medication

Investigations: serum amylase and lipase (levels are ≥ 3 times ULN; elevated lipase indicates pancreatic damage); possible elevated calcium; possible elevated cholesterol; possible elevated ALT (this indicates associated liver inflammation); chest x-ray (this may show left-sided or bilateral pleural effusion; atelectasis); abdominal x-ray (this may show calcifications within pancreatic ducts, calcified gallstones, or localized ileus of a segment of small intestine); US

C

ANXIETY DISORDERS[1(pp189–234)]

Examples of anxiety disorders listed in *DSM-5* include generalized anxiety disorder, panic disorder, separation anxiety disorder, social anxiety disorder, and specific phobia. Anxiety disorders can provoke panic attacks (e.g., exposure to a phobic object). In the case of panic disorder, panic attacks occur spontaneously.

Signs and symptoms: history of anxiety disorder and/or symptoms consistent with a panic attack; history of social or emotional triggers for symptoms (possible); lack of evidence for other causes, including hyperthyroidism (anxiety can mimic other conditions and is therefore a diagnosis of exclusion)

Panic attack: symptoms that peak within minutes; symptoms that can include palpitations, accelerated heart rate, shortness of breath, chest pain, dizziness, numbness or tingling, fear of losing control, fear of dying

CHEST WALL PAIN (E.G., COSTOCHONDRITIS)

Costochondritis

Signs and symptoms: chest wall trauma; consistent pain with specific movements; pain on palpation of the ribs, sternum, and/or sternoclavicular joints

Keys to patient encounter

Key concerns

Exclude life-threatening entities.

Stay alert to red flags for serious causes of chest pain (see the pointer).

POINTER

Red flags for serious causes of chest pain

- Abnormal vital signs
- Signs of hypoperfusion
- Shortness of breath
- Hypoxemia
- Asymmetric breath sounds or pulses
- New heart murmur
- Pulsus paradoxus > 10 mmHg

Airway and hemodynamic status

Check the patient's ABCs. Provide emergency management to stabilize the patient as required. Ensure any unstable patient is in a monitored setting with good peripheral IV access.

History

PAIN HISTORY

Ask when the current episode of chest pain started and what triggered it, and about the character of the pain, its location, and what makes it better and worse. Ask specifically if the pain is present with respiration (this suggests pericarditis or pleuritis), with swallowing (esophageal condition), with exercise (cardiovascular condition), or with changes in position (pericarditis, pancreatitis).

Examples of characteristic pain include:

ACS: unremitting, squeezing chest pain that radiates to the left arm or jaw, and that started with exertion

Pericarditis: sudden-onset stabbing chest pain that radiates to the trapezius muscle, made better by leaning forward

ASSOCIATED SYMPTOMS

Examples of characteristic symptoms include:

Aortic aneurysm: shortness of breath, cough, and difficulty swallowing

PE: shortness of breath and unilateral calf swelling

Pleuritis: shortness of breath and fever

Pancreatitis: shortness of breath, nausea, vomiting, and fever

MEDICATIONS AND DRUGS

Ask about phosphodiesterase inhibitors, triptans, and cocaine.

RISK FACTORS FOR CORONARY ARTERY DISEASE

Ask about hypertension, hyperlipidemia, diabetes, smoking, and a family history of premature cardiovascular disease (onset before age 55 in men and age 60 in women).

RISK FACTORS FOR VENOUS THROMBOEMBOLISM

Ask about immobilization, recent surgery, malignancy, pregnancy, and a family history of venous thromboembolism.

Physical exam

General inspection: Look for pallor, sweating, cyanosis, and anxiety.

Vital signs:

- Measure BP in both arms.
- Check for pulsus paradoxus.

Neck:

- Look for venous distention and increased hepatojugular reflux, and note the carotid pulses.
- Check for an enlarged thyroid and lymphadenopathy.

Cardiovascular:

- Auscultate the heart for splitting, pericardial friction rubs, murmurs, and gallops.
- Palpate pulses in both arms and both legs.

Respiratory: Auscultate the lungs for adventitious sounds.

Abdominal: Look for tenderness, organomegaly, and masses.

Legs: Look for edema and signs of DVT (swollen calf that is erythematous, tender, and > 3 cm larger than the other calf when measured 10 cm distal to the tibial tuberosity).

Investigations

ECG: Look especially for ST elevation.

Pulse oximetry

Chest x-ray

IN POSSIBLE PULMONARY EMBOLISM

D-dimer

IN POSSIBLE ACUTE CORONARY SYNDROME

Serum troponin

Because a single normal set of cardiac markers does not rule out a cardiac cause, patients whose symptoms suggest ACS should have serial measurement of the cardiac marker troponin and ECGs at least 6 hours apart. Some clinicians follow these tests (acutely or within several days) with a stress ECG or a stress imaging test. Drug treatment (acetylsalicylic acid and clopidogrel) is begun while awaiting results of the second troponin level, unless there is a clear contraindication (see the pointer on contraindications). A diagnostic trial of sublingual nitroglycerin or an oral liquid antacid does not adequately differentiate myocardial ischemia from GERD or gastritis. Either drug may relieve symptoms of either disorder.

Troponin will be elevated in all ACS causing cardiac injury, and often in other disorders that damage the myocardium (e.g., myocarditis, pericarditis, aortic dissection involving coronary artery flow, PE, HF, severe sepsis). CK may be elevated due to damage to any muscle tissue, but CK-MB elevation is specific to damage to the myocardium. However, troponin is now the standard marker of cardiac muscle injury. ST-segment abnormality on ECG may be nonspecific or due to antecedent disorders, so comparison with previous ECGs is important.

Management

Treat any identified disorders. Remember the mnemonic "MONA treats MIs." **MONA** stands for **m**orphine, **o**xygen, **n**itrates, and **a**spirin. Begin fibrinolytic therapy within 30 minutes of hospital arrival, and, if available, initiate primary PCI within 90 minutes of hospital arrival. On hospital discharge, ensure the patient is prescribed aspirin, a $P2Y_{12}$ inhibitor, a beta-blocker, an ACE inhibitor or ARB, and a statin. If the patient smokes, counsel the patient on smoking cessation. Refer the patient to a cardiac rehabilitation service.

REFERENCE

1. American Psychiatric Association. Diagnostic and statistical manual of mental disorders. 5th ed. Arlington, VA: American Psychiatric Association; 2013. 59–60. 991 p.

POINTER

Contraindications to fibrinolysis in acute myocardial infarction

- Systolic BP > 180 mmHg, diastolic BP > 110 mmHg
- Aortic dissection
- History of structural CNS disease
- Significant closed head injury or facial trauma in the past 3 months
- Recent stroke
- Intraocular bleeding
- Major trauma, surgery, or GI or GU bleeding in the past 6 weeks
- Bleeding or clotting problems, or taking an oral anticoagulant
- CPR longer than 10 minutes
- Pregnancy
- Advanced or terminal cancer, or severe liver or kidney disease

CARDIAC PRESENTATIONS

Palpitations

Differential diagnosis

SUPRAVENTRICULAR CONDITION

Sinus tachycardia

INCREASED DEMAND (E.G., PREGNANCY, ANEMIA)

PREGNANCY

Signs and symptoms: amenorrhea, especially during childbearing years (some experience spotting); sexual activity, especially without contraception or with inconsistent use of contraception; nausea, vomiting (common early sign); breast enlargement and tenderness; increased frequency of urination without pain or difficulty; fatigue

Investigations: blood or urine β-HCG

ANEMIA

Signs and symptoms: pallor, chest pain, palpitations, weakness, headache, dizziness, shortness of breath

Risk factors: intestinal disorders (Crohn disease, celiac disease), menstruation, pregnancy, chronic disease (e.g., cancer, kidney failure), family history of sickle cell disease

Investigations: CBC; visual examination of RBCs for unusual size, shape, color

METABOLIC CONDITION (E.G., THYROTOXICOSIS, PHEOCHROMOCYTOMA)

THYROTOXICOSIS (INCLUDES HYPERTHYROIDISM)

A thyroid storm may lead to HF.

Signs and symptoms: tachycardia; palpitations; weight loss despite increased appetite; tremor; muscle weakness; sweating; fatigue; anxiety; poor concentration; heat intolerance; neck swelling; depression; eye irritation; eyelid swelling; warm moist skin; hair thinning; AF

Investigations: blood tests (findings: low thyrotropin, elevated free T_3 or T_4); ECG (findings: sinus tachycardia; increased QRS voltages; AF)

PHEOCHROMOCYTOMA

Signs and symptoms: tachycardia; pallor; headaches; shortness of breath; symptoms that occur in brief spells (up to 20 minutes) with no symptoms between (these spells may be mistaken for panic attacks); volatile or therapy-resistant hypertension

Investigations: plasma metanephrines or urinary fractionated metanephrines to measure catecholamines; abdominal and pelvic MRI or CT scan

ANXIETY DISORDERS[1(pp189–234)]

Examples of anxiety disorders listed in *DSM-5* include generalized anxiety disorder, panic disorder, separation anxiety disorder, social anxiety disorder, and specific phobia. Anxiety disorders can provoke panic attacks (e.g., exposure to a phobic object). In the case of panic disorder, panic attacks occur spontaneously.

Signs and symptoms: history of anxiety disorder and/or symptoms consistent with a panic attack; history of social or emotional triggers for symptoms (possible); lack of evidence for other causes, including hyperthyroidism (anxiety can mimic other conditions and is therefore a diagnosis of exclusion)

> Panic attack: symptoms that peak within minutes; symptoms that can include palpitations, accelerated heart rate, shortness of breath, chest pain, dizziness, numbness or tingling, fear of losing control, fear of dying

DRUGS (E.G., COCAINE, CAFFEINE)

Atrial fibrillation or flutter

ATRIAL FIBRILLATION

Signs and symptoms: sustained irregular heart rhythm on pulse palpation or auscultation; shortness of breath; light-headedness or dizziness; focal neurological deficits; variable S1 intensity and absence of S4 on auscultation

Risk factors: hypertension, coronary heart disease, valvular heart disease, diabetes mellitus, sleep apnea

Investigations: ECG

> Findings: absence of P waves; irregular R-R intervals; narrow QRS complex (< 120 milliseconds) if no underlying bundle branch block

ATRIAL FLUTTER

Signs and symptoms: persistent or paroxysmal palpitations

> More severe: dizziness, chest pain, shortness of breath, anxiety

Investigations: AV conduction (findings: ventricular rate 140 to 150 beats per minute; AV conduction 2:1 or 4:1); 12-lead ECG (finding: flutter waves)

Supraventricular tachycardia (atrioventricular reentrant tachycardia), Wolff-Parkinson-White syndrome

SUPRAVENTRICULAR TACHYCARDIA

This is the most common arrhythmia in pediatrics.

Signs and symptoms: tachycardia (regular, fast cardiac rhythm of 150 to 270 beats per minute); episodes that last minutes to days; fatigue; light-headedness; chest pain; shortness of breath; anxiety; syncope

Investigations: ECG

Findings: narrow QRS complex (< 120 milliseconds)

WOLFF-PARKINSON-WHITE SYNDROME

This is caused by congenital cardiac bypass tracts.

Signs and symptoms: young adult male (more common); tachycardia; palpitations; shortness of breath; syncope; fatigue; anxiety; chest pain, tightness; episodes that last seconds to hours, at rest or during exercise

Investigations: ECG (findings: short PR interval; delta waves; increased QRS interval)

Junctional tachycardia

This is a form of supraventricular tachycardia involving the atrioventricular node.

Causes include digitalis toxicity, theophylline, onset of ACS, and HF.

Signs and symptoms: tachycardia (either present or provoked by esophageal stimulation or invasive electrophysiological investigation); ventricular rate of 60 to 100 beats per minute; palpitations; fatigue, light-headedness; chest pain; shortness of breath; anxiety; polyuria; pounding sensation in the neck

Automatic junctional tachycardia: irregular rhythm and heart rate; nonresponsiveness to vagal maneuvers (e.g., gagging, holding breath, coughing)

Investigations: ECG

Findings: P wave that may be inverted in inferior leads (P wave can be before, during or after QRS complex); narrow QRS complex (< 120 milliseconds)

Premature junctional complexes and premature atrial contractions

PREMATURE JUNCTIONAL COMPLEXES

Signs and symptoms: often asymptomatic, palpitations with hypotension (it may occur in healthy patients, or may be due to drug cardiotoxicity, electrolyte imbalance, mitral valve surgery, or cold water immersion)

Risk factors: stress; caffeine, nicotine, alcohol use

Investigations: ECG (findings: normal QRS complex, preceded by an abnormal P wave or no P wave)

PREMATURE ATRIAL CONTRACTIONS

Signs and symptoms: heart "skipping a beat"; occasionally strong heartbeat, fluttering sensation

Risk factors: stress, poor sleep, caffeine use, alcohol use

Investigations: ECG (findings: P wave with different morphology from preceding P waves; premature atrial complex followed by a noncompensatory pause)

VENTRICULAR CONDITION

Ventricular tachycardia

Sudden cardiac death or cardiac arrest is possible.

Causes include cardiomyopathy; structural or ischemic heart disease; HF; and oral macrolide antibiotics.

Signs and symptoms: palpitations, tachycardia, dizziness, syncope, fatigue, shortness of breath, angina, hypotension

Investigations: ECG (findings: $\geq$ 3 continuous beats of wide QRS with a pulse > 100 beats per minute)

Premature ventricular contractions (PVCs)

Signs and symptoms: feeling of heart "skipping a beat," or a strong beat, or chest suction; chest pain; light-headedness; fatigue; hyperventilation after exercise

Risk factors: alcohol, caffeine, cocaine, nicotine use; exercise; hypertension; hypercalcemia; anxiety; underlying heart disease

Investigations: ECG (**but** isolated PVCs may not be detected due to their infrequency); Holter monitor (this is a better detection method)

Ventricular fibrillation

This is associated with CAD.

Sudden cardiac death or arrest is a common initial presentation.

Signs and symptoms: underlying rhythm of cardiac arrest

Risk factors: ST-segment elevation and atrioventricular-conduction block during acute MI

Investigations: ECG

Keys to patient encounter

Key concerns

Identify patients in need of urgent care.

Differentiate intrinsic heart disease from other disorders.

History

Ask when the palpitations happen and how long they last. Ask about symptoms of intrinsic heart disease versus other causes (see the pointer). Ask about anxiety, hyperthyroidism, and heart disease.

Physical exam

Vital signs

Cardiovascular: Note the rate and rhythm of the heart.

Respiratory: Auscultate the lungs.

Investigations

Electrolytes (potassium and magnesium)

ECG

Holter monitor if ECG is not diagnostic

Echocardiogram (consider this)

Thyrotropin (TSH) (consider this)

Management

In intrinsic heart disease, urgently consult a cardiologist. Treat any other underlying disorders. Counsel patients on lifestyle modification, as appropriate (e.g., avoiding stress and stimulants).

POINTER

Features of palpitations

INTRINSIC HEART DISEASE

Chest pain

Tachycardia or bradycardia

Palpitations with syncope

OTHER DISORDERS

Current anxiety disorder or life stressors

Excessive intake of caffeine, alcohol, or nicotine

Heat intolerance (hyperthyroidism)

Palpitations that can be stopped by deep breathing or changing body position

REFERENCE

1. American Psychiatric Association. Diagnostic and statistical manual of mental disorders. 5th ed. Arlington, VA: American Psychiatric Association; 2013. 59–60. 991 p.

CEREBROVASCULAR ACCIDENT AND TRANSIENT ISCHEMIC ATTACK

Cerebrovascular accident and transient ischemic attack

Differential diagnosis

ISCHEMIC STROKE

Thrombotic

Signs and symptoms (these depend on the affected blood vessel): hemiparesis, monoparesis, or (rarely) quadriparesis; hemisensory deficits; vision loss in 1 or both eyes; visual field deficits; double vision; difficulty speaking; facial droop; ataxia; vertigo; aphasia; fever; sudden decrease in level of consciousness

History of hypertension, diabetes, smoking, high cholesterol, CAD, coagulopathies, illicit drug use (especially cocaine), migraines, OC use

Investigations: CT scan, MRI; ECG to detect AF; presence of cardiac markers (troponins, CK-MB); abnormalities on PTT and/or PT/INR

Embolic

Signs and symptoms: symptoms similar to thrombosis (see above)

History of AF, cardiac defects, hypertension, CAD

Investigations: abnormal ECG; presence of cardiac markers (troponins, CK-MB); abnormalities on PTT, and/or PT/INR

HEMORRHAGIC STROKE

Intracerebral and cerebellar

Signs and symptoms: symptoms with sudden onset that gradually become worse (e.g., over hours); symptoms that include neurologic deficits (e.g., weakness or hemiparalysis in the face, arms, or legs), headache, impaired vision, aphasia, dysphasia, nausea, vomiting, sleepiness, loss of consciousness, confusion, delirium, fever

History of head injury or trauma; known cerebral aneurysm or AVM; bleeding disorders or use of blood thinners; bleeding tumors; cocaine use (this can cause severe hypertension)

Investigations: CT scan, cerebral angiogram

Subarachnoid

Signs and symptoms: sudden-onset severe symptoms; symptoms that include: severe headache (this is the most common symptom; it is sometimes called a "thunderclap" headache); neck or shoulder pain; meningismus with nuchal rigidity; photophobia; pain with eye movements; nausea, vomiting; seizures; confusion; fever; syncope (prolonged or atypical); neurological abnormalities

History of congenital berry aneurysm; bleeding from an AVM; bleeding disorders or use of blood thinners

Investigations: CT scan, MRI; cerebral angiogram; transcranial US

Keys patient encounter

Key concerns

Take action in the case of CVA or TIA.

Reduce the risk of CVA and TIA through preventive health care.

History

In the case of acute stroke, the patient will likely be unable to give a history. Seek information from accompanying caregivers.

Ask about risk factors for stroke including hypertension, diabetes, smoking, high cholesterol, CAD, coagulopathies, illicit drug use (especially cocaine), migraines, OC use, and a history of TIA or stroke.

Physical exam

Vital signs: Look in particular for fever.

Neurological: Perform a full exam, looking for deficits.

Cardiovascular: Listen for bruits over the carotid arteries and abdominal aorta.

Investigations

IN SUSPECTED STROKE: IMMEDIATE INVESTIGATIONS

Point-of-care glucose

Emergent CT scan of the head

OTHER INVESTIGATIONS

CBC

Electrolytes (see *Notes on labs and assessments*)

Creatinine

PT/INR

aPTT

Troponin to rule out concurrent or recent heart attack

Serum glucose

ECG to detect AF and/or recent MI

Management

Obtain an emergent referral to a stroke team or acute stroke unit.

Treat ischemic stroke patients presenting within 4.5 hours (or within 3 hours for patients older than 80) with fibrinolytic therapy (see the pointer for inclusion criteria and absolute contraindications). Order patients to have nothing by mouth. Before allowing oral food, liquids, or pills, perform a swallowing assessment.

For patients with a fever > 38°C, administer acetaminophen rectally.

For all patients, consider supplemental oxygen and order a cardiac monitor to assess for ischemic changes and AF.

Treat patients with antihypertensives **only** if systolic BP is > 220 mmHg or if diastolic BP is > 120 mmHg, **except** in the administration of fibrinolytic therapy (where systolic BP > 185 mmHg or diastolic BP > 110 mmHg is a contraindication and so requires treatment). First-line antihypertensive medications include:

- **Labetalol:** 10–20 mg by IV every 10 to 20 minutes
- **Nicardipine:** 5 mg/hour; titrate by 2.5 mg/hour every 5 to 15 minutes; maximum 15 mg/hour

When the target BP is reached, lower the dose of labetalol or nicardipine to 3 mg/hour, or administer enalapril 1.25 mg by IV push.

In patients who do not respond to fibrinolytic therapy or who are not candidates, refer emergently for endovascular therapy (stent placement).

In patients with TIAs, start low-dose acetylsalicylic acid and evaluate for treatable risk factors (hypertension, smoking, diabetes, high cholesterol, carotid stenosis). TIAs confer a 10% risk of stroke in the next 30 days. When stroke occurs after a TIA, 50% occur within the next 48 hours.

Following acute treatment, refer the patient to an occupational therapist and for rehabilitation therapy.

POINTER

Criteria for fibrinolysis with tissue plasminogen activator

INCLUSION CRITERIA

Age 18 or older
Clinical diagnosis of ischemic stroke causing neurologic deficit(s)
Symptom onset over less than 4.5 hours

ABSOLUTE CONTRAINDICATIONS

Significant head trauma or prior stroke in the previous 3 months
Subarachnoid hemorrhage
Noncompressible arterial puncture in the previous 7 days
History of previous intracranial hemorrhage
Intracranial neoplasm, AVM, or aneurysm
Recent intracranial or intraspinal surgery
Systolic BP > 185 mmHg or diastolic BP > 110 mmHg
Active internal bleeding
Acute bleeding diathesis
Blood glucose < 48.6 mg/dL (2.7 mmol/L)
CT demonstrating a multilobar infarction (hypodensity in more than one-third of the cerebral hemisphere)

RELATIVE CONTRAINDICATIONS

Only minor or quickly improving stroke symptoms (clearing automatically)
Pregnancy
Seizure at the onset with postictal residual neurological impairments
Major surgery or trauma within the previous 14 days
GI or urinary tract hemorrhage with in the previous 21 days
Acute MI within the previous 3 months

CONSTIPATION

Adult constipation

Differential diagnosis

DIET, LIFESTYLE

Causes include recent changes in diet; recent decrease in activity level; low-fiber diet; and inadequate hydration.

IRRITABLE BOWEL SYNDROME[1]

Irritable bowel syndrome is commonly diagnosed by applying the Rome criteria.

Signs and symptoms (Rome criteria): at least 2 symptoms, present for ≥ 1 day/week for ≥ 3 months

> Symptoms: pain associated with 1) defecation, 2) change of stool frequency, and/or 3) change in stool consistency

DRUG-INDUCED CONDITION

Drugs known to cause constipation include opioids, iron supplements, antidepressants, antipsychotics, levodopa, antihistamines, and antacids.

NEUROGENIC CONDITION (CENTRAL OR PERIPHERAL)

Spinal cord injury

Signs and symptoms: history of trauma, infection, or malignancy; leg weakness; fatigue; lack of coordination

Amyotrophic lateral sclerosis

Signs and symptoms: onset in a limb or extremity; weakness, cramps, twitching, muscle wasting (lower motor neuron involvement); walking difficulty due to spasticity (upper motor neuron involvement); general fatigue; reduced exercise tolerance; possible language dysfunction

> Bulbar onset, which may precede limb weakness: swallowing difficulty; slurred speech; jaw jerking; increased gag reflex; tongue twitching (very specific for ALS)

Investigations: EMG, nerve conduction study, MRI

Spina bifida

This is congenital and diagnosed at birth.

Multiple sclerosis

Signs and symptoms: variable depending on lesion location

- Spinal cord: sensory or motor dysfunction; Lhermitte sign (paresthesias radiating down the extremities or trunk with neck flexion); bowel, bladder, or erectile dysfunction
- Brainstem: double vision; swallowing, speech difficulties; vertigo; pseudobulbar palsy
- Cerebrum: cognitive impairment; depression; upper motor neuron signs; unilateral motor or sensory deficits
- Cerebellum: problems with balance and coordination; vertigo
- Other symptoms: tonic spasms; fatigue; pain; exercise intolerance; temperature sensitivity; painful unilateral loss of visual acuity

Risk factors: younger than 50, female

Investigations: brain and spinal cord MRI, including advanced MRI techniques, with established occurrence of multiple episodes; CSF fluid analysis

Parkinson disease

Signs and symptoms (mnemonic **TRAP**): **t**remor at rest; **r**igidity of the lower limbs; **a**kinesia, bradykinesia; **p**ostural instability

- Other symptoms: cognitive impairment; dementia; shuffling gait with stooped posture and loss of arm swing; micrographia; hypophonia; masklike facies; "pill rolling"; lack of blinking; orthostatic hypotension
- History of use of antipsychotics, antiemetics; toxin ingestion (e.g., carbon monoxide, cyanide); head trauma; vascular disease; other neurodegenerative disease (e.g., Lewy body dementia, Huntington disease); brain tumor, hydrocephalus; metabolic conditions (e.g., hypoparathyroidism, Wilson disease, chronic liver failure); infections that spread to the brain (HIV/AIDS, syphilis, prion disease, toxoplasmosis, encephalitis lethargica, progressive multifocal leukoencephalopathy)

Stroke

Signs and symptoms: history of stroke, or signs and symptoms consistent with stroke (e.g., unilateral neurologic defects)

Risk factors: hypertension, dyslipidemia, diabetes, coagulopathy

MYOPATHIC CONDITION

Signs and symptoms: child (usual, but still rare); history of long-standing constipation; increased anal tone on physical exam

Investigations: positive for myopathy on rectal biopsy

METABOLIC CONDITION

Hypothyroidism

Signs and symptoms: history of hypothyroidism or symptoms of hypothyroidism (cold intolerance, decreased reflexes, dry skin, weight gain, impaired cognition)

Investigations: elevated thyrotropin (TSH)

Diabetes

Signs and symptoms: personal or family history of diabetes; history of diabetic complications and/or inadequate monitoring; polydipsia, polyuria, and/or weight loss

Investigations: fasting glucose or HbA_{1c}

PREGNANCY

Signs and symptoms: amenorrhea, especially during childbearing years (some experience spotting); sexual activity, especially without contraception or with inconsistent use of contraception; nausea or vomiting (common early sign); breast enlargement and tenderness; increased frequency of urination without other urinary symptoms; fatigue

Investigations: blood or urine β-HCG

OBSTRUCTIVE LESIONS

Signs and symptoms: constitutional symptoms (fever, weight loss, night sweats, fatigue); rectal bleeding or blood in the stool; increased bowel sounds (this can indicate early obstruction; bowel sounds may be decreased in later obstruction); possible enlarged lymph nodes in the groin; possible palpable abdominal mass

> History of colorectal carcinoma (this is a source of intrinsic lesions); carcinoma, sarcoma, lymphoma (these are sources of extrinsic lesions)

Investigations: colonoscopy, x-ray

ANORECTAL DISEASE

Anal fissures or hemorrhoids

Signs and symptoms: history of anal fissures or hemorrhoids; small amounts of bright red blood following bowel movements; anal pain or irritation; anal fissures and/or hemorrhoids on physical exam

Anal fistulas or abscesses

Signs and symptoms: history of inflammatory bowel disease (e.g., Crohn disease, ulcerative colitis); blood in the stool; abdominal pain; weight loss; fever; fatigue; fistulas and/or abscesses on physical exam

Inflammatory bowel disease

Signs and symptoms: younger than 30 (usually); family history of inflammatory bowel disease; fluctuating symptoms with periods of exacerbation and remission; diarrhea (possibly with nocturnal waking); blood in the stool; abdominal pain; weight loss; fever; fatigue; right lower quadrant and periumbilical pain; extraintestinal manifestations (e.g., uveitis, arthritis)

Crohn disease: right lower quadrant mass, uveitis, arthritis

Investigations: elevated CRP (this suggests active inflammation); fecal calprotectin; colonoscopy with biopsy (this is a standard diagnostic procedure); CT scan or MRI (findings: diagnostic structural changes associated with inflammatory bowel disease)

Keys to patient encounter

History

HISTORY OF PRESENT ILLNESS

Ask when the constipation started and how often the patient has a bowel movement. Ask about the size and consistency of the stools. In female patients, ask if digital splinting of the vagina is necessary to have a bowel movement (this indicates pelvic floor dysfunction).

Ask about red-flag symptoms (see the pointer) and constitutional symptoms (these suggest malignancy).

PAST MEDICAL HISTORY

Ask about neurogenic conditions, hypothyroidism, diabetes, cancer (colorectal carcinoma, other carcinoma, sarcoma, lymphoma), hemorrhoids, and irritable bowel syndrome.

MEDICATIONS

Ask about opioids, iron supplements, antidepressants, antipsychotics, levodopa, antihistamines, and antacids. Ask whether the patient uses laxatives.

FAMILY HISTORY

Ask about a family history of bowel cancer and inflammatory bowel disease.

Physical exam

Abdominal: Look for masses, liver enlargement, and a palpable colon.

Perineal: Look for fissures, rectal prolapse, and hemorrhoids.

DRE: Look for masses and fecal impaction.

Investigations

Routine investigations in patients without red flags (see the pointer) are usually not indicated.

IN UNCERTAIN DIAGNOSIS

Chest x-ray

Abdominal x-ray (flat and upright)

IN OTHER CONTEXTS

Suspected anemia: CBC

Older patients: fecal immunochemical test; colonoscopy to rule out colorectal cancer

Ruling out hypothyroidism: thyrotropin (TSH)

Ruling out metabolic cause: electrolytes and calcium

POINTER

Red flags in constipation

- New-onset constipation in an elderly patient
- Anemia (symptoms: fatigue, pallor, dizziness, shortness of breath, tachycardia)
- Rectal bleeding or positive fecal occult blood test
- Family history of bowel cancer or inflammatory bowel disease
- Tenesmus
- Weight loss

POINTER

Risk factors for constipation

- Female
- Older age
- Inactivity
- Low caloric intake and/or low-fiber diet
- Polypharmacy
- Low income

Management

In patients without red flags, provide counseling on increasing dietary fiber and fluid intake, increasing exercise, and using laxatives as needed (magnesium hydroxide, lactulose, polyethylene glycol). If red flags are present, refer the patient to a gastroenterologist or surgeon for colonoscopy.

REFERENCE

1. Lacey B, Mearin F, Chang L, et al. Rome IV functional gastrointestinal disorders: disorders of gut-brain interaction. 4th ed. Vol. 2. Raleigh, NC: Rome Foundation; 2017. Chapter 11, Functional bowel disorders; 1393–1407.

CONSTIPATION

Pediatric constipation

Differential diagnosis

PEDIATRIC CONSTIPATION IN GENERAL

Most pediatric constipation has a nonorganic cause.

NEONATES AND INFANTS

Diet-induced constipation

Signs and symptoms: formula feeding; introduction of solid foods; iron supplementation; possible impacted stool in rectum

Anatomic condition

Signs and symptoms: family history of Hirschsprung disease; passage of meconium > 48 hours after delivery; tight anal sphincter; empty rectum; palpable abdominal fecal mass

Older children: abdominal distention; failure to thrive

Investigations: positive rectal biopsy

OLDER CHILDREN

Diet-induced constipation

The common cause is a diet low in fiber and fluid, and/or high in calcium.

Psychologically induced constipation

Signs and symptoms: excessive worry; loss of interest in friends and usual activities; changes in sleep habits; hallucinations or delusions; suicidal thoughts

History of emotional, physical, or sexual abuse; substance abuse; recent stresses (e.g., death of a friend or family member)

Risk factors: family history of mental health disorders

Anatomic condition (e.g., bowel obstruction)

BOWEL OBSTRUCTION

Signs and symptoms: crampy abdominal pain; nausea, vomiting; change in bowel habits (diarrhea or constipation); abdominal distention; palpable abdominal mass; increased bowel sounds (this can indicate early obstruction: bowel sounds may be decreased in later obstruction); history of colonic diseases (diverticulitis, colon cancer, inflammatory bowel disease)

Risk factors: paralytic ileus (narcotic medications, chronic neuromuscular disease, diabetes), adhesions (abdominal surgery)

Investigations: abdominal x-ray

Neurologic condition

Signs and symptoms: symptoms of spinal cord injury (e.g., history of trauma; leg weakness; fatigue; lack of coordination); decreased anal tone and lack of stool in the rectum (usual); absent cremasteric reflex (in males) (usual); absent anal wink (in both sexes) (usual); decreased muscle tone and reflexes in the lower extremities (usual)

Endocrine or metabolic condition

DIABETES

Signs and symptoms: personal or family history of diabetes; history of diabetic complications and/or inadequate monitoring; polydipsia, polyuria, and/or weight loss

Investigations: fasting glucose or HbA_{1c}

HYPOTHYROIDISM

Signs and symptoms: history of hypothyroidism or symptoms of hypothyroidism (cold intolerance, decreased reflexes, dry skin, weight gain, impaired cognition)

Investigations: elevated thyrotropin (TSH)

Other condition (e.g., celiac disease, cystic fibrosis)

CELIAC DISEASE

Signs and symptoms: family history of celiac disease, or signs and symptoms of celiac disease (chronic abdominal pain, rashes)

Investigations: positive serum anti-tTG (with IgA level); duodenal biopsy to detect villous blunting

CYSTIC FIBROSIS

Signs and symptoms: family history of CF; recurrent pneumonia; shortness of breath; productive cough; failure to thrive; fever; wheezing on lung auscultation

Investigations: positive sweat chloride test

C

Keys to patient encounter

History

HISTORY OF PRESENT ILLNESS

Ask how often the child has a bowel movement, and about the size and consistency of the stools.

Ask about associated symptoms. Examples of characteristic symptoms include:

Psychologically induced constipation: mental health issues
Bowel obstruction: nausea and vomiting
Diabetes: increased thirst and urine production
Celiac disease: chronic abdominal pain and rash
CF: recurrent pneumonia, productive cough, and failure to thrive

PAST MEDICAL HISTORY AND SURGICAL HISTORY

Ask about Hirschsprung disease, mental health issues, abdominal surgery, neuromuscular disease, spinal cord injury, colonic disease, diabetes, hypothyroidism, celiac disease, and CF.

MEDICATIONS

Ask about medications associated with constipation (e.g., opioids).

FAMILY HISTORY

Ask what conditions run in the family.

SOCIAL HISTORY

Ask about diet, especially the patient's intake of dietary fiber, and about toileting behavior (e.g., timing of bowel movements, toilet avoidance).

Physical exam

Vital signs

Height, weight, head circumference: Plot these on a growth chart.

Abdominal: Look for tenderness and palpable stool in the large bowel.

Neurological: Look for decreased anal tone, absent anal wink, and lower limb weakness.

DRE: Look for impacted stool in the rectum.

Investigations

Abdominal x-ray (consider this to confirm constipation if DRE is not possible)

Management

Rule out secondary causes (e.g., CF: pneumonia, failure to thrive; celiac disease: chronic abdominal pain, rash; Hirschsprung disease: bloating, failure to thrive). Stay alert to red flags (see the pointer). Treatment of functional constipation starts with disimpaction by enemas, rectal suppositories, or oral agents (polyethylene glycol, lactulose, mineral oil, senna). This is followed by maintenance medications (polyethylene glycol, lactulose) and increased dietary fiber.

POINTER

Red flags in pediatric constipation

Abnormal anatomy
Signs or symptoms of hypothyroidism
Signs or symptoms of CF
Signs or symptoms of diabetes
Findings on neurological exam
Poor growth
Bilious vomiting
Ileus

POINTER

Incidence of functional constipation

Most patients (95%) have functional constipation characterized by infrequent, large-caliber stools.

CYANOSIS, HYPOXIA

Cyanosis, hypoxia

Differential diagnosis

CENTRAL CYANOSIS OR HYPOXIA

CENTRAL CYANOSIS OR HYPOXIA IN GENERAL

Signs and symptoms: mental status changes; bluing of the lips and mucous membranes; tachycardia (except for opioid overdose); tachypnea (except for opioid overdose)

High alveolar-arterial (A-a) gradient

SHUNTING (E.G., TETRALOGY OF FALLOT, ACUTE RESPIRATORY DISTRESS SYNDROME)

TETRALOGY OF FALLOT

Signs and symptoms: newborn or infant; heart murmur

Investigations: decreased oxygen on ABG; characteristic heart defects on chest x-ray, echocardiogram; right ventricular hypertrophy on ECG

ACUTE RESPIRATORY DISTRESS SYNDROME

Signs and symptoms: recent critical illness (e.g., sepsis; severe pneumonia; major trauma; serious smoke or chemical inhalation); severe shortness of breath

Investigations: decreased oxygen on ABG; bilateral infiltrates on chest x-ray

VENTILATION-PERFUSION MISMATCH (E.G., CYSTIC FIBROSIS, PULMONARY EMBOLUS)

CYSTIC FIBROSIS

Signs and symptoms: family history of CF; recurrent pneumonia; shortness of breath; productive cough; failure to thrive; fever; wheezing on lung auscultation

Investigations: positive sweat chloride test

PULMONARY EMBOLISM

Signs and symptoms: sharp chest pain; shortness of breath; cough (possibly with blood); hypoxia; possible unilateral swelling of the lower limbs (this indicates DVT); elevated pulse and respiratory rate; arrhythmias; lung rales on auscultation; lower-lung dullness on percussion; motor or sensory deficits

Risk factors: HF; cancer; surgery; prolonged immobility (e.g., long plane trips); smoking; estrogen replacement therapy; OCs; current pregnancy; previous DVT, embolism, or stroke; family history of embolism

Investigations: elevated d-dimer level; area of reduced pulmonary perfusion on V/Q scan; CT angiography to detect blocked vessel

DIFFUSION IMPAIRMENT (E.G., RESTRICTIVE LUNG DISEASE)

RESTRICTIVE LUNG DISEASE

Signs and symptoms: dry cough (usual), progressive exertional shortness of breath (usual)

Risk factors: family history of restrictive lung disease; occupational exposure to asbestos or heavy metals (e.g., construction, farming, mining)

Normal A-a gradient

HYPOVENTILATION (E.G., OPIOID OVERDOSE)

OPIOID OVERDOSE

Signs and symptoms: bradycardia; constricted pupils; confusion, stupor, or coma; nystagmus; gait disturbance; history of opioid abuse, or signs of abuse (track marks on the arms)

HIGH ALTITUDE

Signs and symptoms: current or recent exposure to high altitudes; shortness of breath; elevated pulse

PERIPHERAL CYANOSIS OR HYPOXIA (E.G., LOW CARDIAC OUTPUT, COLD EXPOSURE)

PERIPHERAL CYANOSIS OR HYPOXIA IN GENERAL

Definition: cyanosis of ≥ 1 extremities

Low cardiac output

Signs and symptoms: history of CHF; shortness of breath; increased JVP; dependent edema; livedo reticularis; lung rales on auscultation; heart murmurs or extra sounds on auscultation

Investigations: ECG; pulmonary edema on chest x-ray

Cold exposure

Patients suffering from cold exposure have hypothermia.

Keys to patient encounter

Key concern

Determine if hypoxia (low oxygen level in tissues) or hypoxemia (low oxygen levels in blood) is present.

Provide supplemental oxygen.
Determine and treat the underlying cause.

History

HISTORY OF PRESENT ILLNESS

Ask when the patient first noticed the cyanosis, how constant it is, and what parts of the body it affects.

Examples of characteristic features include:

Acute versus gradual onset: Acute onset suggests a recent trigger such as an embolus or overdose.

Intermittent versus constant symptoms: Intermittent symptoms suggest reversible causes such as pulmonary embolus.

Symptoms in the extremities only: This suggests peripheral cyanosis (central cyanosis affects the central body).

PAST MEDICAL HISTORY

Ask about recent critical illness, CVD, and lung disease.

MEDICATIONS

Ask about drugs associated with hypoventilation (opioids), methemoglobinemia (nitrites, topical anesthetics, dapsone, phenytoin, sulfonamides, metoclopramide), and sulfhemoglobinemia (e.g., sulfonamides, sulfasalazine).

SOCIAL HISTORY

Obtain a smoking history.

Physical exam

General inspection: Look for the pattern of cyanosis: central versus peripheral.

Full physical: Pay special attention to the cardiorespiratory system.

Investigations

Pulse oximetry

ABG

Chest x-ray or CT scan

Pulmonary function test

Nocturnal (overnight) oximetry

CALCULATING THE ALVEOLAR-ARTERIAL (A-A) GRADIENT

The A-a gradient is estimated as:

$$[150 \text{ mmHg} - (5/4 \times PaCO_2)] - PaO_2$$

A normal A-a gradient is:

$$(\text{age} \div 4) + 4$$

See the pointer for the differential diagnosis of increased and normal A-a gradients. Consider methemoglobinemia or sulfhemoglobinemia in patients with cyanosis and normal oxygenation. Methemoglobinemia and sulfhemoglobinemia are both diagnosed by cooximetry.

Management

Treat the underlying cause identified. Methemoglobinemia is reversible with methylene blue, with or without ascorbic acid. In cases of sulfhemoglobinemia, or when methylene blue is contraindicated in methemoglobinemia, treatment with hyperbaric oxygen prevents tissue hypoxia.

POINTER

Interpretation of alveolar-arterial (A-a) gradient

INCREASED A-a GRADIENT

- Right-to-left intrapulmonary shunt
- CHF
- Pneumonia
- PE
- Atelectasis
- Obstructive lung disease (e.g., asthma, COPD)
- Pneumothorax
- Interstitial lung disease

NORMAL A-a GRADIENT

- Hypoventilation
- Neuromuscular disorders
- CNS disorders
- Effects of high altitudes

DEVELOPMENTAL PRESENTATIONS

Abnormal pubertal development

Differential diagnosis

DELAYED PUBERTY

DELAYED PUBERTY IN GENERAL

Signs and symptoms:

Girls: no breast development by age 13; no menstruation 5 years after first appearance of breast tissue

Boys: no testicle development by age 14; incomplete development of male organs 5 years after first signs of testicle development

Variant of normal constitutional delay of puberty

This describes the absence of pubertal development before age 14, with evidence of sexual maturation by age 18.

It is more common in males.

It may generate anxiety in adolescents and their families, and contribute to psychosocial difficulties for some children.

Signs and symptoms: family history of delayed sexual development; stature that is small for age, but with normal growth rate

No evidence of growth hormone deficiency; hypothyroidism; systemic conditions interfering with puberty; hypogonadism

Investigations: blood tests to exclude other possible causes

Primary gonadal disorders

CONGENITAL: CHROMOSOMAL (E.G., TURNER AND KLINEFELTER SYNDROMES), CONGENITAL MALFORMATIONS

TURNER SYNDROME

This is the most common chromosomal abnormality in women (45,X).

Signs and symptoms: ovarian insufficiency (no or minor breast development; primary or secondary amenorrhea); short stature with webbed neck and widely spaced nipples; cubitus valgus; Madelung deformity of the forearm and wrist; normal intelligence (usual)

Neonates (possible signs and symptoms): lymphedema of the hands and feet; nail dysplasia; high-arched palate; short fourth metacarpals and/or metatarsals

As girls age: hearing loss, hypothyroidism, liver dysfunction

Adult women: mildly elevated liver enzymes

Investigations: elevated FSH; presence of anti-müllerian hormone; karyotyping

KLINEFELTER SYNDROME

This is the most common congenital abnormality causing hypogonadism in men (most common karyotype: 47,XXY).

Signs and symptoms: small, firm testes or cryptorchidism; small penis; gynecomastia; infertility; decreased virilization; long legs due to long bone abnormality; difficulty with social interactions; learning disabilities; impaired attention without impulsivity

Investigations: low sperm count; elevated FSH and LH; low serum testosterone; karyotyping

CONGENITAL MALFORMATIONS

These result from genetic or environmental factors (half of all cases have an unknown cause). They are either structural or functional. Structural abnormalities are likely identifiable at birth; functional abnormalities can take months or years to identify.

ACQUIRED GONADAL DISORDERS (E.G., GONADAL INFECTION, TRAUMA, NEOPLASM)

Signs and symptoms:

Gonadal infection: history of infection (e.g., mumps orchitis)

Ovarian neoplasm: abdominal pain, palpable mass

Testicular neoplasm: painless scrotal mass

Secondary gonadal disorders

FUNCTIONAL (E.G., CHRONIC ILLNESS, MALNUTRITION)

DIABETES

Signs and symptoms: personal or family history of diabetes; history of diabetic complications and/or inadequate monitoring; polydipsia, polyuria, and/or weight loss

Investigations: fasting glucose or HbA_{1c}

CYSTIC FIBROSIS

Signs and symptoms: family history of CF; recurrent pneumonia; shortness of breath; productive cough; failure to thrive; fever; wheezing on lung auscultation

Investigations: positive sweat chloride test

KIDNEY DISEASE

Signs and symptoms: history of kidney disease, chronic renal failure, and/or current renal dialysis; bilateral lower limb swelling; shortness of breath; paroxysmal nocturnal dyspnea; orthopnea

Risk factors: diabetes, diabetic complications, and/or inadequate monitoring; hypertension; smoking

MALNUTRITION: ANOREXIA NERVOSA[1(pp338–339)]

This causes secondary amenorrhea.

Signs and symptoms: significantly low body weight; intense fear of gaining weight or persistent behavior that interferes with gaining weight; excessive focus on body weight or shape in self-evaluation, or persistent lack of recognition of current low body weight

HYPOTHALAMIC DYSFUNCTION (E.G., HYPERPROLACTINEMIA)

HYPERPROLACTINEMIA

The most common cause is prolactinoma (which usually presents in adulthood).

Signs and symptoms:

Girls: delayed puberty, amenorrhea, galactorrhea

Boys: delayed puberty, gynecomastia, galactorrhea, impaired vision, headaches

PITUITARY DYSFUNCTION (E.G., CENTRAL NERVOUS SYSTEM TUMOR)

CENTRAL NERVOUS SYSTEM TUMOR

Signs and symptoms: headache that gets worse over time (this is a common symptom: 50% of cases); vision impairment; balance problems; personality or behavior changes; seizures; drowsiness

Pituitary adenomas or cysts can press on gonadotrophs, causing disrupted function, decreased prolactin (reduced galactorrhea), and decreased gonadotropins (e.g., LH, FSH).

Risk factors: exposure to radiation (e.g., to treat leukemia in childhood); family history (rare); neurofibromatosis type 1 or type 2; tuberous sclerosis; Von Hippel-Lindau disease; Li-Fraumeni syndrome; immune system disorders

PRECOCIOUS PUBERTY

PRECOCIOUS PUBERTY IN GENERAL

Signs and symptoms:

Girls, before age 6–7 years: breast development, menarche

Boys, before age 9 years: enlarged testicles and penis; facial hair (usually upper lip); voice change

Both sexes: pubic and underarm hair; rapid growth; acne; adult body odor

Central precocious puberty (gonadotropin dependent)

Central precocious puberty is related to the hypothalamus or pituitary gland.

IDIOPATHIC

CENTRAL NERVOUS SYSTEM (E.G., NEOPLASMS, HYDROCEPHALUS)

CENTRAL NERVOUS SYSTEM NEOPLASM

Signs and symptoms: headache, vision impairment

> Hamartoma is the most common type of CNS neoplasm to cause precocious puberty in very young children and infants. It is usually benign, often found incidentally. Pubertal development stops on removal. Signs and symptoms include gelastic seizures; other types of seizures; convulsions; intellectual developmental delay; and behavioral disorders.

Risk factors: exposure to radiation (e.g., to treat leukemia in childhood); family history (rare); neurofibromatosis type 1 or type 2; tuberous sclerosis; Von Hippel-Lindau disease; Li-Fraumeni syndrome; immune system disorders

Investigations: brain MRI

HYDROCEPHALUS

Excess fluid accumulation, and pressure from dilated third ventricle on the hypothalamus, results in accelerated or precocious puberty.

Signs and symptoms: early morning headaches in children with possible nausea and vomiting; changes in behavior (e.g., irritability, unruliness, loss of interest); changes in vital signs (bradycardia, hypertension, altered respiratory rate); dilated or prominent scalp veins; double vision; papilledema; impaired upward gaze; spasticity in the legs, extremities

> As hydrocephalus progresses: lethargy and drowsiness

Peripheral precocious puberty (gonadotropin independent)

This is abnormal development of secondary sex characteristics not related to the hypothalamus or pituitary gland.

Investigations: high serum androgen or estrogen levels

Autonomous gonadal function (e.g., ovarian cysts, Leydig cell tumors of ovaries or testes)

OVARIAN CYSTS

Large functioning follicular ovarian cysts are the most common cause of peripheral precocity in girls. They appear and regress spontaneously. They can cause ovarian torsion.

Signs and symptoms: early breast development; vaginal bleeding once cysts regress

Investigations: pelvic US

LEYDIG CELL TUMORS OF OVARIES OR TESTES (ARRHENOBLASTOMA)

In girls, these produce androgens. They are usually benign (90%). Signs and symptoms include virilization precocity.

In boys, they produce asymmetric testicular enlargement. They are usually benign (90%). Signs and symptoms include feminization (if estrogen-secreting) or pubertal precocity (if androgen-secreting).

Investigations: pelvic US; histology (in boys, biopsy the larger testicle, if present, regardless of the presence of a mass)

ADRENAL PATHOLOGY (E.G., TUMORS, CONGENITAL ADRENAL HYPERPLASIA)

ADRENAL TUMORS

In girls, granulosa cell tumors cause gender-conforming precocity (unlike Leydig cell tumors which cause virilization precocity—see above).

In boys, HCG-secreting germ cell tumors increase testosterone production, which causes increased testicular size.

Investigations: pelvic and adrenal US

CONGENITAL ADRENAL HYPERPLASIA (CAH)

CAH is an enzyme defect in adrenal steroid biosynthesis. The most common cause is deficiency in 21-hydroxylase. Most patients are identified as neonates or infants.

In neonate boys (1 to 4 weeks), severe 21-hydroxylase deficiency can cause salt wasting (signs and symptoms include difficulty feeding, failure to thrive, vomiting, dehydration, volume depletion, hyponatremia, hyperkalemia, and shock).

Signs and symptoms: premature pubic hair growth

- Infant girls: virilization; ambiguous genitals
- Infant boys: undervirilization; normal genitals
- Later in childhood (in cases of mild 21-hydroxylase deficiency): accelerated growth and skeletal maturation; enlarged genitalia

Risk factors: Ashkenazi Jewish descent, Eastern European descent

Investigations for CAH due to 21-hydroxylase: high serum 17-hydroxyprogesterone; elevated adrenal androgens (DHEA-S); genetic testing

EXOGENOUS SEX HORMONE EXPOSURE

Examples include the use by parents or caregivers of estrogen-containing products (e.g., to treat menopause: creams, ointments, sprays with estrogen) and androgen creams (e.g., to treat low testosterone levels). Other sources include food contaminated with hormones and foods high in phytoestrogens (soy, lavender oil, tea tree oil).

Keys to patient encounter

Key concerns

Distinguish normal variants of pubertal development from serious underlying disorders.

Provide supportive counseling on the psychosocial aspects of puberty.

History

Establish whether the issue is delayed or precocious puberty. Make sure, based on the age of the child and the symptoms, that delayed or precocious puberty is really at issue (see the definitions in the differential diagnosis).

SYMPTOMS OF DELAYED PUBERTY

Ask about the specific symptoms of concern.

Examples of characteristic symptoms include:

Turner syndrome (in girls): short stature, webbed neck, widely spaced nipples

Klinefelter syndrome (in boys): small genitals or cryptorchidism

Prolactinoma: galactorrhea

CNS tumor: headache, seizures, abnormal movement, or changes in personality

PAST MEDICAL HISTORY

Ask about mumps, kidney disease, anorexia nervosa, exposure to radiation, and use of steroids (for example, to treat skin conditions).

FAMILY HISTORY

Ask about diabetes and CF.

SYMPTOMS OF PRECOCIOUS PUBERTY

Ask about the specific symptoms of concern.

Examples of characteristic symptoms include:

CNS neoplasm: headaches, vision problems

Hydrocephalus: headaches, nausea, behavior changes, spasticity

FAMILY HISTORY

Ask about the age at which the patient's parents and siblings went through puberty.

SOCIAL HISTORY

Ask about possible exposure to hormone-containing products from adult caregivers (e.g., to treat menopause or low testosterone).

Physical exam

Stage of pubertal development: Compare findings with Tanner staging for normal puberty (see the pointer).

Signs of specific entities: Look for signs of entities you suspect from the history (e.g., cryptorchidism in Klinefelter syndrome; palpable masses in gonadal neoplasm).

Investigations

CNS or pelvic imaging in suspected neoplasm

Karyotyping in suspected genetic abnormality

Other specific investigations as indicated by the results of the history and physical exam

Management

Specialist referral to a pediatrician or endocrinologist is usually indicated.

REFERENCE

1. American Psychiatric Association. Diagnostic and statistical manual of mental disorders. 5th ed. Arlington, VA: American Psychiatric Association; 2013. 991 p.

POINTER

Tanner staging for normal puberty

Tanner staging defines typical development across 5 age spans in girls and boys.

In girls, the stages track growth in height, breast development, development of pubic hair, and menarche.

In boys, the stages track growth in height, testicular length, penis length and width, development of pubic hair, increase in muscle mass, voice changes, and development of facial hair.

DEVELOPMENTAL PRESENTATIONS

Abnormal stature in a child

Differential diagnosis

TALL STATURE

Genetic (e.g., Marfan syndrome)

MARFAN SYNDROME

This is a connective tissue disorder.

Signs and symptoms: tall stature; long arms, legs, fingers (disproportionate); high arched palate, crowded teeth; heart murmurs; severe myopia; curved spine; flat feet

Risk factors: family history of Marfan syndrome

Investigations: bone x-rays to determine maturity and growth potential; echocardiogram to detect cardiac abnormalities

Endocrine disorder (e.g., excess growth hormone)

EXCESS GROWTH HORMONE

The common cause is pituitary tumor (usually benign).

Signs and symptoms: large body stature; delayed puberty; large hands and feet with widening distal phalanges; large forehead, jaw, tongue, nose, lips; underbite; wide teeth spacing

Pituitary tumor (other signs and symptoms): headache, vision impairment

Investigations: IGF-1; growth hormone suppression test; bone x-rays to determine maturity and growth potential; imaging to detect pituitary tumor, if suspected

SHORT STATURE

Short stature is defined as ≥ 2 SD below the mean height for children of the same sex and chronological age in a given population (below the 2.3rd percentile).

Genetic cause (e.g., Down syndrome)

DOWN SYNDROME

Signs and symptoms: characteristic dysmorphic features (small head, flattened facial features, protruding tongue, upward slanting eyes, small hands and feet, short fingers, single crease on the palms of the hands)

Other: ligamentous laxity

Risk factors: older maternal age, siblings with Down syndrome

Investigations: genetic testing (karyotyping will also detect other genetic causes such as Turner syndrome), x-rays of target areas to assess development

Systemic disorder (e.g., chronic disease and treatment complications)

Almost any serious systemic disease can cause growth failure. Typical causes include undernourishment from Crohn disease, celiac disease, CF, and cancer; increased energy expenditure from cancer and cardiac disease; cytokine production from rheumatologic disease; and irregular hormone regulation from renal disease.

Therapies (radiation, chemotherapy, stimulants, glucocorticoids) can have transient or permanent effects on growth.

Investigations: tests for nutritional status and hormones; x-rays for bone assessment

Environmental cause

MALNUTRITION

This includes insufficient nutrition (inadequate food supply; self-imposed restriction; underlying systemic disease that interferes with food intake or absorption, or increases energy needs) and vitamin deficiency.

Signs and symptoms: low weight for height

Investigations: blood and urine tests to determine nutritional status, hormones, and drug use; x-rays (wrist or hand) to detect bone age

TOXINS OR DRUGS

Examples of toxins include lead poisoning (common sources for children are dust in older buildings and lead-based paint), and alcohol and tobacco exposure in utero, which can cause IUGR.

Examples of drugs include glucocorticoids and chemotherapy.

Intrauterine growth retardation

This is in-utero growth below the tenth percentile for a baby's gestational age. After delivery, growth and development depend on the severity and cause of IUGR.

Causes include:

Placental problems: placental insufficiency; placental malformation; abruptio placentae; placental ischemia or infarction

Maternal problems: medical conditions (hypertension, diabetes mellitus, renal disease, autoimmune diseases); medications (anticonvulsants, anticoagulants, heparin, antineoplastics, cyclophosphamide); malnutrition; smoking; use of alcohol or illicit drugs; low prepregnancy weight; poverty; younger than 16 or older than 35; use of assisted reproductive technology; pregnancy complications (e.g., preeclampsia, threatened miscarriage with heavy bleeding)

Fetal problems: genetic syndrome; intrauterine infection (toxoplasmosis, CMV, rubella, VZV, malaria, syphilis, HSV, HIV)

Investigations: US to measure fluid around the baby, and the baby's growth, movements, and blood flow

Keys patient encounter

Key concerns

Determine whether the growth pattern is pathologic or normal.

Determine whether the child has dysmorphic features.

History

PAST MEDICAL HISTORY

Ask about underlying conditions such as chronic illnesses and environmental factors (e.g., toxin exposure, malnutrition).

Ask about the gestational age of the child at birth and a history of IUGR.

FAMILY HISTORY

Ask about abnormal stature and genetic disorders.

Physical exam

General inspection: Look for dysmorphic features and other physical abnormalities.

Height, weight, and head circumference:

- Plot these on a growth chart.
- Interpret your findings with consideration to the height of family members.

Investigations

X-ray of the left wrist and hand for bone age (the left hand is the standard as it is less likely to be injured than the right hand)

Karyotyping

Other tests for specific abnormalities (consider this)

Management

In suspected abnormal stature, refer the patient to a pediatrician or medical geneticist for diagnosis and further management.

DEVELOPMENTAL PRESENTATIONS

Adults with developmental disabilities

Differential diagnosis

GENERAL HEALTH ISSUES AND RISKS

Abuse and neglect

Risk factors: older age; female; noncompliance with medication; mental illness; lack of follow-up with medical appointments; repeated emergency room visits or hospital admissions; lack of a social network; dependence on a caregiver; living alone; inadequate housing; poverty; unexplained weight loss or failure to thrive; poor grooming and/or hygiene

Atypical presentations of serious illness and/or pain (e.g., infection, trauma)

Signs and symptoms: change in mood or personality; irritability; change in appetite; change in sleep habits

COMMON HEALTH ISSUES AND RISKS BY ETIOLOGY

Genetic syndromes (e.g., Down syndrome)

DOWN SYNDROME

Susceptibilities and risks: hearing loss; obstructive sleep apnea; ear infections; cataracts; severe refractive errors; ongoing problems stemming from congenital heart defects; GI atresia; hip dislocation; thyroid disease; risks related to reproductive health

Autism spectrum disorder

Susceptibilities and risks: depression, anxiety, bipolar disorder, psychosis, diabetes, GI disorders, epilepsy, sleep disorders, high cholesterol, hypertension, obesity

Fetal alcohol spectrum disorder

Susceptibilities and risks: health issues linked to poverty and/or homelessness (people with fetal alcohol spectrum disorder often have cognitive and behavioral issues that lead to unemployment and inadequate housing); cognitive issues such as attention and memory deficits; behavioral issues such as poor impulse control

Brain injury (e.g., cerebral palsy)

CEREBRAL PALSY

Susceptibilities and risks: seizures, respiratory infections, GERD, obesity, dental diseases, UTI, osteoporosis

Central nervous system infection

Susceptibilities and risks: seizures, memory problems, cognitive changes

Keys to patient encounter

Key concerns

Identify and manage common health issues in adults with developmental disabilities, with particular attention to atypical presentations of serious illness and complex health issues, both of which are common in adults with developmental disabilities.

Provide care with particular attention to known disparities in health status and health care for adults with developmental disabilities, and to the benefit of interdisciplinary coordination of care.

History

Clear and simple language is useful for every patient, but it is especially important for adults with developmental disabilities. For patients with severe developmental disabilities, ask whether you can speak to family or caregivers. Consider how to phrase questions and ideas clearly and simply (see the pointer).

HISTORY OF PRESENT ILLNESS

Establish the patient's disability and current symptoms. Ask about symptoms of common entities in particular, including arthritis, UTI, dysmenorrhea, constipation, and dental disease (these are all possible causes of decline in function); and about difficulties communicating and/or changes in behavior (these may indicate the presence of pain). Remain aware that complex issues and atypical presentations are likely.

POINTER

Communicating with clear and simple language

Avoid jargon: For example, say *urinary tract infection* instead of *UTI.*

Check for understanding: For example, does the patient know what a urinary tract infection is? If not, give some basic information.

Rephrase: For example, try *pee* instead of *urine.*

Break questions down into concise, single-idea components: For example, don't ask: *What prescription medications do you take?* Instead ask: *Have you seen a doctor before? Has a doctor told you to take medicine? What medicine?*

RISK FACTORS FOR ABUSE AND NEGLECT

Risk factors include frequent trips to emergency (which indicates a lack of coordinated care), living alone, social isolation, and financial and housing insecurity.

Physical exam

Conduct a complete general physical exam to screen for possible multiple health issues, including trauma.

Investigations

CBC to assess for anemia and infection

Urinalysis to look for UTI

Cancer screening (prostate, breast, colon)

- Cancer screening is often missed in patients with developmental disabilities.

IN PATIENTS WITH DOWN SYNDROME

Thyrotropin (TSH)

IN YOUNG MEN WITH DEVELOPMENTAL DISABILITIES

Testosterone to screen for hypogonadism (consider this)

Management

Treat any identified underlying disorder.

Psychiatric disorders are common in patients with developmental disorders, but can be difficult to diagnose. Consider referring the patient to a psychiatrist.

Encourage regular physical activity and supplementation with oral vitamin D.

Patients with developmental disabilities need interdisciplinary care. Aim to create systematic follow-up with these patients to coordinate their care, including:

- up-to-date immunizations for influenza, *S. pneumoniae*, HPV, HAV, and HBV
- regular medication reviews to reduce or eliminate medications that are no longer necessary
- assessment for abuse and neglect (report abuse and neglect to the police, and refer patients to community support agencies as necessary)
- capacity for consent, which needs regular reassessment
- care plans, including advance directives
- regular dental care
- regular vision and hearing assessments

DEVELOPMENTAL PRESENTATIONS

Developmental delay

Differential diagnosis

GLOBAL DEVELOPMENTAL DELAY

Neurological disorders (e.g., fetal alcohol spectrum disorder, cerebral dysgenesis)

Signs and symptoms (in general): neurological abnormalities, growth abnormalities, dysmorphic features

History of seizures; complications during gestation (e.g., toxin exposure such as alcohol) and/or delivery

Genetic and metabolic disorders (e.g., trisomy 21, congenital hypothyroidism)

TRISOMY 21 (DOWN SYNDROME)

Signs and symptoms: characteristic dysmorphic features (small head, flattened facial features, protruding tongue, upward slanting eyes, small hands and feet, short fingers, single crease on the palms of the hands)

Other: ligamentous laxity

Risk factors: older maternal age, siblings with Down syndrome

Investigations: karyotyping, x-rays of target areas to assess development

CONGENITAL HYPOTHYROIDISM

This is generally diagnosed at birth: newborn thyroid screening is a requirement in most of North America.

Signs and symptoms: often asymptomatic at birth, jaundice, frequent choking, large tongue, puffy appearance to the face

Investigations: thyrotropin (TSH), thyroxine

Toxic exposures (e.g., lead)

LEAD EXPOSURE

A common source of lead exposure is deteriorating lead paint in pre-1979 houses.

Signs and symptoms: neurological abnormalities, growth abnormalities

Investigations: elevated serum lead level

Severe psychosocial deprivation

Examples include childhood institutionalization, severe abuse, and/or severe neglect.

SPEECH AND LANGUAGE DELAY

Hearing impairment

Signs and symptoms: problems identifying the sources of sounds; complications during gestation (e.g., toxin exposure such as alcohol) and/or delivery; blocked tympanic membranes (e.g., from impacted wax or mass) or nonmobile tympanic membranes (from chronic effusion) (possible)

Investigations: hearing test

Autism spectrum disorder (when associated with atypical social and behavioral features)[1(pp50–51)]

Signs and symptoms: deficits in social interaction and communication; repetitive, stereotyped behaviors (motor and/or vocal); restricted interests; sensory problems; presence of symptoms in all contexts (e.g., home, school); presence of symptoms from early childhood

Developmental language disorder

Signs and symptoms: impaired language skills for a child's age (e.g., impairments with mastery of vocabulary, sentence structure, conversation); impairments with significant impact on the child's day-to-day life; presence of impairments from early childhood

MOTOR DELAY

Cerebral palsy

Signs and symptoms: history of complications during gestation (e.g., toxin exposure such as alcohol) and/or delivery; abnormal posture and/or physical movement; growth abnormalities

Muscular dystrophies

MUSCULAR DYSTROPHY

Common types of MD include Duchenne (more common in males), Becker, facioscapulohumeral, and myotonic.

Signs and symptoms: frequent falls; difficulty getting up from sitting or lying; difficulty running, jumping; waddling gait; walking on the toes; muscle pain, stiffness; large calf muscles

Risk factors: family history of MD
Investigations: muscle biopsy, increased CK, EMG, genetic testing

Developmental coordination disorder

Signs and symptoms: impaired motor skills for a child's age; impairments with significant impact on the child's day-to-day life; presence of impairments from early childhood

Keys to patient encounter

Key concern

Use a validated developmental screening tool to identify domains of developmental delay (children may have delay in 1 or more domains).

History

A detailed history is key to identifying potential developmental problems.

SYMPTOMS

Ask about symptoms in general, and also about specific symptoms including aggression, self-injury, hyperactivity, inattention, anxiety, depression, sleep problems, unusual or repetitive behaviors, lack of friends, and poor school performance.

PAST MEDICAL HISTORY

Ask about prenatal history, including complications during the pregnancy, prenatal infections, prenatal toxic exposures (e.g., alcohol), and abnormal results from prenatal screening.

Ask about birth history, including complications during delivery, gestational age at birth, Apgar score, and maternal group B streptococcus status.

FAMILY HISTORY

Ask about developmental delay and/or genetic abnormalities.

SOCIAL HISTORY

Assess for poverty and unstable living conditions. Ask whether the family has a history of neglect or abuse (e.g., emotional, physical, sexual), or a history of substance abuse. Ask if there is consanguinity between the parents.

Ask about concerns regarding toxic exposures.

Developmental screening

Use a validated screening tool to assess the child for developmental delay. Free, validated developmental milestones checklists are available online from the Centers for Disease Control and Prevention.

Physical exam

Conduct a complete general physical exam, including a full neurological exam.

Investigations

CBC
Lead
Calcium
CK
Thyrotropin (TSH)
Acylcarnitine profile
Liver function (see *Notes on labs and assessments*)
Hearing
Vision
Karyotyping
Other specific tests for genetic entities (in consultation with a clinical geneticist) and metabolic entities, if indicated
MRI of the head
EEG if indicated

Management

Refer children with any identified delays for diagnostic assessment and intervention. Identify any modifiable conditions (toxic exposure, neglect). Consider referring patients to medical genetics for further investigations.

POINTER

Developmental assessment follow-up

Developmental assessment is an ongoing process involving screening, surveillance, and definitive diagnostic assessment. Screening should occur at each regular pediatric visit using a validated screening tool. Surveillance involves parental interviews and direct observation in the office.

REFERENCE

1. American Psychiatric Association. Diagnostic and statistical manual of mental disorders. 5th ed. Arlington, VA: American Psychiatric Association; 2013. 59–60. 991 p.

DIARRHEA

Acute diarrhea

Differential diagnosis

ACUTE DIARRHEA IN GENERAL

Definition: abrupt-onset disturbance of stool frequency or stool consistency

INFECTION

GASTROENTERITIS IN GENERAL

Signs and symptoms: abrupt-onset diarrhea; crampy abdominal pain; nausea, vomiting; fever (this suggests viral infection); blood in the stool (this suggests bacterial infection)

Viruses

Common viruses include norovirus and rotavirus.

Risk factors: contact with infectious people

Bacteria

Common bacteria include *Campylobacter*, *Salmonella*, *Shigella*, *E. coli*, and *C. difficile*.

Risk factors: ingesting undercooked or contaminated foods, or raw fluids; hospitalization, recent antibiotic use (relevant to *C. difficile*)

Parasites

Common parasites include *Giardia* and *Cryptosporidium*.

Risk factors: contact with infants in day care; AIDS; anal sex with multiple partners; coming from a community with a waterborne parasite outbreak; travel to mountainous regions and/or tropical countries

Investigations: stool examination for ova and parasites

DRUGS OR TOXINS

Drugs

Examples include laxatives; antacids containing magnesium; antibiotics; and NSAIDs.

Shiga toxin

Signs and symptoms of *E. coli* infection: abdominal pain, blood in the stool, **no** fever

Preformed toxins

Signs and symptoms: symptoms that develop within 6 hours of ingesting contaminated food (e.g., undercooked meat, poorly refrigerated food)

Investigations: stool culture to detect enteric pathogens

ISCHEMIC CONDITION

This typically occurs in patients with risk factors for mesenteric ischemia.

Signs and symptoms: abdominal pain, bloody diarrhea, **no** risk factors for infection

Risk factors (mesenteric ischemia): CHF, arrhythmia, atherosclerosis, HF, chronic kidney failure

Investigations: CT scan; sigmoidoscopy, colonoscopy, arteriography (these are the best methods to definitively identify ischemia-related intestinal injury)

INFLAMMATORY BOWEL DISEASE

Signs and symptoms: younger than 30 (usually); family history of inflammatory bowel disease; fluctuating symptoms with periods of exacerbation and remission; diarrhea (possibly with nocturnal waking); blood in the stool; abdominal pain; weight loss; fever; fatigue; right lower quadrant and periumbilical pain; extraintestinal manifestations (e.g., uveitis, arthritis)

Crohn disease: right lower quadrant mass, uveitis, arthritis

Investigations: elevated CRP (this suggests active inflammation); fecal calprotectin; colonoscopy with biopsy (this is a standard diagnostic procedure); CT scan or MRI (findings: diagnostic structural changes associated with inflammatory bowel disease)

METABOLIC DISEASE (E.G., HYPERTHYROIDISM)

Hyperthyroidism

This results in hyperdefecation (not diarrhea per se).

Signs and symptoms: history of hyperthyroidism or symptoms of hyperthyroidism (changes in menstrual patterns, enlarged thyroid, tachycardia, palpitations, diarrhea, muscle weakness, tremor, hyperactive reflexes, weight loss, sweating, thinning hair)

Investigations: decreased thyrotropin (TSH)

Keys to patient encounter

Key concerns

Identify risk factors associated with specific causes.

Assess for complications (volume loss, electrolyte abnormalities).

History

HISTORY OF PRESENT ILLNESS

Ask when the diarrhea started, how many bowel movements the patient has per day, and how many bowel movements per day is usual for the patient. Ask about the consistency of the bowel movements, and whether there is blood or pus.

Ask about systemic symptoms (fever, weight loss, fatigue, night sweats), which could indicate malignancy or chronic infection.

PAST MEDICAL HISTORY

Ask about bowel disease, diseases that cause immunodeficiency (e.g., HIV), and risk factors for mesenteric ischemia (CHF, arrhythmia, atherosclerosis, HF, chronic kidney failure). Ask about recent hospitalization.

SURGICAL HISTORY

Ask about previous bowel surgeries.

MEDICATIONS

Ask about laxatives, antacids containing magnesium, antibiotics, NSAIDs, and medications that can cause immunodeficiency (e.g., steroids).

ALLERGIES

Ask about food allergies and intolerances (e.g., lactose intolerance, gluten intolerance).

SOCIAL HISTORY

Ask about recent travel and exposure to others with diarrhea (e.g., workers in day cares).

Physical exam

Vital signs: Look for fever (this suggests infection) and assess the patient's volume status (hypotension suggests dehydration).

Abdominal: Look for tenderness, masses, and increased bowel sounds.

Investigations

Testing is not necessary for most cases of acute diarrhea in developed countries.

IN SEVERELY DEHYDRATED PATIENTS

Serum creatinine

Electrolytes (see *Notes on labs and assessments*)

IN SPECIFIC CASES

Stool cultures and stool examination for ova and parasites in patients with diarrhea lasting more than 7 days, especially in cases of bloody diarrhea, severe dehydration, immunosuppressed patients, patients who have been camping, or during outbreaks

***C. difficile* toxins** in patients with recent hospitalization and/or recent antibiotic use

Management

Treat dehydration with oral (or if needed parenteral) rehydration. Consider loperamide or simethicone for symptomatic treatment of nonspecific diarrhea. Consider antibiotic treatment for traveler's diarrhea (quinolone or azithromycin, depending on local susceptibility patterns and travel history). Treat other infections based on culture results.

POINTER

Reportable diarrhea

Some causes of infectious diarrhea are reportable to public health authorities, including *Campylobacter*, *Salmonella*, *Shigella*, enterohemorrhagic *E. coli* (EHEC), *Vibrio cholerae*, *Cryptosporidium*, and *Giardia*.

DIARRHEA

Chronic diarrhea

Differential diagnosis

CHRONIC DIARRHEA IN GENERAL

Definition: loose and/or watery stools that occur 3 or more times a day for 4 or more weeks

STEATORRHEA

Luminal

PANCREATIC INSUFFICIENCY

Signs and symptoms: chronic weight loss, nausea, diarrhea; pale or clay-colored stools; fatty or oily stools

Investigations: serum enzyme levels; fecal fat test; abdominal CT scan, MRI, or US to detect damage or injury to the pancreas

CHOLESTASIS

Signs and symptoms: abdominal pain; nausea, vomiting; jaundice; itchiness; palpable, tender liver and/or gallbladder; history of liver disease, gallstones, cancer; current pregnancy

Investigations: abnormal liver enzyme tests; elevated bilirubin; abdominal US

ILEAL DISEASE OR RESECTION

Common reasons for extensive resection are diseases, infarction, and congenital anomalies.

Severe diarrhea and bile acid malabsorption result when > 100 cm of the ileum is resected.

BACTERIAL OVERGROWTH

This is an excess of bacteria in the small intestine, which damages the intestinal mucosa.

Signs and symptoms: abdominal fullness; pain, cramps; bloating; weight loss; watery diarrhea; fatty stools

Investigations: breath test for hydrogen; CBC; blood chemistry; vitamin levels; fecal fat test; biopsy or culture of the small bowel; x-ray of the small bowel

Mucosal

LACTASE DEFICIENCY

Signs and symptoms: abdominal distension; abdominal pain; diarrhea; symptom correlation with eating dairy products

Investigations: hydrogen breath test; lactose tolerance blood test

CELIAC DISEASE

Signs and symptoms: family history of celiac disease, or signs and symptoms of celiac disease (chronic abdominal pain, rashes)

Investigations: positive serum anti-tTG (with IgA level); duodenal biopsy to detect villous blunting

LARGE BOWEL CONDITIONS

Secretory diarrhea (e.g., villous adenoma)

VILLOUS ADENOMA

This is a neoplastic colon polyp.

Signs and symptoms: often asymptomatic; hematochezia with anemia; diarrhea; constipation; flatulence; pencil-thin stools; intense cramping (this indicates torsion or large adenomas); palpable mass on digital rectal exam

Common locations: rectum, rectosigmoid

Risk factors: family history of colon polyps and cancer

Investigations: endoscopy (villous adenomas are cauliflower-like projections); biopsy (larger adenomas are associated with severe dysplasia)

Inflammatory diarrhea

INFLAMMATORY BOWEL DISEASE

Signs and symptoms: younger than 30 (usually); family history of inflammatory bowel disease; fluctuating symptoms with periods of exacerbation and remission; diarrhea (possibly with nocturnal waking); blood in the stool; abdominal pain; weight loss; fever; fatigue; right lower quadrant and periumbilical pain; extraintestinal manifestations (e.g., uveitis, arthritis)

Crohn disease: right lower quadrant mass, uveitis, arthritis

Investigations: elevated CRP (this suggests active inflammation); fecal calprotectin; colonoscopy with biopsy (this is a standard diagnostic procedure); CT scan or MRI (findings: diagnostic structural changes associated with inflammatory bowel disease)

INFECTION

Causes include viruses (e.g., norovirus, rotavirus), bacteria (including *C. difficile*), and parasites.

Signs and symptoms: fever (this suggests viral infection); blood in the stool (this suggests bacterial infection)

Risk factors:

- Viral: contact with infectious people
- Bacterial: ingesting undercooked or contaminated foods, or raw fluids (*C. difficile*: recent or chronic antibiotic use, admission to hospital or long-term care facility)
- Parasitic: contact with infants in day care; AIDS; anal sex with multiple partners; coming from a community with a waterborne parasite outbreak; travel to mountainous regions and/or tropical countries

OTHER (E.G., RADIATION, ISCHEMIC COLITIS)

INTESTINAL LINING INJURY, INFLAMMATION IN GENERAL

Signs and symptoms: excretion of large volumes of water; abdominal pain, cramping

Investigations: x-ray with barium; colonoscopy or sigmoidoscopy to assess the extent of intestinal lining damage

RADIATION

An example is treatment for ovarian cancer.

ISCHEMIC COLITIS

Causes include atherosclerosis; hypotension (e.g., from HF, major surgery, trauma, shock); venous thrombosis; bowel obstruction (hernia, scar tissue, tumor); surgery (cardiac, vascular, GI, gynecological); vasculitis; SLE; sickle cell disease; use of cocaine, methamphetamine

Risk factors: older than 60; clotting disorders (factor V Leiden); high cholesterol; previous abdominal surgery; surgery involving the aorta; heavy exercise (e.g., marathon running)

Motility disorder (e.g., irritable bowel syndrome)

IRRITABLE BOWEL SYNDROME[1]

Irritable bowel syndrome is commonly diagnosed by applying the Rome criteria.

Signs and symptoms (Rome criteria): at least 2 symptoms, present for ≥ 1 day/week for ≥ 3 months

- Symptoms: pain associated with 1) defecation, 2) change of stool frequency, and/or 3) change in stool consistency

SMALL BOWEL CONDITIONS

Osmotic diarrhea

Osmotic diarrhea is primarily a result of unabsorbable, water-soluble solutes remaining in the bowel and retaining water.

It is associated with sugar intolerance and large consumption of sugar substitutes.

Secretory diarrhea

NEUROENDOCRINE TUMOR (E.G., CARCINOID)

INERT NEUROENDOCRINE TUMOR

Signs and symptoms: pain, luminal bleeding, GI obstruction

ACTIVE, MALIGNANT CARCINOID

These may exert carcinoid syndrome (excessive release of serotonin hormone and other chemicals, which dilates blood vessels, accelerates intestinal transit, and has other effects).

Signs and symptoms (carcinoid syndrome): telangiectasias; cutaneous flushing of the head and neck; difficulty breathing; cardiac problems; abdominal cramps; diarrhea

Investigations: blood and urine tests to detect serotonin and other chemicals; imaging of the abdomen, chest, heart

NEOPLASIA (E.G., LYMPHOMA)

LYMPHOMA

Signs and symptoms (non-Hodgkin): constitutional symptoms (fatigue, fever, night sweats, weight loss), enlarged lymph nodes, chest pain, coughing, shortness of breath

> Hodgkin lymphoma (less common): constitutional symptoms (fatigue, fever, night sweats, weight loss); enlarged lymph nodes; itching; pain on drinking alcohol, or increased sensitivity to alcohol

Investigations: blasts or cancer cells on peripheral blood smear; excess blasts or cancer cells on bone marrow examination

MUCOSAL

Examples of causes of damage to the mucosal lining include ulcerative colitis, Crohn disease, infections, bacteria overgrowth, and ischemia.

Signs and symptoms: abdominal pain, cramping; fever; diarrhea; fatigue

Investigations: CBC to detect inflammatory markers; barium x-ray of the small bowel; fecal fat analysis

Motility disorders (e.g., diabetic neuropathy)

DIABETIC NEUROPATHY

Signs and symptoms: personal or family history of diabetes; history of diabetic complications and/or inadequate monitoring; polydipsia, polyuria, and/or weight loss

Autonomic neuropathy: indigestion, nausea, diarrhea, constipation, dizziness, urinating difficulty, erectile dysfunction, vaginal dryness

Motor neuropathy: weakness, fatigue, wasting, cramps, twitching, decreased reflexes, myokymia

Sensory neuropathy: numbness, burning, or stabbing pain; tingling; gait and balance difficulty; temperature intolerance; hyperalgesia

Keys to patient encounter

Key concern

Focus the history on differentiating large bowel diarrhea (generally, more-frequent-than-normal stools often without weight loss) and small bowel diarrhea (often, large-volume stools with weight loss and nutrient deficiencies).

History

This clinical presentation has a wide differential diagnosis. A useful first step is differentiating between large and small bowel diarrhea to narrow the possible entities.

HISTORY OF PRESENT ILLNESS

Ask when the diarrhea started, how many bowel movements the patient has per day, and how many bowel movements per day is usual for the patient. Ask about the consistency of the bowel movements, and whether there is blood or pus.

Ask about associated symptoms. Examples of characteristic symptoms include:

Large bowel diarrhea: frequent smaller-volume stools, which may be accompanied by blood, mucus, pus, and lower abdominal pain

Small bowel diarrhea: voluminous, watery stools possibly with fat

Malignancy or chronic infection: systemic symptoms (fever, weight loss, fatigue, night sweats)

Irritable bowel syndrome: pain with defecation, pain with changes in stool form or frequency

PAST MEDICAL HISTORY

Take a general history: many conditions are relevant, including liver disease, gallstones, celiac disease, bowel disease, and diabetes.

PAST SURGICAL AND PROCEDURAL HISTORY

Ask about major surgeries, and in particular abdominal and/or bowel surgery. Ask about radiation treatment.

MEDICATIONS AND DRUGS

Ask about cocaine and methamphetamine.

FAMILY HISTORY

Ask about celiac disease and bowel disease.

SOCIAL HISTORY

Ask about travel, work history (e.g., work in day cares), sexual history, and strenuous physical exercise. Ask about consumption of sugar substitutes (e.g., diet soda).

Physical exam

Perform a full physical exam, looking for extraabdominal signs of disease.

Eyes: Look for episcleritis (relevant to inflammatory bowel disease) and exophthalmia (hyperthyroidism).

Lymph nodes: Assess for lymphadenopathy (malignancy).

Abdominal: Look for bowel sounds, tenderness, and masses.

DRE: Look for anal fistulae (Crohn disease), masses, and impacted stool. (Keep the sample of stool you extract with your glove for occult blood testing.)

Dermatological: Look for dermatitis herpetiformis (celiac disease).

Investigations

CBC

Albumin

CRP or ESR

Liver function (see *Notes on labs and assessments*)

Electrolytes (see *Notes on labs and assessments*)

Thyrotropin (TSH)

Serum creatinine

Serum protein and albumin to look for protein malnutrition

Stool occult blood

OTHER SPECIFIC INVESTIGATIONS

Consider other investigations as warranted by the history and physical exam.

Anti-tTG antibody (with IgA level) for celiac disease

Fecal pH (< 5.5 suggests lactose intolerance)

Fecal electrolytes to distinguish secretory from osmotic diarrhea

Fecal calprotectin (relevant to inflammatory bowel disease)

***C. difficile* stool toxin**

Stool ova and parasites in patients with travel to endemic areas

Management

Treat any specific entities identified. Refer the patient for colonoscopy and biopsy if no specific diagnosis is identified. Empiric antidiarrheal therapy can be considered in patients when a specific treatment is not available. Irritable bowel syndrome is treated first with diet and lifestyle changes (managing stress, increasing dietary fiber, drinking plenty of fluids, exercising regularly, getting adequate sleep). More severe cases may require opiate receptor agonists; anticholinergics; bile acid-binding resins such as cholestyramine; TCAs or SSRIs; and/or pain medications such as pregabalin or gabapentin.

REFERENCE

1. Lacey B, Mearin F, Chang L, et al. Rome IV functional gastrointestinal disorders: disorders of gut-brain interaction. 4th ed. Vol. 2. Raleigh, NC: Rome Foundation; 2017. Chapter 11, Functional bowel disorders; 1393–1407.

DE

DIARRHEA

Pediatric diarrhea

Differential diagnosis

INFECTION

Viral gastroenteritis

This is a common concern, typically in children 2 months to 2 years.

It resolves within 1 week.

Signs and symptoms: abrupt-onset watery, nonbloody diarrhea; crampy abdominal pain; nausea, vomiting; fever (> 38°C); headache; muscle aches; epigastric tenderness on abdominal exam

Bacterial enteritis

This typically occurs in children older than 2 years due to oral-fecal contamination; exposure to farm animals or reptiles; eating contaminated food; outbreak at a day care center; and antibiotic use within the past 2 months.

Signs and symptoms: diarrhea that is bloody or contains mucus; tenesmus; persistent high fever (> 40°C); severe abdominal pain

DIET-RELATED CONDITION (E.G., MILK PROTEIN INTOLERANCE)

Milk protein intolerance

This includes 2 types of allergic responses: immediate IgE-mediated hypersensitivity and delayed cell-mediated reaction.

It is outgrown in early childhood.

Signs and symptoms: itchy eyes, nose, lips, gums, mouth, throat; blood, mucous in the stool; frequent regurgitation, vomiting; diarrhea; constipation; persistent infantile colic; atopic dermatitis; swollen lips and eyelids; chronic cough, wheezing, runny nose; anaphylaxis (rare); possible umbilical erythema

Investigations: serum IgE antibody test or skin testing; food challenge in controlled environment (this is the gold standard)

ISCHEMIC INTESTINAL DAMAGE (E.G., INTUSSUSCEPTION)

Intussusception

Signs and symptoms: sudden-onset symptoms (patients usually present within a few hours of onset); bilious vomiting; severe, intermittent abdominal pain; blood, mucous in the stool ("currant jelly" stools); lethargy; fever; Dance sign (palpable mass beneath the right ribs and emptiness in the right lower quadrant on abdominal exam)

Investigations: US

MALABSORPTION

Lactase deficiency

Signs and symptoms: symptoms that develop shortly after consuming milk products; abdominal pain, bloating, cramping; diarrhea; flatulence; hyperactive bowel sounds; abdominal distension; family history of lactase deficiency; celiac disease; Crohn disease; autoimmune disease; recent treatment with antibiotics, chemotherapy, or radiation

Investigations (it is usually diagnosed clinically): lactose breath hydrogen test

Cystic fibrosis

Signs and symptoms: family history of CF; recurrent pneumonia; shortness of breath; productive cough; failure to thrive; fever; wheezing on lung auscultation

Investigations: positive sweat chloride test

Celiac disease

Signs and symptoms: family history of celiac disease, or signs and symptoms of celiac disease (chronic abdominal pain, rashes)

Investigations: positive serum anti-tTG (with IgA level); duodenal biopsy to detect villous blunting

OTHER CAUSES

Drugs

Examples include antibiotics, ranitidine, and NSAIDs. Herbal tea is also a possible cause.

Laxative abuse

This includes use of laxatives and/or enemas.

Examples of causes include eating disorders and body image dysphoria.

Inflammatory bowel disease

Signs and symptoms: younger than 30 (usually); family history of inflammatory bowel disease; fluctuating symptoms with periods of exacerbation and remission; diarrhea (possibly with nocturnal waking); blood in the stool; abdominal pain; weight loss; fever; fatigue; right lower quadrant and periumbilical pain; extraintestinal manifestations (e.g., uveitis, arthritis)

Crohn disease: right lower quadrant mass, uveitis, arthritis

Investigations: elevated CRP (this suggests active inflammation); fecal calprotectin; colonoscopy with biopsy (this is a standard diagnostic procedure); CT scan or MRI (findings: diagnostic structural changes associated with inflammatory bowel disease)

Keys to patient encounter

Key concern

Pay particular attention to signs of hypovolemia, dehydration, and electrolyte abnormalities.

History

HISTORY OF PRESENT ILLNESS

Ask when the diarrhea started, how many bowel movements the patient has per day, and how many bowel movements per day is usual for the patient. Ask about the consistency of the bowel movements, and whether there is blood or pus.

Ask about associated symptoms. Examples of characteristic symptoms include:

Milk protein intolerance: itchiness

Intussusception: recent, sudden-onset diarrhea with severe abdominal pain

Celiac disease: chronic abdominal pain and rashes

CF: shortness of breath and productive cough

FACTORS OF DEHYDRATION

Ask how much the child is drinking, whether they are vomiting, and how many times a day the child is urinating.

POSSIBLE CAUSES

Check for possible causes, such as infectious contacts, recent travel, recent use of antibiotics, and any chronic illnesses.

FAMILY HISTORY

Ask about lactase deficiency, CF, celiac disease, and inflammatory bowel disease.

SOCIAL HISTORY

Ask about the impact of the diarrhea on the child's daily life and activities.

Physical exam

Vital signs: Look for fever (this is relevant to infection), and tachycardia and/or hypotension (severe dehydration).

Weight: Compare current weight to previous weight(s), looking for dehydration or failure to thrive (relevant to chronic diarrhea).

General inspection:

- Assess the patient's mental status (lethargy may be a sign of sepsis).
- Look for sources of infection.

Signs of dehydration:

- Examine mucous membranes.
- Assess for abdominal skin tenting and capillary refill of longer than 2 seconds.
- In infants, assess for a flat or sunken anterior fontanelle.

Abdominal: Look for masses and peritonitis.

Investigations

CBC for signs of infection and dehydration

Electrolytes (see *Notes on labs and assessments*)

Creatinine for signs of dehydration

OTHER SPECIFIC INVESTIGATIONS

Consider other investigations as warranted by the history and physical exam.

Stool cultures in febrile children with diarrhea

Stool ova and parasites in children who have traveled to endemic areas

Urinalysis for UTI, which often coexists with diarrhea

C. difficile **stool antigen** in older children with recent use of antibiotics

Imaging in suspected intussusception or other intraabdominal process

POINTER

Acute versus chronic pediatric diarrhea

Acute diarrhea is defined as lasting less than 2 weeks; chronic diarrhea is defined as lasting more than 2 weeks.

Management

Manage any significant dehydration with IV fluids. After the patient is stabilized, treat any specific entities identified. Viral gastroenteritis is treated supportively.

DIZZINESS, VERTIGO

Dizziness, vertigo

Differential diagnosis

VERTIGO

VERTIGO IN GENERAL

Signs and symptoms: feeling that the world is moving or spinning

Peripheral vestibular dysfunction

BENIGN POSITIONAL VERTIGO

Signs and symptoms: female (more common); middle-aged and older (more common); positive Dix-Hallpike maneuver (this has a positive predictive value of 83% and negative predictive value of 52% for benign positional vertigo)

PERIPHERAL VESTIBULOPATHY

This includes acute labyrinthitis and acute vestibular neuronitis (vestibular neuritis).

Signs and symptoms: vertigo following a recent viral or bacterial infection

MÉNIÈRE DISEASE

Signs and symptoms: recurrent episodes of vertigo, hearing loss, tinnitus, or aural fullness

DRUGS (E.G., AMINOGLYCOSIDES)

ACOUSTIC NEUROMA

Signs and symptoms: unilateral hearing loss; unilateral tinnitus; vertigo; feeling as if the body is tilted; veering towards the side of the affected ear; facial weakness

Investigations: CT scan or MRI of the head

CENTRAL VESTIBULAR DYSFUNCTION

Cerebrovascular accident

Signs and symptoms: history of stroke, or signs and symptoms consistent with stroke (e.g., unilateral neurologic defects)

Risk factors: hypertension, dyslipidemia, diabetes, coagulopathy

Multiple sclerosis

Signs and symptoms: variable depending on lesion location

Spinal cord: sensory or motor dysfunction; Lhermitte sign (paresthesias radiating down the extremities or trunk with neck flexion); bowel, bladder or erectile dysfunction

Brainstem: double vision; swallowing, speech difficulties; vertigo; pseudobulbar palsy

Cerebrum: cognitive impairment; depression; upper motor neuron signs; unilateral motor or sensory deficits

Cerebellum: problems with balance and coordination; vertigo

Other symptoms: tonic spasms; fatigue; pain; exercise intolerance; temperature sensitivity; painful unilateral loss of visual acuity

Risk factors: younger than 50, female

Investigations: brain and spinal cord MRI, including advanced MRI techniques, with established occurrence of multiple episodes; CSF analysis

Drugs (e.g., anticonvulsants, hypnotics, alcohol)

OTHER DIZZINESS

DIZZINESS IN GENERAL

Signs and symptoms: light-headedness (versus the world moving or spinning)

Hyperventilation

Signs and symptoms: episodes of rapid breathing (e.g., accompanying a panic attack)

Disequilibrium (e.g., poor mobility, peripheral neuropathy)

DISEQUILIBRIUM IN GENERAL

Disequilibrium involves proprioceptive impairment (e.g., from peripheral neuropathy, or from dysfunction of the dorsal root ganglia or the posterior columns of the spinal cord).

DE

Examples of causes include diabetes, chronic malnutrition, vitamin B_{12} deficiency, and Parkinson disease.

PERIPHERAL NEUROPATHY

Signs and symptoms:

Motor: weakness, fatigue, wasting, cramps, twitching, decreased reflexes, myokymia

Sensory: numbness, tingling; burning or stabbing pain; gait and balance difficulty; temperature intolerance; hyperalgesia

Presyncope

Examples of causes include cardiac abnormalities, diabetes, and anemia.

Signs and symptoms: sensation of impending loss of consciousness

Investigations: ECG, serum glucose, CBC

Anxiety disorders[1(pp189–234)]

Examples of anxiety disorders listed in *DSM-5* include generalized anxiety disorder, panic disorder, separation anxiety disorder, social anxiety disorder, and specific phobia. Anxiety disorders can provoke panic attacks (e.g., exposure to a phobic object). In the case of panic disorder, panic attacks occur spontaneously.

Signs and symptoms: history of anxiety disorder and/or symptoms consistent with a panic attack; history of social or emotional triggers for symptoms (possible); lack of evidence for other causes, including hyperthyroidism (anxiety can mimic other conditions and is therefore a diagnosis of exclusion)

Panic attack: symptoms that peak within minutes; symptoms that can include palpitations, accelerated heart rate, shortness of breath, chest pain, dizziness, numbness or tingling, fear of losing control, fear of dying

Keys to patient encounter

Key concern

Distinguish between vertigo and other causes of dizziness (gait disturbances, orthostatic light-headedness, other disorders).

History

HISTORY OF PRESENT ILLNESS

The first step is to determine if the patient has true vertigo as opposed to a gait disturbance or orthostatic light-headedness.

Ask about symptoms specific to vertigo versus other disorders:

Vertigo: feeling like the room is spinning

Disequilibrium: feeling unsteady on feet

Presyncope: feeling light-headed or faint

Ask when the symptoms started, how constant are they, and what triggers the symptoms. Ask about recent infections or fevers, and other associated symptoms. Examples of characteristic symptoms include:

Ménière disease: recurring symptoms, including aural symptoms

Stroke: neurological impairments

PAST MEDICAL HISTORY

Ask about diabetes, MS, hypertension, other chronic illness, and anxiety.

MEDICATIONS

Ask about aminoglycosides, anticonvulsants, and hypnotics. Ask about recent changes in medications.

SOCIAL HISTORY

Ask about alcohol use.

Physical exam

Eyes: Observe the patient for nystagmus.

Ears: Examine the ears with an otoscope.

Gait: Observe the patient walking to assess for gait disturbance.

Neurological: Pay particular attention to the cranial nerves.

Dix-Hallpike maneuver: This diagnoses benign positional vertigo.

Investigations

Laboratory tests do not generally provide information useful to diagnosing or managing dizziness or vertigo.

MRI in patients with neurologic signs or symptoms, or progressive unilateral hearing loss (this suggests acoustic neuroma), or risk factors for stroke

Management

Treatment depends on the specific entity. The Epley maneuver usually resolves benign positional vertigo. In suspected peripheral causes, consider referring the patient to an ENT specialist. In suspected central causes, consider referral to a neurologist.

POINTER

Urgent management in central vertigo

Some patients with central vertigo require urgent management. Consider urgent referral to an ENT specialist for patients with vertigo associated with headache, ataxia, loss of consciousness, focal neurological deficits, or prolonged, severe symptoms.

REFERENCE

1. American Psychiatric Association. Diagnostic and statistical manual of mental disorders. 5th ed. Arlington, VA: American Psychiatric Association; 2013. 59–60. 991 p.

DYING PATIENT

Dying patient

Keys to patient encounter

Key concerns

Create a plan for palliative care with attention to human dignity; control of pain and other symptoms; and the importance of family and social support.

Management

BREAKING BAD NEWS TO THE PATIENT AND FAMILY

The patient and family may not be aware of the patient's condition. It may be up to you to break the bad news (see the pointer).

POINTER

Mnemonics for breaking bad news

A common mnemonic is **ABCDE**:

A — Advance preparation is key. Arrange for adequate time and privacy, confirm medical facts.

B — Build a therapeutic relationship. Identify patient preferences, ensure the right people are present.

C — Communicate. Determine the family's understanding of the situation, proceed at the family's pace, and answer questions.

D — Deal with the family's reactions. Empathize with the family.

E — Encourage and validate emotions.

Another common mnemonic is **SPIKES**[1]:

S — Setting: Choose a private setting where you can sit down and talk to the patient, and their family, if appropriate, in person.

P — Perceptions: Ask the patient for their understanding of their situation.

I — Invitation: Offer to share what you know about their situation. Wait for acceptance of your offer.

K — Knowledge: Describe what you know about the patient's situation and how you came to know it.

E — Empathy: Acknowledge the difficulty of the situation for the patient.

S — Summary, strategy: Summarize and talk about next steps.

END-OF-LIFE CARE

Discuss the patient's wishes regarding end-of-life care. Ask if a personal directive (sometimes called a living will) is in place, which often covers topics such as use of ventilators, CPR, and artificial feeding; administration of antibiotics, and pain and antinausea medications; continuation of treatments (e.g., chemotherapy or radiation therapy); and organ, tissue or body donation. If the patient has a personal directive, ask for a copy.

SUBSTITUTE DECISION MAKERS

Ask if the patient has a substitute decision maker. A personal directive appoints 1 or more substitute decision makers for medical decisions. A power of attorney appoints 1 or more substitute decision makers for financial decisions. Ask if the patient has a will. Encourage the patient to consider appointing substitute decision makers and making a will if they have not done so.

SYMPTOM MANAGEMENT

Symptom management in palliative care generally falls into 5 categories.

Pain management: NSAIDs may suffice for initial pain management. Manage neuropathic pain syndromes with TCAs. Many patients will require opioids. Start with weak opioids (tramadol, codeine) and move to strong opioids (morphine, hydromorphone, oxycodone, fentanyl, methadone) as needed.

Sedation: This may be a side effect of opioids, but is often multifactorial and may be related to disease progression. If it is related to medication, the patient will often build up a tolerance over time. A main consideration is to balance sedation and pain relief.

Respiratory depression: Like sedation, respiratory depression is often a side effect of opioids. Titration to a dose that balances pain relief and respiratory depression is necessary.

Nausea and vomiting: This is often multifactorial, and may be secondary to medications (steroids, antibiotics, opioids) or constipation. If secondary to opioids, consider giving haloperidol 0.5 mg every 12 hours or metoclopramide 10 mg 4 times per day. Use dimenhydrinate to treat nausea present with movement. Ensure that constipation is treated.

Constipation: This is a very common symptom, and is often a side effect of opioids and decreased mobility. Start laxatives when opioids are started. Options include oral sennosides, 24 mg 2 times per day; oral polyethylene glycol, 17 g 2 times per day; oral lactulose, 30 mL 2 times per day; bisacodyl 10 mg suppository as needed; and Fleet enema as needed.

Consider referring the patient to a palliative care team or service. Palliative care offers symptom control in the context of holistic care: it provides medical, nursing, psychological, social, and spiritual care in a culturally sensitive manner.

REFERENCE

1. Baile WF, Buckman R, Lenzi R, et al. SPIKES—a six-step protocol for delivering bad news: application to the patient with cancer. Oncologist. 2000;5(4):302–311.

DYSPHAGIA

Dysphagia

Differential diagnosis

OROPHARYNGEAL DYSPHAGIA

OROPHARYNGEAL DYSPHAGIA IN GENERAL

Signs and symptoms: difficulty with the initiation of swallowing (transferring food from the mouth to the esophagus)

Structural

INFECTION (E.G., PHARYNGITIS, PERITONSILLAR ABSCESS)

Signs and symptoms (in general): recent pharyngitis; fever; hoarse voice; neck pain; difficulty swallowing; peritonsillar swelling

Investigations: elevated WBCs on CBC; lateral neck x-ray to detect pharyngeal swelling; blood culture to detect causative organisms

TUMOR

Signs and symptoms: onset of dysphagia over months, with or without constitutional symptoms (fever, weight loss, fatigue, night sweats); masses and enlarged lymph nodes on head and neck exam

Risk factors for throat and esophageal cancer: smoking, alcohol use, family history

Investigations: CT scan of the oropharynx, neck, and chest

ZENKER DIVERTICULUM

This is herniation of the esophageal mucosa posteriorly between the cricopharyngeus muscle and the inferior pharyngeal constrictor muscles.

Signs and symptoms: male, elderly (more common); regurgitation of undigested food (common)

Neuromuscular

CENTRAL (E.G., CEREBROVASCULAR ACCIDENT)

CEREBROVASCULAR ACCIDENT

Signs and symptoms: history of stroke, or evidence consistent with stroke (e.g., unilateral neurologic impairments)

Risk factors: hypertension, dyslipidemia, diabetes, coagulopathy

CRANIAL NERVES (E.G., AMYOTROPHIC LATERAL SCLEROSIS)

AMYOTROPHIC LATERAL SCLEROSIS

Signs and symptoms: onset in a limb or extremity; weakness, cramps, twitching, muscle wasting (lower motor neuron involvement); walking difficulty due to spasticity (upper motor neuron involvement); general fatigue; reduced exercise tolerance; possible language dysfunction

Bulbar onset, which may precede limb weakness: swallowing difficulty; slurred speech; jaw jerking; increased gag reflex; tongue twitching (very specific for ALS)

Investigations: EMG, nerve conduction study, MRI

Xerostomia

Signs and symptoms: oral mucosal dryness; use of drugs that cause xerostomia (e.g., TCAs, antipsychotics, antihistamines); history of Sjögren syndrome or evidence consistent with it (dry eyes; dry mouth; history of RA, SLE)

ESOPHAGEAL DYSPHAGIA

ESOPHAGEAL DYSPHAGIA IN GENERAL

Signs and symptoms: difficulty with swallowing after the transfer of food out of the mouth; sensation of food getting stuck

Mechanical obstruction

INTERMITTENT (E.G., LOWER ESOPHAGEAL RING, WEB)

The oropharyngeal region and esophagus are important for the action of swallowing. Physical anatomical abnormalities can impair their ability to function properly.

Investigations: upper endoscopy of the esophagus, barium x-ray

PROGRESSIVE (E.G., CARCINOMA, PEPTIC STRICTURE)

PROGRESSIVE MECHANICAL OBSTRUCTION IN GENERAL

Signs and symptoms: dysphagia that becomes gradually worse; difficulty with solid foods, and eventually soft foods and liquids

Investigations: endoscopy and biopsy; CT scan

CARCINOMA

Signs and symptoms: often asymptomatic until advanced; pain with swallowing; heartburn-like pain; hoarse cough; nausea, vomiting (sometimes with blood)

Risk factors for throat and esophageal cancer: smoking, alcohol use, family history

PEPTIC STRICTURE

This is the most common benign esophageal stricture (90% of cases).

Signs and symptoms: history of chronic reflux esophagitis

FOREIGN OBJECT

Signs and symptoms: sudden-onset dysphagia that correlates with swallowing an object (e.g., a toothpick) or food (especially chicken and fish)

"Classic presentation": adult with dentures who chews their food incompletely (e.g., because of alcohol)

Investigations: x-ray of the esophagus to identify location of the object

Neuromuscular disorder

Causes include a central or peripheral nerve disorder or injury, which can alter the control of muscles in the mouth, throat, and esophagus.

Signs and symptoms: neurological impairments (motor, sensory); history of neuromuscular disorder (e.g., ALS, MD, MS, Parkinson disease), stroke, spinal cord injury, brain injury

Keys to patient encounter

Key concern

Differentiate oropharyngeal causes from esophageal causes.

History

HISTORY OF PRESENT ILLNESS

Ask about the onset and progression of the dysphagia, including when the difficulty with swallowing started, how constant it is, and how it has changed.

Onset over months: possible malignancy

Gradual onset: possible progressive cause such as a progressive neuromuscular disorder

Intermittent symptoms: possible dysfunction of the lower esophageal ring or web

Progressive symptoms: possible tumor, peptic stricture, or progressive neuromuscular disorders

Ask about associated symptoms, which often point to the specific anatomic location of the problem.

Oropharyngeal localization: coughing, choking, and nasal regurgitation

Esophageal localization: food sticking in the throat or chest

Symptoms can also distinguish neuromuscular motility disorders from mechanical obstruction.

Neuromuscular motility disorder: progressive difficulty swallowing both solids and liquids

Mechanical obstruction: difficulty swallowing solids, but not liquids, with regurgitation of undigested food

PAST MEDICAL HISTORY

Ask about stroke and conditions associated with stroke risk (hypertension, dyslipidemia, diabetes, coagulopathy); Sjögren syndrome or conditions associated with it (rheumatic diseases); GERD; and neuromuscular disorders.

MEDICATIONS

Ask about medications that commonly cause dysphagia (NSAIDs, anticholinergics, alpha-blockers, ACE inhibitors, doxycycline, tetracycline, clindamycin, trimethoprim-sulfamethoxazole) and xerostomia (TCAs, antipsychotics, antihistamines).

Physical exam

Mental status: Assess the patient for altered mental status (check their orientation to time, place, and person).

Neurological:

- Perform a full examination, including cranial nerves.
- Assess the patient's gag reflex.

Investigations

Laboratory tests do not usually contribute useful information for diagnosing or managing dysphagia.

Barium swallow (esophagram) to assess motility and for masses

Endoscopy in suspected mucosal abnormalities or masses (note that this does not assess motility)

Manometry to assess esophageal contractions if no diagnosis is made on barium swallow or endoscopy

24-hour pH monitoring in suspected reflux disease (consider this)

POINTER

Dysphagia incidence

Dysphagia is a common medical presentation affecting up to 10% of adults older than 50.

Management

Treat any contributing conditions. Refer patients with masses and obstructive lesions to a surgeon. Refer patients with neuromuscular disorders to a neurologist. Be aware of the common complications of dysphagia: weight loss, malnutrition, dehydration, and aspiration pneumonia.

DYSPNEA

Dyspnea

Differential diagnosis

CARDIAC CONDITIONS

Myocardial dysfunction (e.g., ischemic cardiomyopathy)

Signs and symptoms (in general): chest pain (usual), sweating, pallor, abnormal heart sounds, hypotension

Investigations: elevated serum troponin; ECG; chest x-ray to detect cardiac enlargement and pulmonary edema

Valvular heart disease

Signs and symptoms: chest pain; palpitations; dizziness or fainting; fever; rapid weight gain (from fluid retention); lung rales (this suggests HF); dependent edema

History of rheumatic fever, hypertension, MI, aortic stenosis, bacterial endocarditis

Investigations: ECG (urgent), chest x-ray, echocardiogram

Pericardial disease (e.g., tamponade)

CARDIAC TAMPONADE

Signs and symptoms: history of invasive heart procedures; chest pain, radiating to the neck and jaw; right upper quadrant pain (due to hepatic venous congestion); tachycardia; elevated JVP; pulsus paradoxus

Investigations: abnormal ECG; normal chest x-ray

Increased cardiac output (e.g., anemia)

ANEMIA

Signs and symptoms: pallor, chest pain, palpitations, weakness, headache, dizziness, dyspnea

Risk factors: intestinal disorders (Crohn disease, celiac disease), menstruation, pregnancy, chronic disease (e.g., cancer, kidney failure), family history of sickle cell disease

Investigations: CBC; peripheral blood smear (visual examination of RBCs for unusual size, shape, color)

Arrhythmia

Signs and symptoms: light-headedness, fainting, shortness of breath, tachycardia, bradycardia, hypotension

Investigations: ECG

PULMONARY CONDITIONS

Upper airway (e.g., foreign body, anaphylaxis)

FOREIGN BODY

Foreign body: sudden-onset symptoms correlating with ingestion of food or object; cyanosis; choking; difficulty breathing; loss of consciousness

Investigations: bronchoscopy or laryngoscopy; x-ray of the neck and chest

ANAPHYLAXIS

Signs and symptoms: personal or family history of anaphylaxis; hives; itchiness; peripheral edema; tongue or throat swelling; wheezing; stridor; shortness of breath; tachycardia; cardiovascular collapse; hypotension

Chest wall and pleura (e.g., pleural effusion)

PLEURAL EFFUSION

Some pleural effusions are asymptomatic and discovered incidentally during physical exam or on chest x-ray (they appear as white space at the base of the lung).

Signs and symptoms: pleuritic chest pain; dyspnea; cough (dry or productive); fever; rapid, shallow respiration (this indicates a large-volume effusion)

> Physical exam: absent tactile fremitus; dullness on percussion; decreased breath sounds on the side of the effusion

Investigations: chest x-ray (posteroanterior and lateral), US, CT scan; thoracentesis and pleural fluid analysis (cell count; pH; protein; LDH; glucose; amylase; cholesterol; triglycerides; NT-proBNP; adenosine deaminase; Gram and acid-fast bacilli stain; bacterial and acid-fast bacilli culture; cytology)

Lower airway (e.g., asthma, chronic obstructive pulmonary disease, pulmonary embolism)

ASTHMA

This is diffuse airway inflammation and narrowing caused by a variety of triggering stimuli that results in bronchoconstriction.

Signs and symptoms: episodic symptoms; episodes that involve dyspnea, tachypnea, tachycardia, chest tightness, cough, wheezing; known triggers for episodes (often); impaired pulmonary function on testing with spirometry

> Common triggers: exercise, exposure to workplace irritants (chemicals, dust, smoke), exposure to allergens (e.g., pet dander, pollen), respiratory infections

Risk factors: family history of asthma; other allergic condition (e.g., atopic dermatitis, seasonal allergies); overweight; smoking; chronic exposure to irritants (secondhand smoke, workplace irritants)

CHRONIC OBSTRUCTIVE PULMONARY DISEASE

Signs and symptoms: older than age 40 (usual: symptoms do not appear until significant lung damage has occurred); progressive symptoms; wheezing; chest tightness; chronic productive cough; clubbing of the fingers; cyanosis around the lips and in the extremities; decreased oxygen saturation; impaired pulmonary function on testing with spirometry

Risk factors: smoking, occupational exposure, intrinsic lung disease

Investigations: chest x-ray, CT scan; ABG

PULMONARY EMBOLISM

Signs and symptoms: sharp chest pain; shortness of breath; cough (possibly with blood); hypoxia; possible unilateral swelling of the lower limbs (this indicates DVT); elevated pulse and respiratory rate; arrhythmias; lung rales on auscultation; lower-lung dullness on percussion; motor or sensory deficits

Risk factors: HF; cancer; surgery; prolonged immobility (e.g., long plane trips); smoking; estrogen replacement therapy; OCs; current pregnancy; previous DVT, embolism, or stroke; family history of embolism

Investigations: elevated d-dimer level; area of reduced pulmonary perfusion on V/Q scan; CT angiography to detect blocked vessel

Alveolar (e.g., pneumonia)

PNEUMONIA

Signs and symptoms: shortness of breath; cough; purulent sputum; chest pain on coughing or deep breaths; fatigue; tachypnea; tachycardia; decreased oxygen saturation; lung crackles on auscultation; lung dullness on percussion

Children: fever

Elderly: confusion, low body temperature

Risk factors: very old, very young, smoking, immune compromise (e.g., due to chronic illness), hospitalization

Investigations: chest x-ray to detect consolidation

CENTRAL CONDITIONS (E.G., METABOLIC ACIDOSIS, ANXIETY)

Metabolic acidosis

Signs and symptoms: chest pain; palpitations; headache; altered mental status; severe anxiety; decreased visual acuity; nausea, vomiting; abdominal pain; altered appetite; weight gain; muscle weakness; bone pain; joint pain; deep, rapid breathing (Kussmaul respiration)

Investigations: ECG, electrolytes, glucose, renal function, CBC, urinalysis, arterial blood sampling

Arterial blood sampling findings: decreased pH; decreased $PaCO_2$; decreased HCO_3^-; anion gap (> 12–16 mEq/L [12–16 mmol/L] is high)

Anxiety disorders[1(pp189–234)]

Examples of anxiety disorders listed in *DSM-5* include generalized anxiety disorder, panic disorder, separation anxiety disorder, social anxiety disorder, and specific phobia. Anxiety disorders can provoke panic attacks (e.g., exposure to a phobic object). In the case of panic disorder, panic attacks occur spontaneously.

Signs and symptoms: history of anxiety disorder and/or symptoms consistent with a panic attack; history of social or emotional triggers for symptoms (possible); lack of evidence for other causes, including hyperthyroidism (anxiety can mimic other conditions and is therefore a diagnosis of exclusion)

Panic attack: symptoms that peak within minutes; symptoms that can include palpitations, accelerated heart rate, shortness of breath, chest pain, dizziness, numbness or tingling, fear of losing control, fear of dying

Keys to patient encounter

Airway and hemodynamic status

Respiratory distress is possible in this clinical presentation. Start by checking the patient's ABCs. Provide emergency care to any patient with unstable vital signs. Give supplemental oxygen, obtain IV access, and consider intubation.

History

HISTORY OF PRESENT ILLNESS

Ask how long the patient has felt short of breath, and how the problem has changed since it began.

Listen for:

Acute or episodic shortness of breath versus chronic symptoms: Chronic symptoms suggest chronic underlying disease such as COPD or heart disease.

Worsening symptoms: This could indicate an impending emergency.

Ask about associated symptoms. Examples of characteristic symptoms include:

Fever: valvular heart disease, pleural effusion, and pneumonia

Cough: pulmonary conditions

Chest pain with sweating, dizziness, and/or palpitations: cardiac conditions

PAST MEDICAL HISTORY

Ask about cardiac disease (ischemic heart disease, CHF) and pulmonary disease (asthma, COPD). Ask about a history of gastroesophageal reflux. Ask about a history of anxiety.

SOCIAL HISTORY

Ask whether the patient is or was a smoker, and about occupational and environmental exposures to dust and pollutants.

Physical exam

Mental status: Assess the patient for altered mental status (check their orientation to time, place, and person).

Cardiovascular: Look for heart murmurs or extra sounds. Assess the patient for JVP and dependent edema (relevant to CHF).

Respiratory:

- Auscultate the lungs for wheezing (asthma), stridor (upper airway obstruction), rales (pulmonary edema and pneumonia), and absent breath sounds (pneumothorax).
- Palpate the chest for subcutaneous emphysema (pneumothorax).
- Palpate the trachea for lateral deviation (pneumothorax).
- Percuss the chest for dullness (consolidation or effusions).

Abdominal: Look for organomegaly.

Investigations

CBC

ABG

ECG

Chest x- ray

IN SUSPECTED PULMONARY EMBOLISM

V/Q scan

D-dimer

IF DIAGNOSIS REMAINS UNCERTAIN

CT scan of the chest (consider this)

Management

Management depends on the diagnosis. Tension pneumothorax is treated with needle thoracentesis. Give a nebulized bronchodilator for asthma or COPD. Give IV furosemide if pulmonary edema is present.

REFERENCE

1. American Psychiatric Association. Diagnostic and statistical manual of mental disorders. 5th ed. Arlington, VA: American Psychiatric Association; 2013. 991 p.

EAR PAIN

DE

Ear pain

Differential diagnosis

EXTERNAL EAR PAIN

Infection

OTITIS EXTERNA (E.G., FUNGAL, BACTERIAL)

The most common cause is bacterial infection (90% of cases).

Signs and symptoms: ear pain; ear pruritus (this can occur with chronic infection; it is more common with fungal infection); discharge; hearing loss; feeling of fullness; pain with jaw movement; erythema of the external ear; pain on traction of the pinna or pressure on the tragus (these typically do not cause pain in acute otitis media); normal tympanic membrane on otoscopy; pain on otoscopy

Fungal infection: white, flakey debris

Risk factors: water exposure ("swimmer's ear"), use of ear devices (e.g., headphones, hearing aids), trauma (e.g., Q-tip use), dermatitis

AURICULAR CELLULITIS

Signs and symptoms: rapid-onset painful, red, swollen auricle

Risk factors: laceration, abrasion, insect bite, dermatitis, ear piercing

Trauma (e.g., frostbite, piercings)

FROSTBITE

Signs and symptoms: prolonged exposure to cold and/or exposure to pronounced cold; progressive symptoms; coldness; burning, throbbing pain; skin discoloration; numbness

Before rewarming: reduced skin sensation; white or grey skin color; hard or waxy skin to the touch

After rewarming (depending on the depth of tissue involvement): erythema and mild edema (mild frostbite); bullae and tissue necrosis (severe frostbite)

Other (e.g., foreign body, cerumen impaction)

Signs and symptoms (in general): hearing loss; ear pain; tinnitus; vertigo; feeling of fullness; history of recent mechanical cleaning of ears (e.g., Q-tip use); possible visible trauma; foreign body or cerumen impaction on otoscopy

MIDDLE AND INNER EAR PAIN

Infection or inflammation

ACUTE OTITIS MEDIA

Signs and symptoms: ear pain; fever; hearing loss; tympanic membrane that is not translucent; ear discharge (this indicates perforation of the tympanic membrane); loss of bony landmarks; middle ear effusion with bulging or reduced mobility of tympanic membrane on pneumatic otoscopy

Infants and toddlers: ear tugging, irritability, poor feeding, vomiting, diarrhea

Risk factors: URTI; allergic rhinitis; chronic rhinosinusitis; attending day care (for children); contact with infectious illness; exposure to secondhand smoke; age (the condition peaks at age 6 to 24 months)

SEROUS OTITIS MEDIA

Signs and symptoms: ear pain; hearing loss; feeling of fullness; fluid (yellow or clear) behind a retracted tympanic membrane on otoscopy; reduced mobility of tympanic membrane on pneumatic otoscopy

Children: speech and/or learning difficulties

Risk factors: recurrent acute otitis media, recent URTI, environmental allergies, recent airplane travel

Investigations: audiogram to detect conductive hearing loss; tympanogram to detect flat configuration

MASTOIDITIS

Signs and symptoms: symptoms that occur 2 weeks after inadequately or untreated acute otitis media (typical); fever; headache; hearing loss; discharge from the ear; protruding ear; tenderness, erythema over the mastoid; retroauricular swelling; otitis media on otoscopy

Investigations: CT scan to detect loss of mastoid air cells

Trauma (e.g., perforation, barotrauma)

TYMPANIC MEMBRANE PERFORATION

Signs and symptoms: ear pain; clear, pus-filled, or bloody discharge from the ear; hearing loss; tinnitus; dizziness

History of otitis media infection; barotrauma or head trauma; acoustic trauma; foreign object in the ear (e.g., Q-tip)

Investigations: culture of discharge; tympanometry; audiology assessment

Neoplasms

NEOPLASMS IN GENERAL

Signs and symptoms: ear pain that is nonresponsive to treatment for presumed underlying causes; constitutional symptoms (fever, night sweats, weight loss); lymphadenopathy; abnormalities on cranial nerve exam

Skin cancer lesion: asymmetrical lesion; irregular borders; color that is not uniform; distinctly different appearance from surrounding skin lesions; recent growth; ulceration

Head and/or neck cancers: epistaxis, hoarseness, difficulty swallowing, odynophagia, shortness of breath, stridor, hemoptysis

Investigations: US, MRI, CT scan to detect head and/or neck mass; biopsy (definitive diagnosis)

CHOLESTEATOMA

Signs and symptoms: ear pain; progressive hearing loss; feeling of fullness; fever

Otoscopy findings: retraction pocket in tympanic membrane (this may contain keratin debris); tympanic membrane perforation; granulation tissue; polyps; discharge from the ear

Risk factors for acquired cholesteatoma: acute otitis media, eustachian tube dysfunction (e.g., tympanostomy tubes, history of ear surgery)

REFERRED PAIN (SINUSITIS, DENTAL, TEMPOROMANDIBULAR JOINT DYSFUNCTION)

Sinusitis

Signs and symptoms: purulent nasal discharge (or congestion) and facial pain that persists > 10–14 days or is worsening after 5 days; fever; maxillary toothache; facial swelling; tender paranasal sinuses; erythema or swelling of the nasal mucosa; postnasal drip; periorbital swelling

Dental disease

Signs and symptoms: toothache, or sensitivity of a tooth to cold; fever and/or chills (this suggests infection); abnormalities on dental exam; deep neck space infection on full head and neck exam

DE

Temporomandibular joint dysfunction

Signs and symptoms: pain that is worse with jaw motion (chewing, talking), especially in the morning; pain that may radiate to the ear, cheek, temple, neck, or shoulder; headache; TMJ symptoms (pain, tightness, crepitation, clicking, catching sensation); TMJ symptoms on palpation or applied finger pressure (clicking, limited range of motion, subluxation, deviation of jaw, pain)

Keys to patient encounter

Key concern

Complete a careful head and neck exam, especially when the ear canal, tympanic membrane, and middle ear appear normal.

History

HISTORY OF PRESENT ILLNESS

Ask when the pain started and how constant it is. Ask about recent or current infections (sinus, throat), recent viral illnesses, and possible trauma (e.g., Q-tip use; head trauma; exposure to a loud noise; pressure changes from recent flights or scuba diving).

Ask about associated symptoms. Examples of characteristic symptoms include:

Acute otitis media: sudden-onset constant pain, fever, and hearing loss

Neoplasm: ear pain with constitutional symptoms

TMJ malfunction: headache, and ear pain made worse with jaw motion

ALLERGIES

Ask about a history of allergies (this is common in eustachian tube dysfunction).

Physical exam

Otoscopy

Head, neck:

- Look for sinusitis, dental disease, and TMJ dysfunction.
- Palpate the mastoid process for tenderness (relevant to mastoiditis).

Investigations

CBC to look for elevated WBCs (relevant to infection)

Culture and sensitivity for any ear discharge

Audiogram in patients with hearing loss

Other investigations as warranted by the history and physical exam

> **POINTER**
>
> **Common features of ear pain**
>
> Ear pain from a dental problem is both common and commonly missed. In addition, approximately half of all patients with no identifiable cause experience spontaneous resolution.

Management

Management is directed at the underlying cause. Refer patients with tympanic membrane rupture or malignancy to an ENT specialist.

EDEMA

Generalized edema

Differential diagnosis

INCREASED CAPILLARY HYDROSTATIC PRESSURE

Increased plasma volume due to renal sodium retention

HEART FAILURE

The most common causes are CAD, hypertension, alcohol use, and valve disease.

Common precipitating factors include hypertension; poor medication adherence; dietary indiscretion (eating foods high in salt); anemia; arrhythmia; ischemic heart event; infection; and pulmonary disease.

Signs and symptoms: chest pain, shortness of breath, orthopnea, paroxysmal nocturnal dyspnea, cough, syncope, fatigue, peripheral edema

Left-sided HF: hypotension, reduced capillary refill, peripheral cyanosis, pulsus alternans, mitral regurgitation murmur, S3, pulmonary crackles

Right-sided HF: tricuspid regurgitation murmur, S3, peripheral edema, increased JVP, Kussmaul sign, hepatosplenomegaly

Investigations: chest x-ray to detect interstitial edema (redistribution of Kerley B lines, bronchiolar-alveolar cuffing), cardiomegaly, or pleural effusion; CBC to detect low hemoglobin or elevated WBCs; electrolytes; elevated thyrotropin (TSH) (thyrotoxicosis can precipitate CHF); creatinine, BUN to detect renal insufficiency (due to reduced renal blood flow from reduced cardiac output in more severe CHF); elevated troponin (if cardiac ischemia is present); HbA_{1c}; liver function tests; elevated BNP; urinalysis to detect proteinuria; echocardiogram; ECG

REDUCED SYSTEMIC VASCULAR RESISTANCE (E.G., CIRRHOSIS)

CIRRHOSIS

Signs and symptoms: jaundice; easy bruising, bleeding; itching; ascites; spiderlike blood vessels on the skin; systemic symptoms (anorexia, weight loss, weakness, fatigue)

History of chronic alcohol abuse; chronic infection with HBV or HCV; hemochromatosis; nonalcoholic fatty liver disease

HBV and HCV risk factors: unprotected sex, IV drug abuse, blood transfusions, tattoos, body piercings, imprisonment, workplace exposure to body fluids

Investigations: liver function tests

PRIMARY SODIUM RETENTION (E.G., RENAL DISEASE, DRUGS)

RENAL DISEASE

Signs and symptoms: history of kidney disease, chronic renal failure, and/or current renal dialysis; bilateral lower limb swelling; shortness of breath; paroxysmal nocturnal dyspnea; orthopnea; elevated JVP; pulmonary crackles; peripheral pitting edema

Risk factors: diabetes, diabetic complications, and/or inadequate monitoring; hypertension; smoking

Investigations:

Markers of renal disease: reduced calcium; elevated phosphate; elevated creatinine; elevated BUN; reduced GFR; reduced vitamin D; elevated albumin:creatinine ratio; red cell casts, proteinuria on urinalysis; hyperkalemia; elevated phosphate; anemia on CBC; elevated PTH

Cardiac function: normal echocardiogram once fluid around the heart has been removed (this distinguishes renal etiology from CHF)

DRUGS

These include NSAIDs, glucocorticoids, fludrocortisones, thiazolidinediones (glitazones), insulin, hormone medications (estrogens, progestins, androgens, testosterone, aromatase inhibitors), vasodilators, and CCBs.

PREGNANCY

Signs and symptoms: amenorrhea, especially during childbearing years (some experience spotting); sexual activity, especially without contraception or with inconsistent use of contraception; nausea or vomiting (common early sign); breast enlargement and tenderness; increased frequency of urination without other urinary symptoms; fatigue

Investigations: blood or urine β-HCG

Decreased arteriolar resistance (e.g., calcium channel blockers, idiopathic)

CALCIUM CHANNEL BLOCKERS

This is usually due to a recent start of CCBs or an increase in dose.

IDIOPATHIC

Signs and symptoms: bilateral peripheral edema; normal pulmonary exam; normal cardiac exam (including normal JVP); **no** evidence of pulmonary edema (shortness of breath, paroxysmal nocturnal dyspnea, orthopnea), hepatic disease, renal disease, cardiac disease, or medications associated with edema

Investigations: normal albumin, liver enzymes, liver function, and renal function

DECREASED ONCOTIC PRESSURE (HYPOALBUMINEMIA)

Protein loss (e.g., nephrotic syndrome)

NEPHROTIC SYNDROME

Signs and symptoms: progressive lower extremity edema (ankles and feet); swelling around the eyes; weight gain (from water retention); foamy urine

Risk factors: conditions that damage the kidneys (e.g., diabetes, SLE, amyloidosis); use of NSAIDs, antibiotics; history of HIV, HBV, HCV, malaria

Investigations: urine (proteinuria, spot urine protein:creatinine ratio, lipuria); hyponatremia with low fractional sodium excretion; low serum albumin; high total cholesterol (hyperlipidemia); elevated BUN

Reduced albumin synthesis (e.g., liver disease, malnutrition)

LIVER DISEASE

Patients with compensated cirrhosis may be asymptomatic.

HCV is often asymptomatic.

Signs and symptoms: jaundice; abdominal pain, swelling; palpable, tender liver; swelling in the legs and ankles; systemic symptoms (anorexia, weight loss, weakness, fatigue); itching; easy bruising

History of chronic alcohol abuse; chronic HBV or HCV; hemochromatosis; autoimmune conditions; α_1-antitrypsin deficiency; primary biliary cirrhosis; CHF

HBV and HCV risk factors: unprotected sex, IV drug abuse, blood transfusions, tattoos, body piercings, imprisonment, workplace exposure to body fluids

Investigations: tests for liver enzymes (elevated AST, ALT) and liver function (elevated bilirubin; possible abnormal PT/INR); viral serologic tests to detect HBV, HCV; Doppler US; CT scan; MRI; transient elastography; liver biopsy

MALNUTRITION

Signs and symptoms: weight loss, reduced intake

History of alcohol use disorder, malignancy, diabetes, renal disease, protein-losing enteropathy (e.g., inflammatory bowel disease, Crohn disease, ulcerative colitis)

Investigations: low prealbumin; low albumin

INCREASED CAPILLARY PERMEABILITY (E.G., BURNS, INFLAMMATION)

Signs and symptoms: burns, tissue trauma

Systemic inflammatory response syndrome: temperature < 35°C or > 38°C; heart rate > 90 beats/minute; respiratory rate > 20 breaths/minute or $PaCO_2$ < 32 mmHg; WBC count < 4000/μL (4×10^9/L) or > 12 000/μL (12×10^9/L) or > 10% bands

Allergic reaction: skin or mucosal symptoms (e.g., urticaria, pruritus, angioedema), shortness of breath, hypotension, nausea, vomiting

INCREASED INTERSTITIAL ONCOTIC PRESSURE (E.G., MYXEDEMA)

Myxedema

This is nonpitting edema due to deposition of glycosaminoglycans and is typically a severe presentation of hypothyroidism.

Signs and symptoms: history of hypothyroidism or symptoms of severe hypothyroidism (hypothermia, bradycardia, decreased reflexes, dry skin, weight gain, impaired cognition); hypotension; hypoventilation; generalized edema

Risk factors: infection, cerebrovascular disease, CHF, trauma-induced MI

Investigations: elevated thyrotropin (TSH); hypoglycemia; hyponatremia

Keys to patient encounter

Key concerns

Differentiate between systemic edema and localized edema.

Categorize the general mechanism of edema, because this can affect management.

History

HISTORY OF PRESENT ILLNESS

Ask when the edema started, where the swelling is located, and what makes the swelling better and worse.

Gradual-onset versus sudden-onset edema: Gradual onset suggests an underlying chronic condition.

Unilateral versus bilateral edema: Bilateral edema usually indicates a systemic condition.

Changes in swelling with changes in body position: Edema caused by chronic venous insufficiency often improves with limb elevation; edema associated with decreased oncotic pressure does not.

PAST MEDICAL AND PROCEDURAL HISTORY

Ask about disorders commonly associated with edema: CHF, renal disease, liver disease, sleep apnea, and thyroid disease.

In cases of lower limb edema, DVT is a possibility, especially if the swelling is asymmetrical: use the Wells criteria to guide further history (see the pointer).

MEDICATIONS
Ask about CCBs.

POINTER

Wells criteria for deep vein thrombosis

The Wells criteria assess the risk of DVT by scoring clinical features such as: compromised leg movement (e.g., paralysis, orthopedic casting); recent major surgery; recent extended immobilization; deep-vein tenderness; leg or calf swelling, with or without pitting edema; cancer or recent treatment for cancer; and previous DVT.

Physical exam

Full physical:

- Assess the affected areas for pitting, tenderness, and skin changes.
- Look for signs of HF (rales, increased JVP), liver disease (jaundice, ascites, asterixis), and thyroid disease (hyper- or hypothermia, tachy- or bradycardia, exophthalmos, tremor).
- In cases of lower limb edema, apply the Wells criteria (see the pointer).

Investigations

Creatinine for liver disease
Liver function (see *Notes on labs and assessments*)
Serum albumin for hypoalbuminemia
Urinalysis for renal disease
Chest x-ray for HF
Echocardiography in patients with sleep apnea to detect associated pulmonary hypertension (consider this: it is a common complication)

OTHER SPECIFIC INVESTIGATIONS
In cases of lower limb edema, pursue further investigations based on the Wells criteria (see the pointer).

Management

Treatment is directed toward the underlying etiology. For patients with chronic venous insufficiency, treatment includes emollients, topical steroid creams as needed, and compression stockings.

EDEMA

Localized edema

Differential diagnosis

VENOUS INSUFFICIENCY (INCLUDING POSTPHLEBITIC SYNDROME)

Signs and symptoms: history of DVT (particularly recurrent DVT; this is a major risk factor for the development of postphlebitic syndrome), pain, leg heaviness, ankle and calf swelling (relieved by elevation), tightness, skin irritation, muscle cramps, itching, varicose veins

Skin symptoms: overlying skin changes; dry skin; brown hyperpigmentation (hemosiderin deposits); stasis dermatitis; lipodermatosclerosis (fibrosing dermatitis of subcutaneous fat) if the condition is chronic; ulcers (weeping, painless, with irregular borders) above the medial malleolus

Investigations: duplex US to detect venous reflux (retrograde flow)

DEEP VEIN THROMBOSIS

Signs and symptoms: history of recent stroke or uncontrolled severe hypertension; red, painful, warm, and/or swollen calf (the affected calf is erythematous, tender, swollen; it is > 3 cm larger than the other calf when measured 10 cm distal to the tibial tuberosity)

Symptoms if concurrent with PE: chest pain, shortness of breath

Risk factors: recent surgery; trauma; malignancy; blood disorders; prolonged immobilization; increased estrogen (e.g., pregnant, OC use); antiphospholipid syndrome; CHF; a score of 2 or 3 on Wells criteria

Investigations: positive d-dimer (this should prompt further diagnostic tests); duplex US

D-dimer testing should only be considered in patients with a low pretest probability (e.g., the patient is young, is presenting with their first episode of DVT, and has few medical comorbidities) and the result is only helpful if it is negative.

TRAUMA

An example is an anterior ACL tear.

LYMPHEDEMA (E.G., MALIGNANCY, PRIMARY)

Signs and symptoms (in general): swelling; reduction in mobility; pain; nonpitting edema

Risk factors: history of malignancy, radiation, surgery, infection

INFECTION (CELLULITIS; INFECTION OF SOFT TISSUE OR BONE)

Symptoms (in general): unilateral erythema, tenderness, and warmth (affected areas have poorly demarcated borders); fever and/or malaise (these are severe symptoms); wet or dry wound (if present, a wet wound has purulent discharge)

Risk factors: recent trauma; instrumentation; surgery; lymphedema; diabetes; peripheral vascular disease

Keys to patient encounter

Key concerns

Local edema is most commonly caused by impaired lymphatic drainage. In the lower limbs, this is commonly the result of DVT.

Consider lymphatic filariasis in patients who reside in or have traveled to tropical countries: it is a significant and neglected tropical disease.

Consider lymphatic damage from malignancy or previous surgery.

History

HISTORY OF PRESENT ILLNESS

Determine if the edema is acute or chronic. Acute edema, especially in 1 leg, raises the possibility of DVT, although chronic edema does not exclude DVT.

Use the Wells criteria to guide further history in all cases of lower limb edema (see the pointer).

PAST MEDICAL HISTORY

Ask about a history of cancer, trauma, pelvic surgery (including inguinal lymphadenectomy), axillary surgery (e.g., for breast cancer), and radiation therapy.

SOCIAL HISTORY

Ask about travel to tropical countries (relevant to filariasis).

Physical exam

Swollen extremity: Look for signs of a clot (a palpable clot, tenderness), pitting versus nonpitting edema, and hemosiderin and ulcers (relevant to venous insufficiency).

Investigations

Assess the patient using the Wells criteria (see the pointer) and order further investigations as indicated.

Wells criteria score ≤ 0

- *D-dimer*
- *US* for patients with positive d-dimer (negative US rules out DVT)

Wells criteria score 1–2

- *High-sensitivity d-dimer* (if available) (negative result rules out DVT)
- *US* for patients with positive d-dimer

Wells criteria score ≥ 3

- *Immediate US*
- *On negative US:* second US in 1 week if symptoms persist

POINTER

Wells criteria for deep vein thrombosis

The Wells criteria assess the risk of DVT by scoring clinical features such as: compromised leg movement (e.g., paralysis, orthopedic casting); recent major surgery; recent extended immobilization; deep-vein tenderness; leg or calf swelling, with or without pitting edema; cancer or recent treatment for cancer; and previous DVT.

POINTER

Contraindications to anticoagulant therapy

ABSOLUTE CONTRAINDICATIONS

- Active bleeding
- Severe underlying bleeding disorder or platelet count below 20×10^3/µL (20×10^9/L)
- Intracranial hemorrhage
- Neurosurgery or ocular surgery in the previous 10 days

RELATIVE CONTRAINDICATIONS

- Mild to moderate bleeding disorder or thrombocytopenia
- Brain metastases
- Recent trauma
- Recent GI or GU bleed
- Recent abdominal surgery
- Endocarditis

DE

Management

DVT can be managed on an outpatient basis for most patients. Administer LWMH and start direct oral anticoagulants (see the pointer on contraindications). Overlap these until the patient's PT/INR is higher than 2 for at least 24 hours (this usually takes about 5 days).

Treat venous insufficiency (stasis dermatitis) with emollients, topical steroid creams, and compression stockings (rule out peripheral arterial disease before prescribing compression stockings).

Treat any other underlying associated conditions.

ELECTROLYTE IMBALANCES

Hypercalcemia

Differential diagnosis

HYPERCALCEMIA IN GENERAL

Definition: total calcium ≥ 10.52 mg/dL (2.63 mmol/L) or ionized calcium ≥ 5.6 mg/dL (1.4 mmol/L)

Signs and symptoms: fatigue, depression, constipation, vomiting, bone pain, confusion, history of kidney stones

INCREASED INTESTINAL ABSORPTION

Increased intake (e.g., milk-alkali syndrome)

Causes include use of calcium supplements (milk-alkali syndrome has been associated with ≥ 2 g of elemental calcium per day) and a diet high in calcium (e.g., high in milk and cream).

Investigations: decreased PTH

Vitamin D–mediated condition (e.g., sarcoidosis)

SARCOIDOSIS

Sarcoidosis can cause hypercalciuria and hypercalcemia through calcitriol (the active form of vitamin D).

Signs and symptoms: lymphadenopathy (a mass in the middle of the mediastinum is the most common lesion), fever, fatigue, weight loss, lung symptoms (dry cough, shortness of breath, wheezing, chest pain)

Other (for this context): aggravated hypercalcemia on exposure to the sun; increased intestinal calcium absorption; serum calcitriol that is not reduced on intake of calcium

Risk factors: age 20 to 40, African descent, family history of sarcoidosis

Investigations: decreased PTH; elevated calcitriol

INCREASED BONE RESORPTION

Malignancy

Signs and symptoms: history of cancer, especially cancer of the breast or prostate, or multiple myeloma

Investigations: decreased PTH

Hyperparathyroidism

Signs and symptoms: often asymptomatic; bone pain; nephrolithiasis; fractures; proximal muscle weakness (often in the lower extremities); depression; lethargy; confusion, dementia

Risk factors: postmenopausal woman; CKD; vitamin D deficiency; kidney transplant recipient; elderly with depression; family history of hyperparathyroidism

Investigations: ALP; BUN; creatinine; vitamin D; 24-hour urine collection for calcium; dual-energy x-ray absorptiometry (bone mineral density); US or parathyroid sestamibi scan (for localization)

Primary hyperparathyroidism: elevated serum calcium; normal or elevated PTH

Secondary hyperparathyroidism (this may occur in the context of vitamin D deficiency): normal/low serum calcium; extremely elevated PTH

Tertiary hyperparathyroidism (this may occur in the context of CKD): normal/elevated calcium; elevated PTH after treatment of secondary hyperparathyroidism

Hyperthyroidism

Signs and symptoms: history of hyperthyroidism or symptoms of hyperthyroidism (changes in menstrual patterns, enlarged thyroid, tachycardia, palpitations, diarrhea, muscle weakness, tremor, hyperactive reflexes, weight loss, sweating, thinning hair)

Investigations: decreased thyrotropin (TSH)

Immobilization

Examples of causes include spinal cord injury; stroke; and long-bone fracture, especially in children.

Investigations: decreased PTH

DIMINISHED EXCRETION (E.G., DIURETICS)

Diuretics

The cause is thiazide-type diuretics.

Investigations: decreased urinary calcium, decreased serum PTH, increased serum vitamin D

Keys to patient encounter

History

HISTORY OF PRESENT ILLNESS

The symptoms of hypercalcemia are classically described by the somewhat pejorative mnemonic "stones, bones, abdominal moans, and psychic groans," which correlates with kidney stones, bone pain, abdominal pain, and confusion, lethargy, and impaired concentration and memory.

PAST MEDICAL HISTORY

Ask about pancreatitis, malignancy, hyperthyroidism, Paget disease, sarcoidosis, TB, hepatitis, and AIDS.

MEDICATIONS

Ask about thiazide diuretics, lithium, and theophylline, and about excessive intake of calcium supplements.

Physical exam

Vital signs: Look for hypertension.

Volume status

Neurological

Investigations

Serum total calcium or ionized calcium

Creatinine

Electrolytes (see *Notes on labs and assessments*)

Lipase

Thyrotropin (TSH)

PTH

ECG to look for shortened QT interval

CALCULATING TOTAL CALCIUM

The result for total calcium must be corrected for the patient's serum albumin level, because calcium is tightly bound to albumin in the circulation. The equation to use is:

$$\text{Corrected Ca}^{2+} = \text{Total Ca}^{2+} + [0.02 \times (40 - \text{albumin})]$$

Note that if Ca^{2+} is in mmol/L, albumin must be in g/L.

Management

Most cases of hypercalcemia are due to hyperparathyroidism or malignancy.

Patients with hyperparathyroidism have elevated PTH. Refer these patients to an ENT surgeon for an urgent parathyroidectomy.

In patients with reduced PTH, malignancy is the most common diagnosis (especially lung and breast cancer, and multiple myeloma). In malignancy-related hypercalcemia, begin treatment with IV zoledronate or pamidronate, and monitor the patient's hemodynamic and electrolyte status.

Patients with elevated calcium are often significantly dehydrated. Emergency treatment includes aggressive hydration with IV normal saline. Consider treatment with a loop diuretic once the patient is replete and there is evidence of volume overload.

ELECTROLYTE IMBALANCES

Hypocalcemia

Differential diagnosis

HYPOCALCEMIA IN GENERAL

Definition: total calcium < 8.4 mg/dL (2.1 mmol/L) or ionized calcium < 4.4 mg/dL (1.1 mmol/L)

Signs and symptoms: unusual sensations or loss of feeling in the fingers, toes, and around the mouth; itchy areas on the body; tetany; fatigue; depression; papilledema

DE

LOSS OF CALCIUM FROM THE CIRCULATION

Hyperphosphatemia (e.g., renal insufficiency)

RENAL INSUFFICIENCY

Signs and symptoms: history of kidney disease, chronic renal failure, and/or current renal dialysis; bilateral lower limb swelling; shortness of breath; paroxysmal nocturnal shortness of breath; orthopnea

Risk factors: diabetes, diabetic complications, and/or inadequate monitoring; hypertension; smoking

Investigations: renal function tests (reduced calcium, elevated phosphate, elevated creatinine), reduced vitamin D

Pancreatitis

Signs and symptoms: constant upper abdominal pain that radiates to the back (sitting up and leaning forward may reduce the pain; pain occurs with coughing, vigorous movement, deep breathing); shortness of breath; nausea, vomiting; hypotension; fever; jaundice; abdominal tenderness

History of gallstones or chronic alcoholism (usual); hyperlipidemia; change of medication

Investigations: serum amylase and lipase (levels are ≥ 3 times ULN; elevated lipase indicates pancreatic damage); possible elevated cholesterol; possible elevated ALT (this indicates associated liver inflammation); chest x-ray (this may show left-sided or bilateral pleural effusion and/or atelectasis); abdominal x-ray (this may show calcifications within pancreatic ducts, calcified gallstones, or localized ileus of a segment of small intestine); US

Osteoblastic metastases

Signs and symptoms: history of cancer, especially breast or prostate; point tenderness over bones on physical exam

Investigations: elevated phosphate; x-ray or bone scan to detect metastases

Rhabdomyolysis

Signs and symptoms: use of street drugs (especially cocaine, heroin, and amphetamines), statins, or anesthetics (i.e., during recent surgery); muscle weakness; recent severe trauma; fever and/or hypotension (possible: these are signs of malignant hyperthermia following anesthesia)

Investigations: elevated creatine kinase; elevated serum or urine myoglobin; elevated phosphate

DECREASED VITAMIN D PRODUCTION OR ACTION

Kidney injury—see renal insufficiency, above

Rickets

Signs and symptoms: children younger than 3 years (most common); skeletal abnormalities (bowed legs; thick wrists and ankles); pain in the back, pelvis, legs

History of premature birth; delayed growth; malnutrition; exclusive breastfeeding without vitamin D supplementation

Investigations: reduced serum vitamin D

Malabsorption

Signs and symptoms: muscle wasting (possible)

History of celiac disease, surgical removal of part of the small bowel, chronic diarrhea, weight loss

Investigations: CBC (to detect anemia); tTG antibodies (this is a sign of celiac disease); decreased serum vitamin D

DECREASED PARATHYROID HORMONE PRODUCTION OR ACTION

Signs and symptoms: history of thyroidectomy, parathyroidectomy, autoimmune hypoparathyroidism, or polyglandular autoimmune syndrome

Investigations: decreased PTH; > 1 type of endocrine deficiency (testosterone, FSH, LH, ACTH, thyrotropin) (this is a sign of polyglandular autoimmune syndrome)

LOW MAGNESIUM

Signs and symptoms: history of hypomagnesemia; use of diuretics, especially thiazide diuretics; diet low in green leafy vegetables

Investigations: decreased magnesium

Keys to patient encounter

History

HISTORY OF PRESENT ILLNESS

Note that many patients with hypocalcemia are asymptomatic and the problem is discovered incidentally with blood testing.

The most common etiologies for chronic hypocalcemia are hypoparathyroidism and vitamin D deficiency.

Ask about numbness and tingling, especially in the fingers and toes or around the mouth; muscle cramping, twitching, or stiffness; seizures; spasms in the throat or difficulty breathing (this indicates laryngospasm, bronchospasm); and fatigue or depression.

PAST MEDICAL HISTORY

Ask about risk factors for hypocalcemia: history of neck surgery (hypoparathyroidism), chronic renal disease, and diabetes (this is a risk factor for renal failure). Also ask about hypertension, gallstones, hyperlipidemia, cancer, celiac disease, and conditions that affect parathyroid hormone (see the differential diagnosis).

MEDICATIONS

Ask about bisphosphonates, cisplatin, antiepileptics, aminoglycosides, diuretics, and PPIs.

FAMILY HISTORY

Ask about hypocalcemia, to look for a genetic cause.

Physical exam

Mental status: Confusion or delirium may be manifestations of hypocalcemia.

Eyes: Look for papilledema.

Neurological: Look for increased reflexes, Trousseau sign, and Chvostek sign (see the pointer).

Cardiovascular and respiratory: Look for signs of CHF.

POINTER

Trousseau sign and Chvostek sign

Trousseau sign: Inflate a BP cuff to a pressure above the systolic BP for 3 minutes. This induces carpal spasm.

Chvostek sign: Tap the facial nerve anterior to the earlobe and just below the zygomatic arch. This induces spasm of the facial muscles.

Investigations

Serum total calcium or ionized calcium

- Correct serum total calcium for albumin.

CBC

Creatinine

Phosphorus
Magnesium
Electrolytes (see *Notes on labs and assessments*)
PTH
Vitamin D (25-hydroxyvitamin D)
ECG to look for prolonged QT interval

CALCULATING TOTAL CALCIUM

The result for total calcium must be corrected for the patient's serum albumin level, because calcium is tightly bound to albumin in the circulation. The equation to use is:

$$\text{Corrected } Ca^{2+} = \text{Total } Ca^{2+} + [0.02 \times (40 - \text{albumin})]$$

Note that if Ca^{2+} is in mmol/L, albumin must be in g/L.

INTERPRETING FINDINGS

High PTH, high phosphorus, high creatinine: renal failure

High PTH, low or normal phosphorus, normal creatinine: vitamin D deficiency or pancreatitis

Low PTH, high phosphorus, normal creatinine: hypoparathyroidism or hypomagnesemia

Management

If patients are symptomatic or serum calcium levels fall below 7.6 mg/dL (1.9 mmol/L), or ionized calcium levels are less than 4 mg/dL (1 mmol/L), treat with IV calcium gluconate. Rapid correction of hypocalcemia can cause cardiac arrhythmias, so patients must be on a cardiac monitor.

Chronic (asymptomatic) hypocalcemia is treated with oral calcium (calcium carbonate or calcium citrate) and vitamin D supplementation.

Oral calcium and vitamin D are easily absorbed and essential in management. In addition to treating hypocalcemia, they correct hypomagnesemia, which can result from hypocalcemia. Prescribe 1 g to 2 g of elemental calcium 3 times daily. Start elemental calcium supplements at 500 mg to 1000 mg 3 times daily and titrate upward. Asymptomatic ECG changes usually normalize with calcium and calcitriol supplementation.

Note that hypercalciuria is a complication of vitamin D therapy, particularly for patients with hypoparathyroidism, as the absence of PTH enhances urinary calcium losses.

If hypocalcemia is due to malabsorption of vitamin D, treat the underlying cause (e.g., gluten-free diet in celiac disease). Concurrent hypomagnesemia can be corrected with magnesium supplementation.

ELECTROLYTE IMBALANCES

Hyperkalemia

Differential diagnosis

HYPERKALEMIA IN GENERAL

Definition: serum potassium > 5.5 mEq/L (5.5 mmol/L)

INCREASED INTAKE

Note that hyperkalemia is usually associated with low excretion.

REDISTRIBUTION

Decreased entry into cells (e.g., insulin deficiency, beta 2 blockade)

INSULIN DEFICIENCY: TYPE 1 DIABETES

Low insulin causes hyperglycemia, which moves fluid and potassium into blood circulation and leads to hyperkalemia. Low insulin can also result in diabetic ketoacidosis (DKA), which leads to **apparent** hyperkalemia. In DKA, a total body potassium deficit is present, which means that treatment with insulin can result in profound **hypokalemia** if potassium is not appropriately replaced.

Signs and symptoms: personal or family history of diabetes; history of diabetic complications and/or inadequate monitoring; polydipsia, polyuria, and/or weight loss

Investigations: fasting glucose or HbA_{1c}; in suspected ketoacidosis: tests for blood glucose, electrolytes, blood pH, urine ketones

BETA 2 BLOCKADE

Nonselective beta-blockers decrease cellular potassium uptake, which leads to hyperkalemia. Beta-blockers also suppress catecholamine-stimulated renin release, decreasing aldosterone synthesis, which also leads to hyperkalemia.

Increased exit from cells (e.g., metabolic acidosis, rhabdomyolysis)

INCREASED POTASSIUM EXIT IN GENERAL

Conditions causing potassium exit cells include volume depletion, hyperchloremic metabolic acidosis, anion gap metabolic acidosis, respiratory acidosis, familial hyperkalemic periodic paralysis, rhabdomyolysis, hemolysis, tumor lysis syndrome, and trauma. Lab error (e.g., lysis during sample collection) is also possible.

METABOLIC ACIDOSIS

Signs and symptoms: chest pain, palpitations; headache; altered mental status; severe anxiety; decreased visual acuity; nausea, vomiting; abdominal pain; altered appetite and weight gain; muscle weakness; bone pain; joint pain; deep, rapid breathing

Investigations: ECG; electrolytes; glucose; renal function; CBC; urinalysis; ABG (blood pH and anion gap) to detect renal tubular acidosis

RHABDOMYOLYSIS

Signs and symptoms: use of street drugs (especially cocaine, heroin, and amphetamines), statins, or anesthetics (i.e., during recent surgery); muscle weakness; recent severe trauma; fever and/or hypotension (possible: these are signs of malignant hyperthermia following anesthesia)

Investigations: elevated CK; elevated serum or urine myoglobin; elevated phosphate

REDUCED URINARY EXCRETION

Decreased glomerular filtration rate (e.g., acute or chronic kidney injury)

ACUTE OR CHRONIC KIDNEY INJURY

Kidney-related causes include acute renal failure or kidney injury; CKD; diabetic nephropathy; SLE; and renal tubular acidosis type IV.

Signs and symptoms: often asymptomatic, muscle weakness, flaccid paralysis, paresthesia

Investigations: repeat test to rule out lab artifact (common occurrence); blood tests to assess kidney function and detect hyperglycemia (serum electrolytes, calcium, magnesium, BUN, creatinine, glucose); ECG to detect arrhythmia; spot urine potassium, creatinine; urine osmolality to calculate fractional excretion of potassium

Decreased secretion (e.g., aldosterone deficiency, drugs)

ALDOSTERONE DEFICIENCY

Chronic aldosterone-related hyperkalemia causes include mineralocorticoid (adrenal) deficiency (Addison disease, congenital adrenal hyperplasia, isolated hypoaldosteronism); hyporeninemic hypoaldosteronism (CKD, diabetic nephropathy, lupus nephropathy, HIV nephropathy); and pseudohypoaldosteronism.

Investigations: low aldosterone, low cortisol, high renin, hyponatremia (adrenal insufficiency), low/normal renin, normal cortisol (hyporeninemic hypoaldosteronism)

DRUGS

Medications associated with hyperkalemia (renal tubular acidosis type IV) include ACE inhibitors; NSAIDs (e.g., celecoxib, diclofenac, indomethacin); angiotensin II receptor blockers; potassium-sparing diuretics (e.g., spironolactone, eplerenone, triamterene); immunosuppressives (e.g., tacrolimus, cyclosporine); beta-blockers; digoxin; heparin; antibiotics containing trimethoprim.

Keys to patient encounter

Key concern

Identify the urgent presentation of hyperkalemia associated with ECG abnormalities.

History

HISTORY OF PRESENT ILLNESS

Patients are often mostly or entirely asymptomatic even with significant hyperkalemia, and the condition is often identified on electrolytes ordered for other reasons. Ask about a history of palpitations and syncope. Ask about a history of weakness and fatigue.

PAST MEDICAL HISTORY

Ask about renal conditions, diabetes, aldosterone-related conditions (e.g., Addison disease), and cancer.

Ask about factors relevant to rhabdomyolysis (recent surgery, severe recent trauma, use of street drugs, use of statins).

MEDICATIONS

Ask about beta-blockers, ACE inhibitors, NSAIDs, angiotensin II receptor blockers, diuretics, immunosuppressives, digoxin, heparin, and antibiotics.

Investigations

Serum creatinine

Urine electrolytes

ECG to assess the physiologic severity of the hyperkalemia

Management

Address any underlying causes.

In severe hyperkalemia, or if ECG changes are present (tall peaked T waves with shortened QT interval; lengthened PR interval; wide QRS interval; absent P waves; sine-wave pattern), administer IV calcium to reduce cardiac toxicity. Give IV glucose and insulin infusion to enhance potassium uptake by cells. Correct severe metabolic acidosis with IV sodium bicarbonate; if failure is present, consider nebulized β-adrenergic agonist instead. Increase potassium excretion by administering loop diuretics or GI cation-exchange medications (e.g., sodium polystyrene sulfonate). Provide emergency dialysis for severe hyperkalemia that is unresponsive to more conservative measures or in patients with complete renal failure.

ELECTROLYTE IMBALANCES

Hypokalemia

Differential diagnosis

HYPOKALEMIA IN GENERAL

Definition: serum potassium < 3.5 mEq/L (3.5 mmol/L)

DECREASED INTAKE (E.G., ANOREXIA NERVOSA)

Anorexia nervosa[1(pp338–339)]

Signs and symptoms: significantly low body weight; intense fear of gaining weight or persistent behavior that interferes with gaining weight; excessive focus on body weight or shape in self-evaluation, or persistent lack of recognition of current low body weight

REDISTRIBUTION (E.G., ALKALEMIA, INSULIN, β2-ADRENERGIC STIMULATING DRUGS)

Signs and symptoms (in general): often asymptomatic, muscle weakness, fatigue, anxiety, constipation, syncope, palpitations, respiratory distress, arrhythmias

Alkalemia: ABG pH > 7.42 and arterial $PaCO_2$ < 38 mmHg

Insulin: personal or family history of diabetes; history of diabetic complications and/or inadequate monitoring; signs and symptoms of diabetes (polydipsia, polyuria, and/or weight loss)

Investigations: serum electrolytes, magnesium, glucose, BUN, creatinine

INCREASED LOSSES

Renal losses

Causes include medications (diuretics, mineralocorticoids, glucocorticoids, high-dose antibiotics) and chloride-responsive metabolic alkalosis.

Signs and symptoms: low BP from hypovolemia

Investigations: 24-hour urine potassium excretion to differentiate renal loss (> 30 mmol) and extrarenal loss

Gastrointestinal loss (e.g., vomiting, diarrhea)

Keys to patient encounter

Key concern

Identify the urgent presentation of hypokalemia associated with muscle weakness and/or ECG abnormalities.

History

HISTORY OF PRESENT ILLNESS

Ask about muscle weakness, vomiting, and diarrhea.

PAST MEDICAL HISTORY

Ask about anorexia nervosa and diabetes.

MEDICATIONS

Ask about diuretics, insulin, β2-adrenergic stimulating drugs, mineralocorticoids, glucocorticoids, and antibiotics.

Physical exam

Physical exam does not usually contribute useful information for diagnosing or managing hypokalemia. Take note, however, of obviously low body weight, which may indicate anorexia nervosa.

Investigations

Serum and urine electrolytes

ECG to identify life-threatening conduction abnormalities

Management

Treat any underlying causes (vomiting, diarrhea, thiazide, and loop diuretics), and replace potassium. For potassium levels of 2.5–3.4 mEq/L (2.5–3.4 mmol/L), replace with oral potassium chloride (KCl). Consider potassium-sparing diuretics in patients with normal renal function who are prone to significant hypokalemia.

For severe hypokalemia (< 2.5 mEq/L [2.5 mmol/L]), apply a cardiac monitor and administer 40 mmol KCl in 1 L of normal saline with an infusion rate of 10 mmol/hour. Recheck the patient's serum potassium level after each 40 mmol of KCl. Also check the patient's magnesium ion (Mg^{2+}) level, because low magnesium may make it more difficult to control the potassium level. If the patient has low magnesium, initially give 4 mL of 50% magnesium sulfate ($MgSO_4$, 8 mmol).

REFERENCE

1. American Psychiatric Association. Diagnostic and statistical manual of mental disorders. 5th ed. Arlington, VA: American Psychiatric Association; 2013. 991 p.

ELECTROLYTE IMBALANCES

Hypernatremia

Differential diagnosis

WATER DEPLETION (DEHYDRATION)

DEHYDRATION IN GENERAL

Symptoms: postural dizziness; headache; malaise; muscle weakness; lethargy or somnolence; change in activity or mental status; restlessness; irritability; agitation; reduced urine output; acute weight loss; constipation

Severe: seizures, coma

Signs on physical exam: dry mucous membranes; sunken-appearing eyes; slow capillary refill; hypotension; resting tachycardia; orthostatic changes; flat neck veins in supine position; oliguria; reduced or abnormal skin turgor; recent change of consciousness; increased postural pulse, decreased postural BP

Risk factors: elderly, acute illness, chronic conditions, no intact thirst mechanism, dementia, reduced kidney function, high percentage fat, low muscle mass, dehydrating medication (e.g., diuretics, laxatives, antidiuretic hormone antagonists, lithium, alcohol, narcotics), reduced fluid intake

Investigations:

Blood tests: electrolytes including sodium (> 145 mEq/L [145 mmol/L]), potassium, chloride, HCO_3^-; BUN; creatinine; osmolality; glucose; calcium

Urine tests: spot sodium concentration; specific gravity; osmolality

Decreased intake of water (e.g., impaired thirst)

IMPAIRED THIRST

Patients in long-term care may have a combination of factors, including altered thirst, decreased cognitive function (e.g., delirium, depression, sedation, dementia), and higher fluid losses.

Increased loss

RENAL LOSS (E.G., OSMOTIC DIURESIS)

OSMOTIC DIURESIS

The most common cause is hyperglycemia due to diabetes.

Signs and symptoms: personal or family history of diabetes; history of diabetic complications and/or inadequate monitoring; polydipsia, polyuria, and/or weight loss

Investigations: fasting glucose or HbA_{1c}

GASTROINTESTINAL LOSS (E.G., DIARRHEA)

INCREASED INSENSIBLE LOSS (E.G., PROLONGED EXERCISE)

SODIUM GAIN (E.G., HYPERTONIC FLUID REPLACEMENT)

Hypertonic fluid replacement

Examples include hypertonic dialysis and administration of hypertonic saline.

Keys to patient encounter

Key concern

In the frail elderly, the cause of hypernatremia is usually water depletion.

History

HISTORY OF PRESENT ILLNESS

Ask whether the patient feels thirsty (hypernatremia with lack of thirst suggests impaired thirst mechanism).

Ask about common triggers and risk factors: recent illness, recent prolonged exercise, diabetes, and diarrhea.

MEDICATIONS

Ask about dehydrating medications and hypertonic fluid replacement.

ELDERLY PATIENTS

Ask about habitation in a long-term care facility (where they may rely on others to get water) and medications that impair cognition.

Physical exam

Vital signs

Volume status

Mental status: Dehydration can lead to changes in mental status.

Neurological: Neurological findings suggest an impaired thirst mechanism, or may be secondary to the hypernatremia itself.

> POINTER
>
> **Correcting hypernatremia**
>
> Overly rapid correction of hypernatremia carries the risk of convulsions and cerebral edema. The rate of correction should not exceed 1 mEq/L (1 mmol/L) per hour. Over a 24-hour period, the rate of correction should not exceed 10–12 mEq/L (10–12 mmol/L).

Investigations

Electrolytes to measure sodium and estimate the level of water deficit

Blood glucose

Brain imaging to detect conditions that impair the thirst mechanism, such as lesions on the hypothalamus

Management

Management depends on the specific entity identified. Consider referral to an endocrinologist or nephrologist.

ELECTROLYTE IMBALANCES

Hyponatremia

Differential diagnosis

HYPONATREMIA IN GENERAL

Signs and symptoms: anorexia, nausea, malaise (early); decreased reaction times, slow cognition, ataxia (moderate to chronic); headache, muscle cramps, irritability, drowsiness, confusion, weakness (worse than moderate); coma, respiratory arrest (severe)

HYPONATREMIA WITH NORMAL SERUM OSMOLALITY (E.G., HYPERLIPIDEMIA)

Hypertriglyceridemia

Signs and symptoms: usually asymptomatic; recurrent pancreatitis

Skin: eruptive xanthomas (yellow papules on the back, chest, proximal extremities); palmar xanthomas (yellow creases on the palms); tuberous xanthomas (red/orange shiny nodules on finger extensors); tendinous xanthomas (Achilles tendon); xanthelasma (yellow plaques on the eyelids)

Contributing medications: atypical antipsychotics; beta-blockers; estrogens; immunosuppressives; isotretinoin; protease inhibitors; thiazide-type diuretics; tamoxifen; clomiphene; herbal or botanical supplements

Risk factors: diabetes; history of CHD or noncoronary atherosclerosis (e.g., AAA); family history of cardiovascular disease; smoking; hypertension; obesity

Investigations: fasting serum triglycerides (< 150 mg/dL [1.7 mmol/L] is normal; 203–495 mg/dL [2.3–5.6 mmol/L] is high; > 495 mg/dL [5.6 mmol/L] is very high)

Hypercholesterolemia

Signs and symptoms: usually asymptomatic

Risk factors: diet high in processed foods and fat; obesity; large waist circumference; lack of exercise; smoking; diabetes

Contributing medications: progestins, anabolic steroids, corticosteroids, protease inhibitors

Investigations: total cholesterol (< 200 mg/dL [5.2 mmol/L] is normal; > 239 mg/dL [6.2 mmol/L] is high); LDL (< 100 mg/dL [2.59 mmol/L] is optimal; > 189 mg/dL [4.90 mmol/L] is very high)

HYPONATREMIA WITH HIGH SERUM OSMOLALITY (E.G., HYPERGLYCEMIA)

Hyperglycemia

Serum sodium decreases by 2.4 mEq/L (2.4 mmol/L) for each increase of 101 mg/dL (5.6 mmol/L) serum glucose. Sodium correction in hyperglycemia is:

$$\text{Na} = \text{Measured Sodium} + 0.016 \times (\text{Glucose} - 100)$$

Risk factors: personal or family history of diabetes; history of diabetic complications and/or inadequate monitoring

Investigations: serum and urine osmolality; serum glucose and lipids

HYPONATREMIA WITH LOW SERUM OSMOLALITY

Low total body water volume, elevated ADH (e.g., gastrointestinal loss, diuretic use)

Signs and symptoms: history of diarrhea or diuretic use

Normal total body water volume (e.g., syndrome of inappropriate ADH secretion, hypothyroidism, adrenal insufficiency)

SYNDROME OF INAPPROPRIATE ADH SECRETION

Signs and symptoms: general symptoms of hyponatremia (see above)

Investigations: hyponatremia; hypoosmolality; urine osmolality $>$ 100 mOsm/kg (100 mmol/kg); urine sodium $>$ 40 mEq/L (40 mmol/L); normal serum potassium; no acid-base disturbance; low serum uric acid (often)

HYPOTHYROIDISM

Signs and symptoms: history of hypothyroidism or symptoms of hypothyroidism (cold intolerance, decreased reflexes, dry skin, weight gain, impaired cognition)

Investigations: elevated thyrotropin (TSH)

ADRENAL INSUFFICIENCY

Signs and symptoms: symptoms that develop slowly (often over several months); hyperpigmentation; fatigue; weight loss; dizziness; muscle and/or joint pain; salt craving

Investigations: serum sodium, potassium, cortisol, ACTH; ACTH stimulation test (this involves artificial stimulation of the adrenal gland) to determine adrenal gland function; CT scan of the adrenal gland

High total body water volume, elevated ADH level (e.g., congestive heart failure, nephrotic syndrome, cirrhosis)

CONGESTIVE HEART FAILURE

Signs and symptoms: history of heart disease (or risk factors for heart disease: diabetes, hypertension, hyperlipidemia, and smoking) or hepatic vein thrombosis (Budd-Chiari syndrome); severe shortness of breath; elevated JVP; edema in the abdomen and legs; pink phlegm; heart murmurs and extra cardiac sounds

Investigations: chest x-ray to detect pulmonary edema; NT-proBNP level; echocardiogram to distinguish forms of HF; cardiac stress testing, either with exercise or pharmacological agent

NEPHROTIC SYNDROME

Signs and symptoms: progressive bilateral lower extremity edema (ankles and feet); swelling around the eyes; weight gain (from water retention); foamy urine

Risk factors: conditions that damage the kidneys (e.g., diabetes, SLE, amyloidosis); use of NSAIDs, antibiotics; history of HIV, HBV, HCV, malaria

Investigations: urine (proteinuria; spot urine protein:creatinine ratio; lipuria); hyponatremia with low fractional sodium excretion; low serum albumin; high total cholesterol (hyperlipidemia); elevated BUN

CIRRHOSIS

Signs and symptoms: jaundice; easy bruising, bleeding; itching; ascites; spiderlike blood vessels on the skin; systemic symptoms (anorexia, weight loss, weakness, fatigue)

> History of chronic alcohol abuse; chronic HBV or HCV infection; hemochromatosis; nonalcoholic fatty liver disease
>
> HBV and HCV risk factors: autoimmune conditions, unprotected sex, IV drug abuse, blood transfusions, workplace exposure to body fluids, tattoos, body piercings, imprisonment

Investigations: liver function tests

Keys to patient encounter

Key concern

Identify severe hyponatremia, which can be life-threatening.

History

HISTORY OF PRESENT ILLNESS

Ask about nausea and vomiting. Ask about mental status changes: altered personality, confusion, irritability, restlessness, and drowsiness. Ask about headache, loss of energy, muscle weakness, spasms, cramps, and seizures.

PAST MEDICAL HISTORY

Ask about renal failure and CHF. Ask about conditions that cause severe vomiting or diarrhea. Ask about excessive thirst (relevant to primary polydipsia).

MEDICATIONS

Ask about diuretic use, and use of antidepressants and pain medications (relevant to sweating and diuresis).

Physical exam

Vital signs

Volume status

Mental status: Severe hyponatremia may lead to confusion.

Investigations

Serum and urine electrolytes (see *Notes on labs and assessments*)

Serum and urine osmolality

Serum creatinine

BUN

Other specific investigations as warranted by the history and physical exam

Management

General management involves restricting water intake and promoting water loss. Any sodium deficit must be replaced (see the pointer). Treat the underlying disorder. Consider referral to an endocrinologist or nephrologist.

POINTER

Correcting hyponatremia

Overly rapid correction of hyponatremia can lead to central pontine myelinolysis. Risk factors for central pontine myelinolysis include alcoholism, liver disease, malnutrition, and a baseline serum sodium of < 120 mEq/L (120 mmol/L). Do not correct by more than 6–8 mEq/L (6–8 mmol/L) over 24 hours.

Erectile dysfunction

Differential diagnosis

ERECTILE DYSFUNCTION IN GENERAL

Definition: difficulty getting or keeping an erection that's firm enough for sex

NEUROLOGIC CONDITION (E.G., DIABETES MELLITUS)

Diabetes

Signs and symptoms: personal or family history of diabetes; history of diabetic complications and/or inadequate monitoring; polydipsia, polyuria, and/or weight loss

Investigations: fasting glucose or HbA_{1c}

CARDIOVASCULAR DISORDER

Signs and symptoms: history of atherosclerosis, hyperlipidemia, hypertension, venoocclusive dysfunction

DRUGS

These include antidepressants and other psychiatric medications; antihistamines; antihypertensives; diuretics, beta-blockers; medications for Parkinson disease; chemotherapy; opiate analgesics; and recreational drugs (alcohol, amphetamines, barbiturates, cocaine, marijuana, methadone, nicotine, opiates).

HORMONAL DISORDER (E.G., TESTOSTERONE DEFICIENCY)

Testosterone deficiency

This is reversible with testosterone treatment.

Signs and symptoms: older age (more common), poor morning erection, decreased sexual libido

Other symptoms: irritability; mood changes; fatigue; decreased muscle bulk and strength; decline in cognitive function; hot flashes

Investigations: serum testosterone < 300 ng/dL (10 nmol/L)

PSYCHOLOGICAL OR EMOTIONAL CONDITION (E.G., PERFORMANCE ANXIETY)

PSYCHOLOGICAL CONDITION IN GENERAL

Signs and symptoms: personal or family history of psychiatric conditions (e.g., anxiety, major depressive disorder); excessive worry; loss of interest in friends and usual activities; changes in sleep habits; hallucinations or delusions; suicidal thoughts; history of adverse experience (emotional, physical, or sexual abuse; recent stress such as death of a friend or family member), or substance abuse

Performance anxiety

Signs and symptoms: maintenance of erections during masturbation or sleep; inability to maintain erections during intercourse

Keys patient encounter

History

HISTORY OF PRESENT ILLNESS

Ask whether the patient has a new sexual partner, how often the patient is sexually active, when the erectile dysfunction began, whether it happens every time the patient has sex, and whether the patient has nighttime erections.

PAST MEDICAL HISTORY

Ask about heart disease, diabetes, peripheral vascular disease, hyperlipidemia, and hypertension.

MEDICATIONS

Ask about hypertension medications, antihistamines, sedatives, and antidepressants.

SOCIAL HISTORY

Ask about smoking, alcohol use, use of recreational drugs, and lack of exercise.

Physical exam

Vital signs: Look for hypertension.

Height and weight: Calculate the patient's BMI (see *Notes on labs and assessments*).

GU: Examine the penis, testicles, and perform a DRE.

Investigations

There is no diagnostic test for erectile dysfunction. Testing is directed toward identifying comorbidities.

Morning serum testosterone

Fasting blood glucose or HbA_{1c}

Lipids (see *Notes on labs and assessments*)

Thyrotropin (TSH)

POINTER

Erectile dysfunction incidence

Erectile dysfunction is very common, affecting a third of men over their lifetimes.

Management

If applicable, counsel the patient on lifestyle changes (weight loss, exercise, smoking cessation). Optimize diabetes management. Consider stopping or substituting contributing medications.

First line therapy is inhibitors of phosphodiesterase type V. The primary contraindication is concurrent treatment with nitrates.

Second-line therapy is intraurethral or intracavernosal alprostadil and vacuum pump devices.

EYE REDNESS

Eye redness

Differential diagnosis

LIDS, LASHES, ORBITS, OR LACHRYMAL SYSTEM

Blepharitis

Signs and symptoms: usually bilateral; red, swollen, and/or itchy eyelids; gritty, burning sensation in the eyes; tearing; crusted eyelashes on wakening; flaky, greasy eyelid skin; loss of eyelashes; eyelashes growing at abnormal angles (misdirected eyelashes); malposition of eyelids from chronic inflammation

History of seborrheic dermatitis (common), rosacea (common), acne, eczema, smoking, allergies, retinoid use

CONJUNCTIVA, SCLERA

Conjunctivitis

Signs and symptoms: red eye; eye discharge; gritty, burning sensation in the eye

Bacterial: unilateral symptoms that progress to bilateral symptoms; purulent discharge; infectious contacts

Viral: unilateral symptoms that progress to bilateral symptoms; watery discharge; URTI (usual) or infectious contacts; pruritus

Allergic: bilateral symptoms; pruritus (this is a distinguishing feature); mucosal discharge; history of atopy (allergic rhinitis, eczema, asthma)

Subconjunctival hemorrhage

This may be spontaneous in elderly patients, but always check for traumatic injury.

Signs and symptoms: painless, well-demarcated area of conjunctival erythema with no visual disturbances; use of anticoagulants (possible contributing factor)

Risk factors: trauma; recent coughing, sneezing; recent heavy lifting

Episcleritis

Signs and symptoms: possibly asymptomatic; abrupt-onset redness, tearing, and/or irritation

History of associated conditions: RA, inflammatory bowel disease, vasculitis, SLE, infection (e.g., Lyme disease, herpes zoster ophthalmicus), atopy, rosacea

Investigations: blanching of vessels with application of phenylephrine (this differentiates episcleritis from scleritis)

Orbital cellulitis

This is an ocular emergency.

Signs and symptoms: fever; malaise; pain with eye movement; reduced vision, double vision; red eye; swelling and/or redness of the eyelid and surrounding skin; proptosis; relative afferent pupillary defect; mucormycosis (this is a severe and destructive fungal orbital cellulitis); history of diabetes

Risk factors: preseptal cellulitis; sinus, face, or tooth infection; trauma

Investigations: leukocytosis on CBC; elevated CRP, ESR; CT scan or MRI of the head

CORNEA

Keratitis

This is inflammation of the cornea, commonly caused by infection. Other causes include neurotrophic, interstitial, fungal, and viral keratitis.

Signs and symptoms: use of contact lenses (common), including wearing lenses too long, not cleaning lenses properly, and/or not replacing lenses regularly; redness; eye pain; feeling of something in the eye; excessive tearing; photophobia

Herpes keratitis: history of herpes infection (e.g., cold sores); branching pattern on fluorescein stain (possible)

Dry eye

This is due to insufficient tear production or poor quality tears.

Signs and symptoms: redness, scratchy feeling in the eyes, eye pain, eye discharge

Corneal abrasion

Signs and symptoms: unilateral (usually); sensation of a foreign object in the eye; pain; redness

ANTERIOR CHAMBER, IRIS

Iritis

Signs and symptoms: typically unilateral; photophobia; redness; pain; globe tenderness or ache; ciliary flush; lacrimation; history of connective tissue disease (e.g., reactive arthritis, psoriatic arthritis, inflammatory bowel disease, ankylosing spondylitis, juvenile idiopathic arthritis), infection (HSV, toxoplasmosis, HIV, syphilis, TB, Lyme disease)

Investigations: tonometry (intraocular pressure is usually reduced unless there is severe or infectious etiology that can lead to inflammatory glaucoma); slit-lamp exam (anterior chamber cells are visible)

Acute angle-closure glaucoma

This is an ocular emergency.

Signs and symptoms: fixed, middilated pupil; exquisitely painful red eye (usually unilateral); reduced, blurry vision; halos seen around lights; nausea, vomiting; photophobia

Investigations: tonometry to detect increased intraocular pressure (> 40 mmHg); slit-lamp exam to detect cloudy cornea, shallow anterior chamber

Endophthalmitis

This is an ocular emergency.

Signs and symptoms: swollen eyelid; pain; redness; photophobia; eye discharge; reduced vision; proptosis; possible globe rupture, hypopyon

Risk factors: immunosuppression, systemic infections (endogenous factors); intraocular surgery, small ocular procedures, penetrating eye injury (exogenous factors)

Investigations: slit-lamp exam (findings: cells in the anterior chamber, corneal edema, hypopyon, reduced red reflex)

Hypopyon (pus in anterior chamber)

This is an ocular emergency: it can be associated with infectious keratitis and endophthalmitis.

Signs and symptoms: history of blunt-force trauma; history of ocular disease (corneal ulcer, iritis, posterior uveitis, endophthalmitis, vitreitis)

Investigations: slit-lamp exam to detect WBCs in the anterior chamber

TRAUMA

Keys to patient encounter

Key concern

Distinguish benign causes from those that require prompt referral to an ophthalmologist to prevent significant vision loss.

History

HISTORY OF PRESENT ILLNESS

Ask when the eye redness started, which eye is involved, and what associated symptoms the patient has.

Examples of characteristic symptoms include:

Blepharitis: eyelash loss or abnormalities

Allergic conjunctivitis: bilateral itchy eyes with discharge

Acute angle-closure glaucoma: recent-onset extreme unilateral eye pain with nausea, impaired vision, photophobia, and perceived halos around lights

Ask about contact lens use, eye trauma, allergies, and systemic disease.

Ask about red flags (see the pointer).

Physical exam

Eyes:

- Examine the eyes and eyelids.
- Record pupil sizes and reaction to light.
- Test visual acuity.
- In cases of corneal abrasion, check for a retained foreign body under the upper eyelid.
- Perform a slit-lamp exam (including fluorescein staining in suspected abrasion or herpes infection).
- Consider measuring intraocular pressure.

Head and neck: Look for lymphadenopathy.

POINTER

Red flags in eye redness

The following findings require immediate ophthalmology referral:

Severe pain not relieved with topical anesthetics
Vision loss
Traumatic eye injury
Herpes infection
Recent ocular surgery
Corneal involvement
Distorted pupil
Copious purulent discharge

Investigations

Laboratory investigations do not generally provide information useful to diagnosing or managing eye redness.

Management

Identify patients who require immediate ophthalmology referral (see the pointer).

Management for common conditions includes:

Blepharitis: eyelid scrubs

Allergic conjunctivitis: topical antihistamines or histamine H_1 receptor antagonist agents

Bacterial conjunctivitis: topical antibiotics

Viral conjunctivitis: supportive therapy, handwashing (viral conjunctivitis is highly contagious)

Corneal abrasion: topical antibiotics

Dry eye: artificial tears

Episcleritis: supportive therapy (episcleritis is self-limiting); in cases of recurrent episodes, referral to an ophthalmologist

Subconjunctival hemorrhage: supportive therapy

FATIGUE

Fatigue

Differential diagnosis

FATIGUE IN GENERAL

Fatigue is a very common presenting complaint. Causes often include medication side effects, sleep disturbances, lifestyle issues, sleep apnea or snoring, chronic medical conditions, and mental disorders.

IATROGENIC OR PHARMACOLOGIC CONDITIONS

Prescription medications

Examples include sedatives or hypnotics such as barbiturates and benzodiazepines; antidepressants such as MAOIs, SSRIs, SNRIs, and TCAs; antipsychotics; and antihypertensives.

Drugs of abuse

Examples include cocaine, heroin, alcohol, amphetamines, and sedatives.

IDIOPATHIC

Chronic fatigue syndrome

Signs and symptoms: extreme fatigue unexplainable by any underlying medical condition; symptoms that do not improve with rest; symptoms for ≥ 6 months

Key symptoms: loss of memory or concentration; sore throat; enlarged lymph nodes (neck, armpits); muscle pain; pain that moves among joints without swelling or redness; headache of a new type, pattern, or severity; unrefreshing sleep; extreme exhaustion lasting > 24 hours after mental or physical exertion

Fibromyalgia

This is a diagnosis of exclusion.

Signs and symptoms: female (more common); chronic, widespread pain for ≥ 3 months; pain that is bilateral, and above and below the waist; aching pain; fatigue; long sleep; restless leg syndrome; sleep apnea; impaired concentration, memory; dizziness; cramping (e.g., menstrual, abdominal); morning stiffness; numbness, tingling in the extremities; tender points; urinary symptoms (difficult or painful urination, irregular urination); sensitivity to noise, light, temperature

Coexisting conditions (often): headaches, irritable bowel syndrome, interstitial cystitis

OTHER

Psychiatric condition

Signs and symptoms: personal or family history of psychiatric conditions (e.g., anxiety, major depressive disorder); excessive worry; loss of interest in friends and usual activities; changes in sleep habits; hallucinations or delusions; suicidal thoughts; history of adverse experience (emotional, physical, or sexual abuse; recent stress such as death of a friend or family member), or substance abuse

Endocrine-metabolic condition

DIABETES

Signs and symptoms: personal or family history of diabetes; history of diabetic complications and/or inadequate monitoring; polydipsia, polyuria, and/or weight loss

Investigations: fasting glucose or HbA_{1c}

HYPOTHYROIDISM

Signs and symptoms: history of hypothyroidism or symptoms of hypothyroidism (cold intolerance, decreased reflexes, dry skin, weight gain, impaired cognition)

Investigations: elevated thyrotropin (TSH)

HYPERCALCEMIA

Signs and symptoms: constipation, polyuria, polydipsia, dehydration, anorexia, nausea, muscle weakness, altered sensory status

History of sarcoidosis, malignancy, hyperparathyroidism, immobilization, use of diuretics (thiazide)

Investigations: blood test (hypercalcemia is total calcium ≥ 10.52 mg/dL [2.63 mmol/L] or ionized calcium ≥ 5.6 mg/dL [1.4 mmol/L]); albumin; PTH

KIDNEY DISEASE

Signs and symptoms: history of kidney disease, chronic renal failure, and/or current renal dialysis; bilateral lower limb swelling; shortness of breath; paroxysmal nocturnal dyspnea; orthopnea

Risk factors: diabetes, diabetic complications, and/or inadequate monitoring; hypertension; smoking

Investigations: renal function tests (reduced calcium; elevated phosphate; elevated creatinine); reduced vitamin D

LIVER DISEASE

Patients with compensated cirrhosis may be asymptomatic.

HCV is often asymptomatic.

Signs and symptoms: jaundice; abdominal pain, swelling; palpable, tender liver; swelling in the legs and ankles; systemic symptoms (anorexia, weight loss, weakness, fatigue); itching; easy bruising

> History of chronic alcohol abuse; chronic HBV or HCV; hemochromatosis; autoimmune conditions; α_1-antitrypsin deficiency; primary biliary cirrhosis; CHF
>
> HBV and HCV risk factors: unprotected sex, IV drug abuse, blood transfusions, tattoos, body piercings, imprisonment, workplace exposure to body fluids

Investigations: tests for liver enzymes (elevated AST, ALT) and liver function (elevated bilirubin; possible abnormal PT/INR); viral serologic tests to detect HBV, HCV; Doppler US; CT scan; MRI; transient elastography; liver biopsy

Cardiopulmonary condition

CONGESTIVE HEART FAILURE

Signs and symptoms: history of heart disease (or risk factors for heart disease: diabetes, hypertension, hyperlipidemia, and smoking) or hepatic vein thrombosis (Budd-Chiari syndrome); severe shortness of breath; elevated JVP; edema in the abdomen and legs; pink phlegm; heart murmurs and extra cardiac sounds

Investigations: chest x-ray to detect pulmonary edema; NT-proBNP level; echocardiogram to distinguish forms of HF; cardiac stress testing, either with exercise or pharmacological agent

CHRONIC OBSTRUCTIVE PULMONARY DISEASE

Signs and symptoms: older than age 40 (usual: symptoms do not appear until significant lung damage has occurred); progressive symptoms; wheezing; chest tightness; chronic productive cough; clubbing of the fingers; cyanosis around the lips and in the extremities; decreased oxygen saturation; impaired pulmonary function on testing with spirometry

Risk factors: smoking, occupational exposure, intrinsic lung disease

Investigations: chest x-ray; CT scan; ABG

Infectious condition (e.g., mononucleosis)

MONONUCLEOSIS

Signs and symptoms (classic triad): fever, pharyngitis, lymphadenopathy (usually posterior cervical)

> Additional signs and symptoms: fatigue and malaise; headache; abdominal pain; nausea, vomiting; rash; splenomegaly; palatal exanthems or petechiae

Investigations: CBC, lymphocytosis (> 50%); peripheral blood smear to detect atypical lymphocytes; heterophile antibody test (e.g., Monospot); EBV-specific serology testing (definitive)

Sleep disturbance

Examples of causes include poor sleep environment, irregular work schedule (e.g., shift work), and insomnia.

> Poor sleep environments may have too much light, too much noise, uncomfortable temperatures (too hot or too cold), or cosleepers with sleep disorders (e.g., snoring).
>
> Insomnia may be due to pain, sleep apnea, snoring, GERD, pregnancy, and postpartum routines.

Neoplastic-hematologic condition

ANEMIA

Risk factors: intestinal disorders (Crohn disease, celiac disease), menstruation, pregnancy, chronic disease (e.g., cancer, kidney failure), family history of sickle cell disease

Investigations: CBC; visual examination of RBCs for unusual size, shape, color

LEUKEMIA

Signs and symptoms: fever; chills; persistent fatigue and weakness; frequent or severe infections; weight loss; pallor; swollen lymph nodes; enlarged liver or spleen; easy bleeding and bruising; recurrent nosebleeds; petechiae; excessive sweating; bone pain or tenderness

Investigations: CBC; peripheral blood smear; flow cytometry; bone marrow aspiration and biopsy

LYMPHOMA

Signs and symptoms (non-Hodgkin): constitutional symptoms (fatigue, fever, night sweats, weight loss), swollen lymph nodes, chest pain, coughing, shortness of breath

> Hodgkin lymphoma (less common): constitutional symptoms (fatigue, fever, night sweats, weight loss); swollen lymph nodes; itching; pain on drinking alcohol, or increased sensitivity to alcohol

Investigations: blasts or cancer cells on peripheral blood smear; excess blasts or cancer cells on bone marrow examination

MALIGNANCY
Signs and symptoms: history of solid organ cancer (e.g., breast, lung, kidney, colon); easy bruising or bleeding; nodules or lumps anywhere on the body; constitutional symptoms (fever, weight loss, night sweats)

Investigations: x-ray, CT scan, MRI; biopsy

Keys to patient encounter

History

HISTORY OF PRESENT ILLNESS

FATIGUE CHARACTERISTICS

Ask when the fatigue started, how constant it is, and how it has changed since it started. Ask how rest affects it, and how mental or physical exertion affects it.

Examples of characteristic features include:

Infection: recent-onset fatigue

Chronic conditions: progressive fatigue

Chronic fatigue syndrome: extreme intermittent fatigue after mental or physical effort that is unrelieved by rest

Ask about the impact of the fatigue on the patient's quality of life and daily functioning.

ASSOCIATED SYMPTOMS

Ask about constitutional symptoms (these suggest malignancy: weight loss, fever, night sweats); excessive thirst and urination (diabetes); GI symptoms, steatorrhea, and weight loss (celiac disease); intolerance to cold (hypothyroidism); shortness of breath (HF, COPD); chest pain (CAD); and anxiety and depression (psychiatric condition).

RISK FACTORS FOR INFECTION

Screen the patient for a history of immunosuppression (this is relevant to CMV); exposure to unpasteurized dairy products (brucellosis); exposure to areas where Lyme disease is endemic; IV drug use and/or unprotected sex (HIV, HBV, HCV); and contact with cat feces (toxoplasmosis).

SLEEP ROUTINES

Ask how regular the patient's sleep is, and how much sleep they get. Listen for evidence of disrupted sleep.

MEDICATIONS

Ask about antidepressants, antiepileptics, antihistamines, antihypertensives, neuroleptics, corticosteroids, and diuretics. Ask about recreational drug use and substance abuse.

SOCIAL HISTORY

Ask about possible exposure to heavy metals, such as work in demolition (lead exposure) and artisanal glass manufacture (arsenic, cadmium).

Physical exam

General inspection: Look for pallor.

Cardiovascular: Look for tachycardia, and a systolic ejection murmur (relevant to anemia).

Abdominal: Look for masses and signs of liver disease (hepatomegaly, splenomegaly, caput medusa, spider nevi).

Lymph notes: Look for lymphadenopathy.

Investigations

UNDERLYING ORGANIC ILLNESS

In the absence of localizing features, investigations may have limited success in diagnosing a specific entity. However, a major role of testing is to rule out underlying organic illness.

- **CBC**
- **ESR or CRP**
- **Fasting blood glucose or HbA_{1c}**
- **Liver function** (see *Notes on labs and assessments*)
- **Electrolytes** (see *Notes on labs and assessments*)
- **Creatinine**
- **CK**
- **Calcium**
- **Thyrotropin (TSH)**
- **Urinalysis**
- **β-HCG** in women of childbearing age

OTHER SPECIFIC INVESTIGATIONS

Consider other investigations as warranted by the history and physical exam.

POINTER

Causes of fatigue in older versus younger patients

Fatigue in patients older than 60 usually has an organic cause. Fatigue in younger patients (especially younger than 40) is more likely to have an unidentifiable cause.

Management

Treat any conditions identified. In the absence of an apparent organic cause, strongly consider depression. It is acceptable practice to follow most patients without apparent cause and with negative workups, and to suggest lifestyle modifications (e.g., avoid triggers for fatigue as much as possible). Regular physical activity should be recommended for all patients. Consider cognitive behavioral therapy for patients with chronic fatigue.

FEVER

Fever and hyperthermia

Differential diagnosis

INFECTIOUS CAUSES

Bacteria (e.g., group A streptococcus, *E. coli*)

GROUP A STREPTOCOCCUS

When this infection occurs with fever, it is typically centered in the throat ("strep throat").

Signs and symptoms: sudden-onset fever and sore throat; enlarged lymph nodes in the neck; swollen tonsils, possibly with white spots or pus; red spots at the top of the mouth

Investigations: rapid antigen test, throat culture

E. COLI

Signs and symptoms: abdominal cramping, diarrhea, nausea, vomiting, fever

Investigations: stool analysis

MENINGOCOCCAL MENINGITIS

Signs and symptoms: fever, headache, Kernig sign (flexing the patient's hip 90 degrees, then extending the knee, causes pain), Brudzinski neck sign (flexing the patient's neck causes flexion of hips and knees)

> Neonates: poor feeding, lethargy, irritability, apnea, listlessness, apathy, hypothermia, seizures, jaundice, bulging fontanelle, pallor, shock, hypotonia, hypoglycemia
>
> Infants and children: nuchal rigidity, opisthotonos, convulsions, photophobia, alterations of the sensorium, irritability, lethargy, anorexia, nausea, vomiting, coma

Investigations: positive culture in CSF; meningeal inflammation (increased pleocytosis, low glucose in CSF); CSF absolute neutrophil count ≥ 1000/μL (1×10^9/L); CSF protein level ≥ 80 mg/dL (0.8 g/L); peripheral blood absolute neutrophil count ≥ 10 000/μL (10×10^9/L); CT scan, MRI

URINARY TRACT INFECTION

Signs and symptoms: frequent urination; painful urination; pelvic pain and/or flank pain; fever; tenderness over the bladder

Investigations: urinalysis, urine culture

Viruses (e.g., influenza, measles)

INFLUENZA

Signs and symptoms: fever, muscle aches, fatigue, chills, sweats, dry cough

Investigations: throat or nose swab for antigens

MEASLES

Signs and symptoms: fever, dry cough, sore throat, runny nose, inflamed eyes (conjunctivitis), light sensitivity, rash (large flat blotches), Koplik spots (these are pathognomonic: tiny white spots with blue-white centers inside the cheek lining that are present before the rash appears)

> Progression from exposure: asymptomatic during incubation (10–14 days); followed by mild fever, nonspecific symptoms (2–3 days); followed by acute illness and rash, beginning with the face (4 days)

Risk factors: unvaccinated for measles; international travel; vitamin A deficiency

Investigations: blood or saliva IgM test

Parasites (e.g., malaria)

MALARIA

Signs and symptoms: travel to an endemic area (equatorial tropical and subtropical regions, including sub-Saharan Africa, Asia, Central America, South America); recurrent symptoms that begin a few weeks after a bite from an infected mosquito (but some types remain dormant for up to a year); shaking chills, high fever, sweating (common); headache; vomiting; diarrhea

Investigations: blood smears to detect malaria parasites

Fungi (e.g., *Cryptococcus*)

CRYPTOCOCCOSIS

Signs and symptoms: history of immune-system compromise (e.g., HIV/AIDS, lymphoma, use of steroids, splenectomy), fever, pulmonary symptoms (cough, shortness of breath, chest pain)

Later symptoms (cryptococcal meningitis): headache, neck pain, cognitive changes

Investigations: chest x-ray, cryptococcal antigen testing (blood, CSF, sputum)

INFLAMMATORY AND MALIGNANT CONDITIONS (E.G., SYSTEMIC LUPUS ERYTHEMATOSUS, LYMPHOMA)

Systemic lupus erythematosus

Signs and symptoms: personal or family history of SLE; malar rash; arthritis; cytopenias

Investigations: elevated ANA titer; elevated dsDNA level

Lymphoma

Signs and symptoms: constitutional symptoms (weight loss, fever, night sweats), enlarged lymph nodes

Investigations: blasts or cancer cells on peripheral blood smear; excess blasts or cancer cells on bone marrow examination

DRUGS (E.G., BLEOMYCIN, INTERFERON)

Fever is a common short-term side effect of these cancer therapies.

INCREASED HEAT LOAD (E.G., HEAT STROKE)

This is a multisystem illness characterized by CNS dysfunction (encephalopathy), additional organ and/or tissue damage, and high body temperature.

Examples of causes include heat exposure and extreme exertion.

Signs and symptoms:

Two criteria: core temp > 40°C; CNS dysfunction

CNS dysfunction: disorientation; headache; irritability; irrational behavior; emotional instability; confusion; altered consciousness; collapse (usually from hypertrophic cardiomyopathy in younger athletes) or coma; seizure

Other signs and symptoms: tachycardia, hypotension, hyperventilation, dehydration, dry mouth, thirst, muscle cramps, loss of muscle function, ataxia

Investigations: chest x-ray (to detect pulmonary edema); ECG (to detect dysrhythmia; conduction disturbance; nonspecific ST-T wave changes; heat-related myocardial ischemia and/or infarction); CBC; serum electrolytes; BUN; creatinine; hepatic transaminases; PT; PTT; ABG; toxicologic screening (to detect medication effects)

DIMINISHED HEAT DISSIPATION (E.G., MEDICATIONS, ILLICIT DRUGS)

Drugs and medications that cause hyperthermia include psychotropic medications such as SSRIs, MAOIs, and TCAs; stimulants such as amphetamines, cocaine, phencyclidine (PCP), LSD, and 3,4 methylenedioxymethamphetamine (MDMA); common anesthetic agents (e.g., halothane) or paralytic agents (e.g., succinylcholine); anticholinergics (muscarinic antagonists); and drugs that decouple oxidative phosphorylation (e.g., 2,4-dinitrophenol, used as a weight-loss drug).

FACTITIOUS FEVER

Patients generally have complex medical histories, health care experience or knowledge, and an underlying psychiatric disorder (e.g., somatic symptom disorder).

Keys to patient encounter

Key concern

Rule out life-threatening conditions, such as meningococcal meningitis.

History

HISTORY OF PRESENT ILLNESS

Ask when the patient's symptoms started. Ask about sudden-onset symptoms following exertion, heat exposure, or drug use;

infectious symptoms (e.g., cough, dysuria, diarrhea, rash); and constitutional symptoms (these suggest malignancy: weight loss, night sweats).

Ask about immune compromise (e.g., HIV/AIDS, splenectomy, corticosteroid use), and about relevant immunizations (e.g., measles).

MEDICATIONS

Ask about relevant medications and street drugs (see the differential diagnosis).

FAMILY HISTORY

Ask about cancer and SLE.

SOCIAL HISTORY

Ask about travel to malaria-endemic areas.

Physical exam

Vital signs

Full physical: Look in particular for sources of infection.

Investigations

CRP

LDH

CK

Thyrotropin (TSH)

Electrolytes (see *Notes on labs and assessments*)

Liver function (see *Notes on labs and assessments*)

ANA

Rheumatoid factor

EBV

CMV

HIV

TB (purified protein derivative skin test)

Urinalysis

Blood cultures

CSF analysis and culture

Chest x-ray

Pelvic US or CT scan

IN CHILDREN

Consider tests for common pediatric infections (see the pointer).

POINTER

Common infections in infants and children

NEONATES YOUNGER THAN 3 DAYS	NEONATES OLDER THAN 3 DAYS	INFANTS UP TO 3 MONTHS OF AGE	CHILDREN AGED 3 MONTHS TO 6 YEARS
Group B streptococci *E. coli* *S. aureus* *Klebsiella* *Enterococcus* *Streptococcus* *L. monocytogenes* Fungi HSV	Coagulase-negative *staphylococci* *Pseudomonas* *Enterobacter* *Citrobacter* *Serratia* *Klebsiella* *Salmonella* *H. influenzae*	RSV Influenza A *Enterobacter* Group B streptococci *L. monocytogenes* *Salmonella enteritidis* *E. coli* *N. meningitidis* *Pneumococcus* *H. influenzae type b* *S. aureus*	Viruses *Pneumococcus* *H. influenzae type b* *N. meningitidis* *Salmonella*

Management

Unstable patients (septic shock) require resuscitation and admission to ICU. Administer acetaminophen or ibuprofen for symptom management, and consider evaporative cooling. Treat any treatable underlying cause (e.g., administer antibiotics or antifungals). Adjust antimicrobial therapy based on culture and sensitivity. In cases of infection, consider referring the patient to an infectious disease specialist. In cases of malignancy, refer the patient to a surgeon or oncologist.

FEVER

Fever in the immune-compromised host or recurrent fever

Differential diagnosis

HOST DEFENSE DEFECTS

Cellular (e.g., HIV, steroids)

HIV

The most common cause of fever in HIV patients is bacterial infection, especially *S. pneumoniae* and *S. aureus*.

Other causes: viral illnesses; focal or systemic bacterial infections; occult bacteremia; HIV-associated opportunistic infections; malignancy; acute retroviral syndrome (in adolescents)

Investigations: WBCs; blood culture; urinalysis and urine culture; chest and sinus x-rays; LP (CSF: cell counts; protein; glucose; bacterial, mycobacterial, fungal, viral studies; cryptococcal and other fungal antigen tests; cytology)

Prolonged fever (> 8 days) with no apparent diagnosis requires more extensive testing.

STEROIDS

The degree of immunocompromise depends on dose.

Signs and symptoms: fever; chills; sore throat; cough; frequent urination; increased thirst; pain (muscles, back, ribs, arms, legs, hips, shoulders, stomach, throat); swollen feet or lower legs; redness; sores

Investigations: neutrophilic leukocytosis; decreased IgG levels with high doses or chronic use (possible)

Humoral (e.g., congenital)

CONGENITAL HUMORAL DEFECTS

Signs and symptoms: recurrent upper and lower respiratory tract infections including otitis media (common in children, less common in adults), sinusitis, pneumonia

Other infections: GI infections (e.g., giardiasis), bacterial meningitis, viral encephalitis, severe HBV

Investigations: IgG, IgA, IgM tests to detect antibody deficiencies; T cells and B cells to detect deficiencies

Neutropenia (e.g., medication induced)

NEUTROPENIA IN GENERAL

Agranulocytosis is an acute and severe leukopenia, most commonly of neutrophils, causing neutropenia in circulation.

Neutropenia: absolute neutrophil count < 1500/μL (1.5×10^9/L)

Signs and symptoms: female (twice as common as males); age 50 or older (50% of cases)

MEDICATION-INDUCED

The most common medications include methimazole, sulfasalazine, and trimethoprim-sulfamethoxazole.

Other: bone marrow suppressors (e.g., methotrexate, cyclophosphamide, colchicine, azathioprine, ganciclovir); calcium dobesilate (Doxium); psychotropic drugs and anticonvulsants (clozapine, olanzapine); deferiprone; thioamides; ticlopidine; rituximab; quinine; cocaine; heroin

Signs and symptoms: onset 3 to 6 days after taking drug; oral ulcerations with or without fever; possible sepsis

Investigations: CBC; WBC differential; peripheral smear; low absolute neutrophil count (neutrophil count recovers after drug cessation); negative for anemia, thrombocytopenia; bone marrow aspiration and biopsy (hypocellular with low granulocytic precursors)

Keys to patient encounter

Key concerns

Determine whether a patient with recurrent fever is immunocompromised and the likely nature of the immune defect.

Perform appropriate investigations to diagnose the source of infection.

Manage, based on the type and severity of the immunosuppression.

History

HISTORY OF PRESENT ILLNESS

Ask when the fever started, how often the patient gets a fever, and how high the fever is.

PAST MEDICAL HISTORY

Ask about immunosuppression (HIV, malignancy, immunosuppressant medications), chronic illnesses, and recurrent infections.

IN HIV PATIENTS

Ask if the patient has a recent CD4 count.

Ask about ART and how consistent the patient has been with the therapy.

Physical exam

Vital signs: Look for a current fever and hypotension (this is a possible sign of septic shock).

Full physical: Look for signs of focal infection and inflammation.

Investigations

CBC to look for neutropenia

IN PATIENTS WITH FEBRILE NEUTROPENIA

Febrile neutropenia is defined as: 1) a fever higher than 38.3°C **or** higher than 38.0°C for more than 1 hour; 2) in a patient who has received chemotherapy in the past month; 3) with an absolute neutrophil count of less than 500/µL (0.5×10^9/L).

Patients with febrile neutropenia require:

CBC

Electrolytes (see *Notes on labs and assessments*)

Creatinine

Liver function (see *Notes on labs and assessments*)

Blood cultures

Urinalysis and urine cultures

Sputum Gram stain and culture if there is a productive cough

Nasopharyngeal swab for respiratory virus testing if respiratory symptoms are present

Chest-x-ray

LP in suspected CNS infection (this is otherwise not routinely performed)

Management

Start immediate empiric antibiotic treatment for all febrile neutropenic patients (modify treatment, as appropriate, based on culture results). A common initial empiric treatment is IV piperacillin-tazobactam at 4.5 g IV every 8 hours. Hospitalize all unstable patients, and patients with abnormal liver or renal function. Other patients can generally be treated as outpatients, unless their fever began in hospital. Prescribe oral ciprofloxacin, and amoxicillin and clavulanic acid, as first-line empiric treatment. In patients with a history of fungal infection or significant mucosal damage, add empiric antifungal treatment with oral posaconazole, fluconazole, or itraconazole. In patients who are seropositive for HSV with stem cell transplants, or in those who had an HSV reactivation with previous chemotherapy, add oral acyclovir or valacyclovir. Continue treatment until the absolute neutrophil count is > 500–1000/µL (0.5×10^9/L to 1.0×10^9/L), or until cultures identify a specific etiology.

Consult an infectious disease specialist.

GENETIC DISORDERS

Congenital anomalies, dysmorphic features

Differential diagnosis

TERATOGENIC DISORDERS (E.G., FETAL ALCOHOL SPECTRUM DISORDER, CONGENITAL CYTOMEGALOVIRUS INFECTIONS)

Fetal alcohol spectrum disorder

Signs and symptoms: history of exposure to alcohol in utero

Pathognomonic dysmorphic features: small eye openings; thin upper lip; smooth philtrum; maxillary hypoplasia; small lower jaw; short upturned nose; flat nasal bridge; abnormal ear position or formation

Other features: growth deficits before and after birth (at birth: low weight; short length; head circumference ≤ tenth percentile); defects in the heart, kidneys, bones; deformities in the joints, limbs, extremities; neurobehavioral impairments

Congenital Cytomegalovirus infections

Infection usually occurs by vertical transmission. The mother may not be aware she has CMV if the virus is dormant.

Most neonates infected with CMV do not have symptoms and do not develop symptoms later in life.

Signs and symptoms:

Neonatal: retinal inflammation; jaundice; large spleen and liver; mineral deposits in the brain; seizures; small head size; rash; low birth weight

Later life: neurologic abnormalities (difficulty with movement, physical activity; vision impairment, blindness; deafness)

Investigations: antibody titer against CMV (maternal and infant); CBC; liver function tests; urine culture to detect CMV in the first 2 to 3 weeks of life; TORCH screen; CT scan or US of the head; chest x-ray; funduscopy

GENETIC DISORDERS (E.G., DOWN SYNDROME, FRAGILE X SYNDROME)

Down syndrome

Signs and symptoms: characteristic dysmorphic features (small head, flattened facial features, protruding tongue, upward slanting eyes, small hands and feet, short fingers, single crease on the palms of the hands)

Other: ligamentous laxity

Risk factors: older maternal age, siblings with Down syndrome

Investigations: genetic testing, x-rays of target areas to assess development

Fragile X syndrome

This is the most common type of inherited disability. Fathers pass it on to all their daughters; mothers have a 50% chance of passing it on to all their children.

Signs and symptoms: possibly asymptomatic; learning disabilities; speech and language problems (these are usual in boys and include unclear speech, stuttering, leaving out parts of words; some children are nonverbal); behavioral problems (hyperactivity, anxiety, aggression); sensitivity to bright light, loud noises, texture of clothing

Physical symptoms (common): onset during puberty; narrow face, large head, prominent forehead, large ears, flexible joints, flat feet

MECHANICAL FORCES (E.G., CONSTRICTION BAND SYNDROME)

Constriction band syndrome

This is a group of birth defects that result from strands of detached amniotic sac wrapping around parts of the fetus.

Signs and symptoms: facial cleft; legs and arms that are partially or completely missing; permanent band or indentation around a leg, arm, toe, finger; defects in the abdomen and chest

Keys to patient encounter

Key concerns

Determine the severity of the immediate presentation.

Identify patients requiring early referral for specialized care.

Provide supportive counseling for parents.

History

Take a 3-generation family history of congenital anomalies and dysmorphic features. Get details on which family members (including age and sex) were affected, when they were diagnosed, what their symptoms were, and when they died. Be sure to establish if there was consanguinity with the current patient.

Obtain a prenatal history of the patient. Listen for evidence of unusual symptoms or circumstances. Ask specifically about possible toxic exposures during the pregnancy.

Physical exam

Full physical: Pay particular attention to cardiovascular abnormalities, ambiguous genitalia, and phenotypic patterns suggestive of a particular disorder (e.g., Down syndrome).

Investigations

X-ray for skeletal assessment

CT scan of internal organs

Chromosome analysis and genetic testing (consider this)

Management

Consult a medical geneticist. The specific diagnosis and pattern of inheritance (either the known pattern for a particular disorder or the observed pattern in the family history) are important for discussion of recurrence risk. Refer the family for genetic counseling, for any specialized medical care needed, and for family support.

POINTER

Indicators of genetic conditions

Dysmorphic features, multiple anomalies, unexplained neurocognitive impairment, and/or a family history of recurrent or unexplained disorders all suggest the presence of genetic conditions. Remember to perform a full examination, including imaging, even if there is an obvious abnormality.

GENETIC DISORDERS

Family planning and genetic disorders

Differential diagnosis

CHROMOSOMAL ABNORMALITIES (E.G., ANEUPLOIDY, REARRANGEMENTS)

Autosomal anomalies (e.g., Down syndrome) are more common than sex-linked anomalies (e.g., Klinefelter syndrome, Turner syndrome).

Chromosomal abnormalities are either numerical or structural. Numerical abnormalities involve an extra chromosome (trisomy; e.g., Down syndrome, Klinefelter syndrome) or a missing chromosome (monosomy; e.g., Turner syndrome). Structural abnormalities involve translocations, or deletions and duplications, of genetic material.

Risk factors:

Down syndrome: older maternal age; other children with Down syndrome

Klinefelter syndrome, Turner syndrome: none known

Investigations: noninvasive prenatal screening; US; amniocentesis; chorionic villus sampling

SINGLE-GENE ABNORMALITIES

Mendelian (e.g., autosomal dominant)

Examples include Huntington disease, Marfan syndrome, neurofibromatosis type 1, Charcot-Marie-Tooth disease type 1, and familial Mediterranean fever.

Risk factors: family history

Either parent can transmit the mutation. A parent with an autosomal dominant disease has a 50% chance of transmitting the mutation to their children.

Children of either sex can be affected. Children who do not inherit the disorder do not have the mutation.

Ethnicity is a risk factor for some entities, including familial Mediterranean fever, which is more common among people of Mediterranean descent (e.g., Turkish, Greek, north African, Italian, Arab).

Nonmendelian (e.g., mitochondrial, epigenetic)

MITOCHONDRIAL

Examples include Leber hereditary optic neuropathy; myoclonic epilepsy with ragged red fibers; and MELAS.

Risk factors: mothers with mitochondrial disorders

Only females can transmit mitochondrial mutations.

Children of either sex can be affected. Children who inherit the mutation may be phenotypically normal.

EPIGENETIC

These are environmental factors that modify genotype-phenotype correlations in monogenic (single gene mutation) and complex diseases.

Risk factors: smoking; alcohol use; obesity; asbestos exposure; carcinogenic exposures (e.g., sun tanning, radon)

PRENATAL EXPOSURE

Drugs or toxins (e.g., fetal alcohol spectrum disorder)

FETAL ALCOHOL SPECTRUM DISORDER

This results from maternal alcohol consumption during pregnancy. No safe limit of alcohol consumption is known, but it is known that the risk increases with consumption.

Signs and symptoms:

Pathognomonic dysmorphic features: small eye openings; thin upper lip; smooth philtrum; maxillary hypoplasia; small lower jaw; short upturned nose; flat nasal bridge; abnormal ear position or formation

Other features: growth deficits before and after birth (at birth: low weight; short length; head circumference ≤ tenth percentile); defects in the heart, kidneys, bones; deformities in the joints, limbs, extremities; neurobehavioral impairments

Infectious exposure (e.g., congenital rubella)

CONGENITAL RUBELLA INFECTION

This is rare in developed countries due to rubella vaccination programs. Cases in North America generally occur in families who have emigrated from countries without rubella vaccination programs.

Infection risks: fetal death in utero, preterm delivery, congenital defects

First trimester infection: high incidence of defects

Infection after 18 to 20 weeks gestation: little to no incidence of defects

Third trimester infection: fetal growth restriction

Infants with congenital rubella infection are asymptomatic at birth but develop manifestations over time.

Neonates: fetal growth restriction, meningoencephalitis, microcephaly, deafness or hearing impairment, infantile glaucoma, cataracts, retinopathy, cardiac defects (patent ductus arteriosus, pulmonary artery stenosis), hepatosplenomegaly, radiolucent bones

Infants and children: deafness (bilateral and sensorineural), cardiac and vascular anomalies, CHD, eye lesions, cataracts, CNS abnormalities (microencephaly)

Late manifestations: permanent hearing loss (bilateral, sensorineural); cataracts; glaucoma; pigmentary retinopathy; endocrine disorders (diabetes, thyroid disease); coronary, cerebral, and peripheral vascular diseases; immune deficiencies (hypogammaglobulinemia); learning disabilities; ataxia

Investigations: antibody titers (rubella-specific IgG and IgM in infants aged 6 to 12 months suggests chronic rubella infection); viral cultures (nasopharynx sample; urine; CSF; buffy coat from blood collection; conjunctiva sample)

Maternal disease (e.g., maternal diabetes)

MATERNAL DIABETES

The outcome for an infant (fetal, neonatal, and long-term complications) exposed to maternal diabetes depends on the mother's onset, duration, and severity of glucose intolerance and diabetes during pregnancy.

Fetal complications from first-trimester onset (including time of conception): diabetic embryopathy, congenital malformations (cardiovascular, CNS), spontaneous abortions; from second- and/or third-trimester onset: fetal hyperglycemia, hyperinsulinism, macrosomia

Neonatal complications: increased risk of prematurity, larger-than-average size, birth injury, respiratory distress, perinatal asphyxia, hypoglycemia, hypocalcemia, hyperbilirubinemia, cardiomyopathy

Long-term complications: increased risk of postnatal diabetes, obesity, impaired glucose metabolism; increased incidence of neuropsychiatric morbidity

FG

MULTIFACTORIAL CONDITION (E.G., NEURAL TUBE DEFECTS)

Neural tube defects

Types of defects include spina bifida (spine), anencephaly (brain), encephalocele (skull), and iniencephaly (neck).

Outcomes for infant: bladder and/or bowel dysfunction; partial or complete paralysis; deformities (weakness in the feet, hips, legs)

Maternal risk factors (gene-environment interaction): folate antimetabolites (e.g., methotrexate); diabetes; obesity; mycotoxins in contaminated cornmeal; arsenic; hyperthermia; radiation; smoking, secondhand smoke

Investigations: prenatal screening for AFP; US; amniocentesis; postnatal US, MRI, CT scan

Keys to patient encounter

Key concern

Recognize when an individual or population is at risk of a genetic or epigenetic condition.

History

Generally, genetic concerns arise in the context of patients who are planning to have children.

OBSTETRICAL HISTORY

Ask how many pregnancies the patient has had (or has fathered), and how many pregnancies ended in miscarriage. A history of repeated spontaneous abortions suggests genetic factors.

Ask whether the patient has children with health issues. Listen for issues that have hereditary characteristics.

PAST MEDICAL HISTORY

Ask about hereditary conditions (e.g., Marfan syndrome), diabetes, and conditions treated with folate antimetabolites (e.g., psoriasis, RA). In women, ask about rubella vaccination.

FAMILY HISTORY

Take a 3-generation family history of inherited disorders. Ask the patient who in their family has had an inherited disorder. Draw a 3-generation pedigree noting affected individuals. Pay particular attention to consanguinity. Ask about the ethnic origin of the family.

SOCIAL HISTORY

In women, ask about drug and alcohol use, and smoking (including exposure to secondhand smoke).

Physical exam

Physical exam does not generally provide useful information.

Investigations

Depending on the history, consider investigations for specific entities listed in the differential diagnosis, including:

Genetic testing

Karyotyping

Imaging studies

Management

In the context of a known hereditary disorder, provide genetic counseling and information on reproductive options (in the case of an already pregnant patient, this means evaluating the fetus with the possibility of terminating the pregnancy). In the context of suspected hereditary disorders, consider referral for specialized evaluation and genetic testing. For all patients, consider referral to community resources, and for social and psychological support services.

POINTER

Inheritance patterns of common genetic disorders

Autosomal dominant: Huntington disease, polycystic kidney disease, Marfan syndrome

Autosomal recessive: CF, sickle cell disease Tay-Sachs disease

Multifactorial: heart disease, diabetes, most cancers, alcoholism, obesity, mental illness, Alzheimer disease

Chromosome disorders: Down syndrome (trisomy 21), Prader-Willi syndrome (absence or nonexpression of a group of genes on chromosome 15), chronic myeloid leukemia (translocation 9;22)

GERIATRIC PRESENTATIONS

Falls

Differential diagnosis

FALLS IN GENERAL

Recurrent falls are defined as more than 2 falls in a 6-month period.

MEDICAL CONDITIONS (E.G., VERTIGO, GAIT DISTURBANCES, SYNCOPE)

Vertigo

Signs and symptoms: positive Dix-Hallpike maneuver (this suggests benign positional vertigo); recent viral or bacterial infection (this suggests peripheral vestibulopathy); recurrent episodes of vertigo, hearing loss, tinnitus, or aural fullness (this suggests Ménière disease); use of aminoglycosides; facial weakness, and ear or mastoid pain (this suggests acoustic neuroma)

Gait disturbances

Signs and symptoms: poor balance; ataxia; antalgic gait; Trendelenburg sign; waddling; knee failing to lock; toe scuffing with steps; spastic gait; high stepping, stamping; decreased stride length; festinating gait (this is a symptom of Parkinson disease); impaired braking and acceleration (stumbling, lurching, staggering, slow pace, wide base, reeling); veering gait; cautious gait; difficulty initiating or maintaining gait

Syncope

Signs and symptoms: fainting; use of antihypertensives; history of cardiovascular condition (arrhythmia, aortic stenosis, MI), carotid artery disease, stroke, hypoglycemia, panic attacks

PSYCHIATRIC CONDITIONS (E.G., COGNITIVE IMPAIRMENT, SUBSTANCE ABUSE)

Cognitive impairment

Causes include Parkinson disease, Huntington disease, paraneoplastic syndrome, dementia (Alzheimer disease, frontotemporal dementia, vascular dementia, Lewy body dementia), depression, delirium, sleep disorders, infection (e.g., prion disease, HIV, chronic meningitis), chronic brain injury, medications (anticholinergics, antihistamines), metabolic conditions (vitamin B_{12} deficiency, hypothyroidism, hypoglycemia), SDH, tumor, and normal pressure hydrocephalus.

Substance abuse

Examples include abuse of cocaine, heroin, alcohol, amphetamines, and prescription medications (opioids, sedatives, stimulants).

Signs and symptoms: personal or family history of substance abuse; excessive worry; loss of interest in friends and usual activities; adverse experience (e.g., emotional, physical, or sexual abuse; death of a friend or family member); physical evidence (track marks on the arms, nasal septum perforation); tachycardia; tremor and/or sweating

MEDICATIONS

Examples include antipsychotics, anticonvulsants, benzodiazepines, narcotics, opioids with codeine, TCAs, diuretics, SSRIs, and antihypertensives.

Polypharmacy (> 4 medications) increases the risk of complications such as falls.

ENVIRONMENTAL OR BEHAVIORAL FACTORS (E.G., WALKING SURFACES, CHOICE OF FOOTWEAR)

Examples include loose area rugs or frayed carpets; slippery floors; uneven walking surfaces; stairs, especially if steep or shallow; poor lighting; footwear that is too large, unstable, or damaged; walking in stockings or bare feet, instead of in shoes; lack of grab bars or railings; and unfamiliar environments.

OTHER CONTRIBUTORS (E.G., DECREASED VISION, URINARY URGENCY)

Decreased vision

Signs and symptoms: falls while walking or doing routine tasks (often); use of multifocal lenses; decreased visual acuity, depth perception, contrast sensitivity

Urinary urgency

Signs and symptoms: frequent or urgent urination; difficult or painful urination; hematuria; incontinence; fever (this suggests UTI)

History of recurrent or recent UTI; atrophic urethritis; vaginitis; prostate enlargement; use of pharmaceuticals (diuretics, benzodiazepines, alcohol, caffeine); endocrine disorders (e.g., hypercalcemia, diabetes mellitus); restricted mobility; stool impaction

Investigations: urinalysis to detect WBCs, nitrites; urine culture

Keys to patient encounter

Key concerns

Identify patients who are at risk of falling.

Identify contributing factors.

Formulate a prevention plan.

History

HISTORY OF PRESENT ILLNESS

Ask what the patient was doing before they fell, where the fall occurred, what injuries the patient sustained, how many times the patient has fallen in the past, and how similar the circumstances of this fall were to previous falls. Ask about specific risk factors for falls (see the pointer).

If a caregiver is present and saw the fall, ask for details.

PAST MEDICAL HISTORY
Ask about chronic or acute illnesses.

MEDICATIONS
Ask about drugs associated with an increased risk of falls (antidepressants, sedatives, anticholinergic drugs, hypoglycemic agents, benzodiazepines, antihypertensive drugs, corticosteroids) and polypharmacy (more than 4 prescription medications).

POINTER

Risk factors for falls in the elderly

Older than 75
Housebound
Cane or walker use
Falling in the past
Polypharmacy
Living alone
Vision impairment
Cognitive impairment
Physical disability
Difficulty rising from a chair

SOCIAL HISTORY
Ask about alcohol and illicit drug use, and about environmental risk factors for falls at home (e.g., poor lighting; unsafe stairways; loose floor mats; irregular or slippery floor surfaces; lack of grab bars for toilets and tubs).

Physical exam

Perform a full physical exam, with particular emphasis on the following:

Vital signs: Measure the patient's BP sitting and standing to look for postural hypotension.

Mental status: Consider using a mini–mental status exam; otherwise, check for orientation to person, place, and time.

Vision

Neurological: Assess for vertigo, balance, and strength.

Feet: Assess for sensation.

Investigations

Specific lab and imaging studies do not usually contribute information useful to diagnosing or managing the cause of falls.

Management

Multifactorial interventions are effective in preventing falls.

Treat any identified underlying conditions. Consider scheduling a home visit, which can be helpful in identifying and modifying environmental factors. Consider referring the patient to a falls clinic, if available, and for a geriatric medicine evaluation. Always consider patient safety and the feasibility of the patient continuing in their current living conditions.

GERIATRIC PRESENTATIONS

Frailty in the elderly

Differential diagnosis

MEDICATIONS

Signs and symptoms: poor adherence to current medications, recent dose changes, sensitivity to adverse effects of medications

ENVIRONMENTAL OR SOCIAL FACTORS (E.G., ISOLATION, POVERTY, ELDER ABUSE, NEGLECT)

Isolation, poverty

Signs and symptoms: living alone; lack of family or social supports; restricted income

Elder abuse, neglect

Signs and symptoms: disclosed abuse (physical, sexual, psychological, financial, neglect); resistance by a caregiver to having the patient interviewed alone (usual); fear of the patient towards a caregiver; isolation; depression; unexplained changes in financial situation; bruising, scars, healed fractures; poor hygiene; sudden weight loss, malnutrition

Note: victims do not always disclose abuse.

Risk factors:

Victim: female; advanced age (especially older than 80); vulnerability due to a chronic disorder, functional impairment, or cognitive impairment

Perpetrator: substance abuse, psychiatric disorder, history of violence, cohabitation, dependence on the elderly person for support

MEDICAL DISEASE

Always consider illnesses that are more likely to occur at the extremes of age among vulnerable populations. For example, seniors living in isolation and poverty are at risk for HUS, which may be overlooked because it is often considered a pediatric condition.

Common medical conditions associated with frailty include depression, malignancy, rheumatic disease, cardiovascular disease, endocrine disease, renal insufficiency, hematological disease, nutritional deficiency, and neurological disease.

Signs and symptoms (in general): weight loss; fatigue; weakness; reduced physical activity and walking pace; increased burden of symptoms; reduced ability to adapt to or recover from medical interventions

Investigations: CBC, creatinine, electrolytes, ALT, AST, GGT, ALP, PT/INR, bilirubin; albumin, vitamin B_{12}, thyrotropin (TSH), urinalysis

MALNUTRITION (E.G., FROM POOR DENTITION, MALABSORPTION, DYSPHAGIA)

Poor dentition

Signs and symptoms: missing teeth, dental caries, swollen gums

Malabsorption

Signs and symptoms: diarrhea; steatorrhea; weight loss despite adequate food intake; fatigue; edema; easy bruising, bleeding; pathological fractures; anorexia; flatulence; abdominal distention

History of PUD, bowel resection, alcohol abuse, autoimmune conditions

Investigations: low electrolytes, calcium, and magnesium; prolonged PT/INR; low triglycerides, cholesterol; low vitamin B_{12}, ferritin, folic acid; hypoalbuminemia; elevated CRP (this suggests an inflammatory condition)

Dysphagia

Several medical conditions at the end of life can contribute to dysphagia (e.g., patients with end-stage COPD may have profound weakness, which impairs the coordination of breathing and swallowing).

Symptoms: choking on fluid intake; prolonged mealtime; nasal regurgitation; difficulty initiating swallowing; dry mouth; solids getting stuck in the throat; drooling; regurgitation after swallowing; painful swallowing; recurrent pneumonia; abnormalities of cranial nerves V, VII, IX, X, XII

History of malignancy of upper GI tract and brain; progressive neurological disorders (e.g., ALS, Parkinson disease, MS, dementia); cerebrovascular event

Investigations: barium swallow, esophagogastroduodenoscopy

PSYCHIATRIC CONDITION (E.G., MILD COGNITIVE IMPAIRMENT, DEMENTIA, DEPRESSION, PSYCHOSIS)

Major or mild neurocognitive disorder

Signs and symptoms: gradual impairment of ≥ 1 cognitive areas (complex attention; executive function; learning and memory; language; perceptual-motor skills; social interaction); **no** evidence that the cognitive impairment occurs only with delirium; **no** evidence of depression

Mild cognitive impairment: deficits that **do not** significantly interfere with day-to-day life

Major cognitive impairment (dementia): deficits that interfere with day-to-day life (e.g., ability to pay bills)

Major depressive disorder[1(pp160–161)]

Signs and symptoms: symptoms that are present most of the time for ≥ 2 weeks; symptoms with significant impact on day-to-day life

Key symptoms: depressed mood and/or loss of interest in usual activities

Other symptoms: significant weight change; sleep disturbance; slowed or agitated mental processes; loss of concentration; recurrent thoughts of death or suicide

Risk factors: family history of mental health disorders (depression, anxiety, suicide); personal history of other mental health disorders; substance abuse; chronic illness (e.g., cancer, stroke, chronic pain)

Psychosis

Schizophrenia is the most common primary disorder associated with psychosis, but it is very uncommon as a new disorder in the elderly. Psychotic symptoms in the elderly are more likely caused by delirium, dementia, or drug-induced depression.

CHANGES IN VISUAL ACUITY

CHANGES IN AUDITORY ACUITY

DECREASED MOBILITY

Causes include history of falls; lower extremity weakness; underlying cognitive impairment; balance problems; polypharmacy,

FG

particularly psychotropic medication; pain (e.g., osteoarthritis, lumbar radiculopathy); history of stroke; orthostatic symptoms; anemia; and dizziness.

Keys to patient encounter

Key concerns

Assess the patient's level of function and cognition.

Manage with a multidisciplinary approach.

History

HISTORY OF PRESENT ILLNESS

Ask about friends and family whom the patient sees regularly, the patient's financial situation, and their use of alcohol. Listen for evidence of social isolation, poverty, and alcohol abuse. Ask about elder abuse.

Ask about unintended weight loss, and for details of the patient's usual diet, looking for malnutrition.

Ask if the patient needs help with ADLs and whether the patient is still driving.

PAST MEDICAL HISTORY

Ask about chronic illnesses and psychiatric conditions.

MEDICATIONS

Ask about drugs associated with an increased risk of falls (antidepressants, sedatives, anticholinergic drugs, hypoglycemic agents, benzodiazepines, antihypertensive drugs, corticosteroids) and polypharmacy (more than 4 prescription medications).

> **POINTER**
>
> **Risk factors for frailty**
>
> Older age
> Polypharmacy
> Alcohol abuse
> Poverty
> Social isolation
> Unintended weight loss (> 5 kg in the past year)
> Chronic medical conditions
> Psychiatric conditions

Physical exam

Perform a full physical exam, with particular emphasis on the following:

Vital signs

Mental status: Consider using a mini–mental status exam; otherwise, check for orientation to person, place, and time.

Mouth: Look for dental problems such as missing teeth, dental caries, and swollen gums.

Gait-speed test: Ask the patient to walk 12 feet (4 meters); a completion time longer than 5 seconds suggests frailty.

Chair-stand test: Ask the patient to stand up from a chair, walk 3 meters, turn around, walk back to the chair, and sit down; a completion time longer than 10 seconds suggests frailty.

Investigations

CBC

Electrolytes

Creatinine

OTHER SPECIFIC INVESTIGATIONS

Order additional investigations to assess the status of any acute or chronic conditions. These conditions and tests commonly include:

Rheumatic disease: serum autoantibodies of rheumatoid factors and/or anticitrullinated peptide/protein antibodies; thrombocytosis; ESR (note that ESR values increase with increasing age); CRP

Cardiovascular disease: lipids (see *Notes on labs and assessments*)

Endocrine disease: fasting blood glucose or HbA_{1c}, and thyrotropin (TSH)

Hematological disease: serum ferritin and iron levels, and folate level

Management

Consider referring the patient to home care and community care agencies, if self-care, including nutrition, is an issue. Consider referring the patient for a geriatric medicine evaluation.

Discuss health goals with the patient, including their desire for CPR. If this is not desired, provide the patient with a form or letter stating "no CPR (do not resuscitate)," and tell family and caregivers about its location.

Refer the patient for counseling if there are financial concerns. Report abuse to adult protection services or the police.

Consider steps to prevent falls (e.g., modifying medications; recommending proper footwear, walking aids, and grab bars in the bathroom).

Consider referring the patient for a road safety test if driving competency is an issue.

REFERENCE

1. American Psychiatric Association. Diagnostic and statistical manual of mental disorders. 5th ed. Arlington, VA: American Psychiatric Association; 2013. 991 p.

GLUCOSE ABNORMALITIES

Diabetes mellitus

Differential diagnosis

TYPE 1 DIABETES MELLITUS

Autoimmunity

Signs and symptoms: family history of type 1 diabetes, autoimmune disease; age 4 to 14 years (peak incidence); polydipsia; polyuria; new-onset bed wetting; extreme hunger; weight loss; blurry vision; vaginal yeast infection

Investigations: blood tests (elevated glucose; HbA_{1c}); urine tests (glucose and ketones)

TYPE 2 DIABETES MELLITUS

Obesity

Signs and symptoms: BMI ≥ 30 (see *Notes on labs and assessments*); family history of type 2 diabetes, obesity; polydipsia; polyuria; fatigue

Investigations: blood and urine tests to detect indicators of metabolic disorder associated with obesity (lipid profile, uric acid, liver enzymes); HbA_{1c}

Other (e.g., genetic predisposition, medications)

GENETIC PREDISPOSITION

Signs and symptoms: family history of type 2 diabetes; African, Hispanic, First Nations, Asian descent; personal history of polycystic ovary syndrome

MEDICATIONS

These include medications to reduce cardiovascular risks (thiazide diuretics, beta-blockers, statins); glucocorticoids; antipsychotics (clozapine, olanzapine, risperidone); and protease inhibitors, which are part of HAART.

GESTATIONAL DIABETES MELLITUS

Gestational diabetes involves the onset of glucose intolerance during pregnancy.

Signs and symptoms: usually asymptomatic (it is detected by routine screening during pregnancy)

Risk factors: aged 35 or older; family history of type 2 diabetes; previous gestational diabetes; previous baby > 4.1 kg at birth; history of unexplained stillbirth; obesity; African, Hispanic, First Nations, or Asian descent; history of prediabetes; polycystic ovary syndrome; use of corticosteroids

Investigations: oral glucose challenge, oral glucose tolerance test

FG

Keys to patient encounter

Key concerns

Pay particular attention to early detection of disease.

Recognize medical emergencies (acute hypoglycemia, diabetic ketoacidosis, hyperosmolar nonketotic coma).

History

PATIENTS WITHOUT A DIABETES DIAGNOSIS

Use the FINDRISC tool to direct the history, which is widely used to assess patients' risk of diabetes. It stratifies patients into risk groups and informs the frequency of recommended screening.

PATIENTS WITH KNOWN DIABETES

Ask about sweating, nausea, tremulousness, palpitations, headache, blurred or double vision, anxiety, confusion, seizures, and difficulty speaking (these symptoms indicate hypoglycemia).

In type 1 diabetics, ask about concurrent illness (pneumonia, UTI) and missed insulin treatments (relevant to diabetic ketoacidosis).

In type 2 diabetics, ask about acute febrile illness or infection (especially pneumonia and UTI); and altered consciousness, focal or generalized seizures, and transient hemiplegia (these symptoms suggest nonketotic hyperosmolar syndrome). Obtain a complete medical history and medication history, and ask about compliance with diabetic medications.

Physical exam

Vital signs: Look for dehydration and fever.

Weight: Calculate the patient's BMI (see *Notes on labs and assessments*).

Full physical:

- Look especially for sources of infection and diabetic complications (neuropathy, retinopathy).
- Look for Kussmaul respirations (rapid and deep breathing to compensate for metabolic acidosis) in patients with possible diabetic ketoacidosis.

Investigations

Testing has 4 purposes: 1) assess glycemic status, 2) detect intercurrent disease (infection), 3) detect acute complications, and 4) detect long-term complications (end organ damage).

Glycemic status: serum glucose or HbA_{1c}

Infection: CBC, CRP, chest x-ray, urinalysis

Acute complications: ABG, electrolytes (see *Notes on labs and assessments*), serum ketone, serum osmolality

End organ damage: creatinine and urine protein (nephropathy); electrocardiogram and serum lipid levels (cardiovascular risk and damage)

Management

Manage any acute conditions (diabetic ketoacidosis, nonketotic hyperosmolar syndrome, hypoglycemia); admit these patients to hospital and treat any underlying causes (e.g., infection).

The first-line management for newly diagnosed type 2 diabetes involves diet modification, regular exercise, and weight reduction. If these steps prove ineffective, or in patients with pronounced lack of glycemic control, consider medical therapy. First-line oral therapy is metformin; second-line agents depend on the presence of CVD. In the event of metabolic decompensation, insulin is the first-line therapy.

Counsel the patient regarding the long-term risk and prevention of complications: heart disease, vascular disease, peripheral neuropathy (including erectile dysfunction), nephropathy, eye damage (potentially blindness), infection (e.g., in feet due to poor circulation), and pregnancy complications (eclampsia, pre-eclampsia, birth defects). Discuss management of other risk factors (hypertension, smoking, sedentary lifestyle, hyperlipidemia).

GLUCOSE ABNORMALITIES

Hypoglycemia, hyperglycemia

Differential diagnosis

GLUCOSE ABNORMALITIES IN GENERAL

The common clinical problem is diabetes mellitus.

HYPOGLYCEMIA

The most common cause is diabetes treatment.

Signs and symptoms: palpitations, pallor, sweating, nightmares, fatigue, hunger

> Severe: confusion, disorientation, blurred vision, seizures, coma

Investigations: low plasma glucose (symptoms typically develop at concentrations ≤ 54 mg/dL [3.0 mmol/L])

Postprandial

Signs and symptoms: symptom onset after meals

Fasting

SECONDARY TO MEDICATION (E.G., SULFONYLUREAS)

Sulfonylurea use has a high risk of hypoglycemia (symptomatic within 2 hours of ingestion). Insulin therapy can also lead to hypoglycemia.

SECONDARY TO IMPAIRED GLUCOSE PRODUCTION (E.G., ADRENAL INSUFFICIENCY)

Signs and symptoms: symptoms that develop slowly (often over several months); hyperpigmentation; fatigue; weight loss; dizziness; muscle and/or joint pain; salt craving

Investigations: fasting plasma glucose; serum sodium, potassium, cortisol; ACTH stimulation test (artificial stimulation of the adrenal gland) to determine adrenal gland function; CT scan of the adrenal gland

HYPERGLYCEMIA

HYPERGLYCEMIA IN GENERAL

Signs and symptoms: often asymptomatic

> Mild to moderate: polydipsia, polyuria, weight loss, hunger, blurred vision, fatigue, weakness, unconsciousness
>
> Severe (e.g., diabetic ketoacidosis): abdominal pain, coma, dehydration, hypokalemia, hypotension, lethargy, metabolic acidosis, Kussmaul respiration, fruity breath

Investigations: high blood glucose levels (> 300 mg/dL [16.7 mmol/L] is a medical emergency); high anion gap, low pH, low HCO_3^-, elevated ketones (in diabetic ketoacidosis); high serum osmolality

Diabetes mellitus

Signs and symptoms: personal or family history of diabetes; history of diabetic complications and/or inadequate monitoring; polydipsia, polyuria, and/or weight loss

Presence of diabetes on screening: fasting glucose or HbA_{1c}

Endocrine condition

DIABETES MELLITUS (COMMON) — SEE ABOVE

HYPERCORTISOLISM (CUSHING DISEASE)

Signs and symptoms: history of glucocorticoid therapy; cushingoid features (round, red face; pronounced abdominal weight; hump on the upper back; thin arms and legs; hypertension; stretch marks; acne)

Investigations: high cortisol levels on either a 24-hour urine cortisol test or dexamethasone suppression test

Drug-induced condition (e.g., steroids)

This includes medications to reduce cardiovascular risks (thiazide diuretics, beta-blockers, statins); glucocorticoids; antipsychotics (clozapine, olanzapine, risperidone); and protease inhibitors, which are part of HAART.

Keys to patient encounter

Key concerns

Manage emergent situations.

Prevent complications.

History

HISTORY OF PRESENT ILLNESS

Mild hyperglycemia is usually occult, but symptoms can be present with long-standing diabetes or with high sugars.

Autonomic symptoms of hypoglycemia occur below about 59 mg/dL (3.3 mmol/L) and can include sweating, nausea, anxiety, tremulousness, palpitations, hunger, and paresthesias. Neurologic symptoms occur below about 50 mg/dL (2.8 mmol/L) and can include headache, blurred or double vision, confusion, difficulty speaking, seizures, and coma.

In patients with hypoglycemia, ask about the timing of symptom onset in relation to meals.

In patients with hyperglycemia, ask about increased thirst and a dry mouth, fatigue, increased urination, blurred vision, recurrent infections, and unintentional weight loss.

PAST MEDICAL HISTORY

Ask about diabetes, CNS tumors, adrenal disease, hepatic failure, chronic infection, and, in women, gestational diabetes.

MEDICATIONS

Ask about insulin, oral hypoglycemic agents, beta-blockers, disopyramide, and antibiotics.

FAMILY HISTORY

Ask about diabetes.

SOCIAL HISTORY

Ask about diet and exercise.

Physical exam

Vital signs: Look for tachycardia and hypotension (relevant to dehydration).

Mental status: Assess for confusion by asking about orientation to person, place, and time.

Height and weight:

- Calculate the patient's BMI (see *Notes on labs and assessments*).
- Measure the patient's waist circumference.

Neurological: Look for focal neurologic signs (these may occur in both hyperglycemia and hypoglycemia).

Dermatological:

- Examine the skin for poor skin turgor (relevant to dehydration), and infections or nonhealing ulcers (these suggest hyperglycemia).
- Look for signs of insulin resistance (acanthosis nigricans, skin tags).

Investigations

Glucose tolerance test in cases of impaired glucose tolerance

48-hour or 72-hour fast in unclear etiology of hypoglycemia (a 48-hour fast is usually sufficient for diagnosis; measure blood glucose at regular intervals and whenever symptoms occur)

C-peptide and serum insulin to distinguish endogenous (pancreatic production of insulin) from factitious hypoglycemia

OTHER SPECIFIC INVESTIGATIONS

Consider other investigations as warranted by the history and physical exam.

Management

Hyperglycemia is managed the same way as diabetes mellitus.

The main task in hypoglycemia is to distinguish between true hypoglycemia, pseudohypoglycemia, artifactual hypoglycemia, and factitious hypoglycemia (see the pointer). Pseudohypoglycemia is demonstrated by a normal blood glucose level during symptoms. Artifactual hypoglycemia can be confirmed by repeating the test. Factitious hypoglycemia secondary to insulin use can be confirmed by looking at C-peptide and serum insulin levels: exogenous insulin use results in a low C-peptide level and a high level of insulin. Symptoms within 2 to 3 hours after eating suggest hyperinsulinemia.

POINTER

Types of hypoglycemia

Pseudohypoglycemia: This involves symptoms of hypoglycemia (e.g., palpitations, sweating, fatigue, hunger) **without** abnormal glucose levels.

- In addition to pseudohypoglycemia, many people with actual low glucose levels have no symptoms.

Artifactual hypoglycemia: This is a lab error caused by allowing whole blood to stand too long before separation (glucose metabolism continues in the blood tube).

Factitious hypoglycemia: This is hypoglycemia caused by taking insulin or another hypoglycemic drug (this can be intentional or due to improper dosing).

FG

GYNECOLOGICAL PRESENTATIONS

Amenorrhea, oligomenorrhea

Differential diagnosis

PRIMARY

Definition: absence of menstruation (i.e., menstruation has not started) in girls age 15 or older, with or without the appearance of other signs of puberty

Central

HYPOTHALAMUS (E.G., FUNCTIONAL)

FUNCTIONAL HYPOTHALAMIC AMENORRHEA

Causes include stress; weight loss (e.g., dieting) or being underweight (e.g., anorexia nervosa); and excessive exercise (e.g., training for a sport).

PITUITARY

PROLACTINOMA

This is the most common type of functioning pituitary tumor.

Signs and symptoms (microprolactinoma):

- General: galactorrhea; clinical signs of estrogen deficiency (vaginal dryness, painful intercourse, decreased bone density in the lower spine and forearm)
- Reproductive-age women: menstrual disturbance (oligomenorrhea, amenorrhea, irregularity) and/or infertility
- Younger women: delayed menarche
- Prepubertal females: hyperprolactinemia

Signs and symptoms (macroprolactinoma): headaches when stretching; vision problems (bitemporal hemianopsia)

Investigations: elevated serum prolactin (> 20 ng/mL [20 μg/L]); MRI of the head to detect mass in the sella turcica

Ovary (e.g., ovarian dysgenesis, polycystic ovary syndrome)

OVARIAN DYSGENESIS

An example is congenital lack of ovaries.

POLYCYSTIC OVARY SYNDROME

Signs and symptoms: symptom onset after puberty, with increased rate of hair growth and male-pattern hair growth; irregular menstruation; infertility; obesity; acne

Investigations: LH:FSH ratio (elevated: 2:1 or 3:1) (usual); elevated testosterone; US to detect ovarian cysts; normal prolactin levels; normal thyroid function

Vaginal, outflow tract (e.g., imperforate hymen)

IMPERFORATE HYMEN

This is a structural abnormality of the vagina preventing visible menstrual bleeding by blocking the outflow of blood, without changes in hormone levels or impairment in the development of sexual characteristics.

Signs and symptoms: feeling of fullness in the lower abdomen; pelvic, abdominal, back pain

Investigations: pelvic US

SECONDARY

Definition: absence of menstruation (sudden cessation) for ≥ 6 months in women who have otherwise experienced normal menstrual cycles

Pregnancy

This is the most common cause.

Signs and symptoms: amenorrhea, especially during childbearing years (some experience spotting); sexual activity, especially without contraception or with inconsistent use of contraception; nausea, vomiting (common early sign); breast enlargement and tenderness; increased frequency of urination without pain or difficulty; fatigue

Investigations: blood or urine β-HCG

Central

HYPOTHALAMUS (E.G., FUNCTIONAL, EXOGENOUS HORMONES)

FUNCTIONAL HYPOTHALAMIC AMENORRHEA—SEE ABOVE

EXOGENOUS HORMONES

An example is glucocorticoid therapy.

PITUITARY (E.G., PROLACTINOMA)

PROLACTINOMA—SEE ABOVE

Other endocrine condition (e.g., thyroid disorders)

THYROID DISORDERS

HYPOTHYROIDISM

Signs and symptoms: history of hypothyroidism or symptoms of hypothyroidism (cold intolerance, decreased reflexes, dry skin, weight gain, impaired cognition)

Investigations: elevated thyrotropin (TSH)

HYPERTHYROIDISM

Signs and symptoms: history of hyperthyroidism or symptoms of hyperthyroidism (changes in menstrual patterns, enlarged thyroid, tachycardia, palpitations, diarrhea, muscle weakness, tremor, hyperactive reflexes, weight loss, sweating, thinning hair)

Investigations: decreased thyrotropin (TSH)

Ovary (e.g., oophorectomy, chemotherapy)

Uterus (e.g., Asherman syndrome)

ASHERMAN SYNDROME

This is scarring of the endometrial or myometrial layers of the uterine wall, preventing the normal buildup and shedding of the uterine lining.

Signs and symptoms: history of uterine surgery (e.g., dilation and curettage; cesarean section; treatment for uterine fibroids)

Investigations: US of the pelvis; hysteroscopy

Keys to patient encounter

Key concerns

Rule out pregnancy first.

In amenorrhea, differentiate between primary and secondary conditions.

History

HISTORY OF PRESENT ILLNESS

Ask when the patient's last period was and how regular their menstrual cycle is.

Ask about other symptoms. Examples of characteristic symptoms include:

Hyperthyroidism: enlarged thyroid, weight loss, palpitations

Hypothyroidism: dry skin, weight gain, impaired cognition

Prolactinoma: vaginal dryness, galactorrhea

Ask about recent weight changes and changes in exercise routines.

SURGICAL AND PROCEDURAL HISTORY

Ask about gynecological procedures and surgeries (e.g., dilation and curettage, cesarean section, treatment for uterine fibroids, oophorectomy).

MEDICATIONS

Ask about glucocorticoid therapy and chemotherapy.

Physical exam

Height and weight: Calculate the patient's BMI (see *Notes on labs and assessments*).

General inspection: Look for hirsutism, acne, and acanthosis nigricans (hyperpigmentation that is often found in the armpits, groin, and folds of the neck).

Pelvic exam: Look for uterine masses.

Investigations

β-HCG

IF THE PATIENT IS NOT PREGNANT

Thyrotropin (TSH)

LH

FSH

Estradiol

Testosterone

Serum prolactin and an MRI of the head to evaluate the pituitary gland (consider this)

Pelvic US or CT scan (consider this)

Management

Manage any underlying conditions. Consider referral to an endocrinologist or gynecologist. The approach to treatment of functional hypothalamic amenorrhea includes medical, dietary, and mental health support.

GYNECOLOGICAL PRESENTATIONS

Dysmenorrhea

Differential diagnosis

PRIMARY/IDIOPATHIC (NO PELVIC ABNORMALITY)

Primary dysmenorrhea involves no underlying medical condition, and no identifiable uterine or pelvic cause.

Signs and symptoms: constant, throbbing, dull or intense pain in the lower abdomen that radiates to the back and thighs, usually just before or during menstruation

SECONDARY (ACQUIRED) (E.G., INFECTION, ENDOMETRIOSIS, ADNEXAL ABNORMALITIES)

Infection (pelvic inflammatory disease)

Signs and symptoms: lower abdominal and pelvic pain; pain during intercourse; fever; urinary symptoms; vaginal discharge; irregular menstruation; pelvic tenderness and pain associated with 1 or both adnexa

History of gonorrhea, chlamydia, or risk factors for them (multiple partners, unprotected sex); IUD; childbirth; gynecologic procedure

Investigations: cultures for gonorrhea and chlamydia; US (this has normal findings)

Endometriosis

Signs and symptoms: pelvic pain associated with menstruation (very common); excessive bleeding during menstruation; pain during intercourse; pain during urination or bowel movements; tenderness on pelvic exam; normal findings on abdominal exam (common)

Risk factors: family history of endometriosis; nulliparity; personal history of PID

Investigations: US to detect ovarian cysts (common finding); laparoscopy with biopsy

Adnexal abnormalities

OVARIAN CANCER

Signs and symptoms: postmenopausal female (more common); asymptomatic in early stage (usual); abdominal bloating, discomfort, distention (ascites); ovarian or pelvic mass; frequent urination and urge to urinate; abnormal vaginal bleeding; fatigue; GI symptoms (nausea, heartburn, diarrhea, constipation, early satiety); shortness of breath

Investigations: transvaginal and abdominal US; CA 125; pelvic or abdominal CT scan; analysis of ascitic fluid; biopsy

Keys to patient encounter

Key concern

Differentiate primary from secondary dysmenorrhea.

History

HISTORY OF PRESENT ILLNESS

Ask how closely the pain coincides with menstruation or bleeding, and what the pain is like. Ask about associated symptoms. Examples of characteristic features include:

Primary dysmenorrhea: pain that radiates to the thighs

Endometriosis: heavy menstruation

Infection: fever and/or vaginal discharge

Ovarian cancer: GI symptoms

PAST MEDICAL HISTORY

Ask whether the patient has given birth (this is relevant to endometriosis). Ask about risk factors for PID (history of STIs, IUD use, multiple sexual partners, gynecological procedures).

FAMILY HISTORY

Ask about endometriosis.

Physical exam

Pelvic exam: Look for pelvic tenderness and pelvic masses, to exclude possible causes of secondary dysmenorrhea.

Investigations

β-HCG

Pap smear

Cultures for gonorrhea and chlamydia

Endometrial biopsy

Pelvic US to exclude uterine and ovarian masses

POINTER

Incidence of dysmenorrhea

Among gynecological disorders, dysmenorrhea is the most common disorder, regardless of age or ethnicity. It affects up to 95% of women.

Management

Consider referral to a gynecologist. Start management with analgesics and NSAIDs, which are effective in up to 70% of women. Consider prescribing OCs. Some alternative therapies (heat, thiamine, magnesium, vitamin E) may be beneficial for some women.

GYNECOLOGICAL PRESENTATIONS

Menopause

Differential diagnosis

Menopause usually occurs around age 50. It is marked by the last period a woman has: 1 year after the last period the woman is considered "postmenopausal."

Keys to patient encounter

Key concerns

Educate patients about menopause.

Manage the undesirable effects of menopause.

History

HISTORY OF PRESENT ILLNESS

Ask when the patient's last period was and how old the patient is. Ask about the patient's symptoms. Typical symptoms of menopause include vaginal dryness, chills, hot flashes, night sweats, sleep disturbance, weight gain, and irritability.

Ask about possible symptoms of hypothyroidism, which can mimic menopause (e.g., dry skin, weight gain, impaired cognition).

FAMILY HISTORY

Ask about the age of menopause in the patient's mother and sisters.

Investigations

Investigations are usually not indicated. In uncertain diagnosis, consider:

FSH

Estrogen (estradiol)

Thyrotropin (TSH)

Management

Patient education is a key first step. Menopausal hormone therapy (MHT) is the most effective therapy for vasomotor symptoms and urogenital atrophy, and as such may improve both sexuality and overall quality of life. However, MHT should always be combined with the lifestyle strategies discussed below.

Mild vasomotor symptoms (hot flashes) may be managed with lifestyle strategies alone, including:

- healthy diet
- regular exercise
- light clothes, cool ambient temperatures
- quitting smoking
- avoiding alcohol

Hormone therapy should be recommended to women with early menopause (before age 45).

The decision to initiate hormone therapy depends on the individual, taking into account the patient's preferences and expectations, need for disease prevention, personal and family history, and severity of symptoms. Women without a uterus can be prescribed systemic estrogen-alone therapy. Women with a uterus can be prescribed combined systemic estrogen and progestogen therapy, or a tissue-selective estrogen complex (conjugated equine estrogens and bazedoxifene).

The decision to continue hormone therapy should be reexamined annually, but there is no mandatory limitation on the duration of therapy. However, in general, the initiation of hormone therapy should occur before age 60 or no later than 10 years past menopause.

GYNECOLOGICAL PRESENTATIONS

Premenstrual dysphoric disorder (premenstrual syndrome)

Indicators[1(pp171–172)]

Signs and symptoms: symptoms synchronous with the menstrual cycle (present in the week before menstruation, improving during menstruation, resolved in the week after menstruation); symptoms during most menstrual cycles for ≥ 1 year; symptoms with significant impact on day-to-day life

- Key symptoms: mood swings, irritability, depressed mood, anxiety
- Other symptoms: loss of interest in usual activities; loss of concentration; fatigue; changes in eating and sleeping routines; a sense of loss of control; physical symptoms (e.g., breast tenderness; joint or muscle pain; "bloating" or weight gain)
- **No** evidence of thyroid disorder, anemia, or exacerbation of a preexisting mental disorder (e.g., major depressive disorder)

Keys to patient encounter

Key concern

Differentiate premenstrual dysphoric disorder from normal premenstrual symptoms, or from other causes of physical and mood changes.

History

Determine if the patient's symptoms are cyclical. Ask the patient to complete a symptom diary if there is uncertainty about the timing of symptoms.

Ask about symptoms of major depressive disorder (e.g., mood symptoms that persist for 2 or more weeks, significant weight change, recurrent thoughts of death or suicide) and risk factors for major depressive disorder (e.g., family history of depression, anxiety, and/or suicide; personal history of substance abuse).

Physical exam

Physical exam does not usually contribute useful information for diagnosing or managing premenstrual dysphoric disorder.

Investigations

Hypothyroidism and anemia may have similar symptoms to premenstrual dysphoric disorder. Exclusion of these conditions is key.

CBC

Thyrotropin (TSH)

Management

Counsel the patient on lifestyle modifications (diet, exercise, stress reduction). Consider prescribing OCs to suppress ovulation. Consider an SSRI to help manage symptoms.

REFERENCE

1. American Psychiatric Association. Diagnostic and statistical manual of mental disorders. 5th ed. Arlington, VA: American Psychiatric Association; 2013. 59–60. 991 p.

GYNECOLOGICAL PRESENTATIONS

Uterine prolapse, pelvic relaxation

Differential diagnosis

UTERINE PROLAPSE, PELVIC RELAXATION IN GENERAL

Signs and symptoms: feeling of heaviness or pressure in the area of the vagina; feeling that the uterus, bladder, or rectum is dropping out; problems with urination (urinary incontinence, urinary retention) or with bowel movements; pelvic organs or small intestine that drop down and protrude into the vagina (or outside the body with severe symptoms); symptoms that occur when upright, straining, or coughing; symptoms that disappear when lying down or relaxing

Prolapsed rectum (rectocele): difficult bowel movements and constipation (women may be unable to empty their bowels completely)

Prolapsed small intestine (enterocele): generally asymptomatic; feeling of fullness, pressure, or pain in the pelvis or lower back

Prolapsed bladder (cystocele): coincident prolapsed urethra (urethrocele) (usual); stress incontinence (e.g., passage of urine during coughing, laughing); overflow incontinence (passage of urine when bladder becomes too full); urinary retention; problems with completely voiding the bladder; UTI; urge incontinence (an intense, irrepressible urge to urinate, resulting in passage of urine)

Prolapsed uterus: uterus that bulges into the upper part of the vagina, or into the opening of the vagina, or partly through the opening, or all the way through the opening (total uterine prolapse); often asymptomatic; pain in the lower back or over the tailbone (total uterine prolapse can cause pain during walking, difficulty with bowel movements; sores may develop on the protruding cervix and cause bleeding, discharge, and infection; possible uterine kink may hide urinary incontinence or make urinating painful)

Risk factors: multiple pregnancies and deliveries; obesity; advanced age

DAMAGE TO VAGINA AND PELVIC FLOOR SYSTEM: VAGINAL BIRTH, PRIOR PELVIC SURGERY, CHRONIC INCREASE IN INTRAABDOMINAL PRESSURE (E.G., CHRONIC COUGH)

Risk factors: multiple pregnancies and deliveries; prolonged labor; bearing down before full dilation; forceful delivery of the placenta

NEUROGENIC DYSFUNCTION OF PELVIC FLOOR

Signs and symptoms: personal or family history of neurologic disease or related conditions; abnormalities in speech or gross motor function; sensory abnormalities of the lumbosacral dermatomes on exam for light and sharp touch (performed with a small cotton swab and a sharp point)

Risk factors: spina bifida, diabetic neuropathy

CONNECTIVE TISSUE DISEASE

Signs and symptoms: personal or family history of connective tissue disease (e.g., Ehlers-Danlos syndrome, Sjögren syndrome)

GENETIC PREDISPOSITION

Signs and symptoms: family history of pelvic prolapse

Keys to patient encounter

History

HISTORY OF PRESENT ILLNESS

Ask about symptoms consistent with uterine prolapse or pelvic relaxation (e.g., problems with urination, feeling that pelvic organs are dropping out).

PAST MEDICAL HISTORY

Ask how many children the patient has, and about the method of delivery and birth weight for each child. Ask about spina bifida, diabetes, and connective tissue disease.

FAMILY HISTORY

Ask about pelvic prolapse.

Physical exam

Pelvic: To make abnormalities more obvious, ask the patient to stand with 1 foot on a stool, and to cough or bear down.

Investigations

Investigations do not usually contribute useful information for diagnosing or managing uterine prolapse or pelvic relaxation.

Management

Discuss the benefits and limitations of treatment options (these include pelvic floor exercises, pessary, or surgery). Refer the patient to a gynecologist or, if appropriate, for surgery.

GYNECOLOGICAL PRESENTATIONS

Vaginal bleeding: excessive, irregular, abnormal

Differential diagnosis

PREMENARCHAL CONDITION (E.G., TRAUMA, SEXUAL ABUSE)

Trauma

Most vaginal trauma in girls is unintentional and due to blunt, nonpenetrating, minor vaginal injuries that commonly occur in car accidents, falls in the bathroom at home, and accidents from bicycles, the playground, or swimming pool.

Penetrating injuries that lacerate the vaginal wall can cause life-threatening hemorrhage. Causes of these injuries include: high pressure water jets from water slides or fountains; water- or jet-skiing accidents; and intercourse.

Child sexual abuse

Signs and symptoms: disclosed abuse (victims do not always disclose abuse); resistance by the parent or caregiver to having the child interviewed alone (usual); coexisting signs of physical or emotional abuse (bruising, scars, healed fractures; developmental delay and/or behavioral problems)

Risk factors: history of substance abuse by the parents or caregiver; unstable living situation of the parents or caregiver; dysfunctional domestic dynamics

PREMENOPAUSAL CONDITION

Ovulatory condition

INTERMENSTRUAL CONDITION (E.G., ORAL CONTRACEPTIVES, BENIGN GROWTHS)

ORAL CONTRACEPTIVES

Symptoms differ by type of OC:

- Progestin-only: irregular uterine bleeding or amenorrhea
- Estrogen-progestin: unscheduled bleeding, especially in the first 3 months of use

BENIGN GROWTHS (E.G., LEIOMYOMA, ADENOMYOSIS, CERVICAL POLYPS)

LEIOMYOMA

This is the most common pelvic tumor in women (usually in reproductive-age women).

Signs and symptoms: commonly asymptomatic; premenopausal (usual); heavy or prolonged menstrual bleeding; pelvic, abdominal pressure; pain on intercourse; urinary symptoms (incontinence; frequent urination; difficulty emptying the bladder); constipation; pelvic mass or enlarged, irregular uterus on bimanual palpation

Risk factors: family history of leiomyoma; African descent

Investigations: US to detect mass ≥ 1 cm in diameter

ADENOMYOSIS

This is often diagnosed by microscopic examination of the uterus at the time of hysterectomy.

Signs and symptoms: asymptomatic (often: a third of cases); parity (more common than nulliparity); heavy and prolonged menstrual bleeding; dysmenorrhea; enlarged uterus; pelvic pain

Investigations: US and MRI (T2) (this is increasingly used for clinical decision making)

CERVICAL POLYPS

Signs and symptoms: older than 40 (common); if symptomatic, bleeding and excessive discharge

Investigations: histology (cervical polyps rarely become malignant, but this should be confirmed)

MENORRHAGIA

Signs and symptoms: change from a woman's normal menstrual cycle that interferes with her quality of life; pain during menstruation; containment problems; anemia (fatigue, pallor, dizziness, shortness of breath, tachycardia)

Investigations: CBC with platelets; tests for coagulation disorders (rare); thyrotropin (TSH); transvaginal or transabdominal US; endometrial biopsy

NEOPLASMS OR COAGULATION DISORDERS

NEOPLASMS—SEE BELOW

COAGULATION DISORDERS

Signs and symptoms: use of anticoagulants; easy bruising or bleeding

OTHER (E.G., ENDOMETRITIS, HYPOTHYROIDISM)

ENDOMETRITIS

Signs and symptoms: pelvic pain associated with menstruation (very common); excessive bleeding during menstruation; pain during intercourse; pain during urination or bowel movements

Risk factors: family history of endometriosis; nulliparity; personal history of PID; tenderness on pelvic exam; normal findings on abdominal exam (common)

Investigations: US to detect ovarian cysts (common finding); laparoscopy with biopsy

HYPOTHYROIDISM

Signs and symptoms: history of hypothyroidism or symptoms of hypothyroidism (cold intolerance, decreased reflexes, dry skin, weight gain, impaired cognition)

Investigations: elevated thyrotropin (TSH)

Anovulatory condition

AGE-RELATED ENDOCRINE OR METABOLIC CONDITION (E.G., THYROID)

HYPOTHYROIDISM—SEE ABOVE

HYPERTHYROIDISM

Signs and symptoms: changes in menstrual patterns; history of hyperthyroidism or symptoms of hyperthyroidism (weight loss, tremor, weakness, diarrhea)

Investigations: decreased thyrotropin (TSH)

NEOPLASM (E.G., PROLACTINOMA, OVARIAN TUMOR)

PROLACTINOMA

This is a benign tumor.

Signs and symptoms of microprolactinoma:

- General: galactorrhea; clinical signs of estrogen deficiency (vaginal dryness, painful intercourse, decreased bone density in the lower spine and forearm)
- Reproductive-age women: menstrual disturbance (oligomenorrhea, amenorrhea, irregularity) and/or infertility
- Younger women: delayed menarche
- Prepubertal females: hyperprolactinemia

Signs and symptoms of macroprolactinoma: headaches when stretching, vision problems (bitemporal hemianopsia)

Investigations: elevated serum prolactin (> 20 ng/mL [20 μg/L]); MRI of the head to detect mass in the sella turcica

OVARIAN TUMOR

Signs and symptoms: child, adolescent, or postmenopausal female (usual); asymptomatic in early stage (usual); abdominal bloating, discomfort, distention (ascites); ovarian or pelvic mass; urinary urgency, frequency; abnormal vaginal bleeding; fatigue; GI symptoms (nausea, heart burn, diarrhea, constipation, early satiety); shortness of breath

Investigations: transvaginal and abdominal US; CA 125; pelvic or abdominal CT scan; analysis of ascitic fluid; biopsy

OTHER (E.G., POLYCYSTIC OVARY SYNDROME; WEIGHT LOSS, EXERCISE, OR STRESS; STRUCTURAL DISEASE)

POLYCYSTIC OVARY SYNDROME

Signs and symptoms: symptom onset after puberty, with increased rate of hair growth and male-pattern hair growth; irregular menstruation; infertility; obesity; acne

Investigations: LH:FSH ratio (elevated: 2:1 or 3:1) (usual); elevated testosterone; US to detect ovarian cysts; normal prolactin levels; normal thyroid function

WEIGHT LOSS, EXERCISE, OR STRESS

Signs and symptoms: history of recent weight loss, prolonged exercise, or personal stress (e.g., death of a friend or family member, divorce, job loss)

STRUCTURAL DISEASE

ENDOMETRIAL POLYPS

Signs and symptoms: intermenstrual bleeding in premenopausal women, usually light; incidence increases with age

FG

Pregnancy-related condition

FIRST TRIMESTER BLEEDING

SPONTANEOUS ABORTION

Signs and symptoms: uterine bleeding, from spotting to heavy bleeding; pelvic pain (severe or dull cramping); uterus that is small for gestational age of the fetus

Risk factors: maternal age; family history of genetic disorders; medication, drug, or substance use; low folate level; high maternal BMI (see *Notes on labs and assessments*); maternal fever, celiac disease, previous miscarriages

Investigations: decrease in β-HCG by at least 21%

ECTOPIC PREGNANCY

Signs and symptoms: symptoms of pregnancy and/or positive pregnancy test; pelvic pain; vaginal bleeding; painful intercourse; shoulder pain; palpable tubal mass; pelvic tenderness and pain associated with 1 or both adnexa

Severe symptom: syncope

Risk factors: previous ectopic pregnancy, PID, pregnancy during IUD use

Investigations (pathognomonic): β-HCG above discriminatory zone (> 1500–2000 mIU/mL [1500–2000 IU/L]) **with** transvaginal US findings of a lack of intrauterine gestational sac, complex (mixed solid and cystic) masses in the adnexa, and free fluid in the cul-de-sac

IMPLANTATION

Signs and symptoms: spotting or minimal bleeding 10 to 14 days after fertilization

PATHOLOGY OF THE CERVIX, VAGINA, OR UTERUS—SEE NEOPLASM, STRUCTURAL DISEASE, GENITAL TRACT DISEASE

SECOND AND THIRD TRIMESTER BLEEDING

This is not as common as first trimester bleeding.

PLACENTA PREVIA

Signs and symptoms: bleeding before or after 20 weeks gestation (any time in the second half of the pregnancy); uterine contractions without abdominal pain, but with vaginal bleeding

Investigations: US

ABRUPTIO PLACENTAE

Signs and symptoms: symptom onset before 20 weeks gestation; bleeding, cramping, placental separation

Investigations note: US not helpful

POSTMENOPAUSAL DISORDER: STRUCTURAL, SYSTEMIC

Genital tract disease (excluding trauma)

ENDOMETRIAL POLYPS—SEE ABOVE

VAGINAL ATROPHY

Signs and symptoms: light bleeding or spotting; vaginal epithelium that is pale, dry, shiny, smooth; patchy erythema, petechiae, bleeding, discharge (if there is inflammation)

ENDOMETRIAL HYPERPLASIA OR CARCINOMA

Signs and symptoms: spotting or heavier bleeding

Endometrial hyperplasia: uterus not enlarged

Endometrial carcinoma: pelvic mass, uterus possibly enlarged

Investigations: biopsy

Neoplastic systemic disease

LEUKEMIA

Signs and symptoms: fever; chills; persistent fatigue and weakness; frequent or severe infections; weight loss; pallor; swollen lymph nodes; enlarged liver or spleen; easy bleeding and bruising; recurrent nosebleeds; petechiae; excessive sweating; bone pain or tenderness

Investigations: CBC; peripheral blood smear; flow cytometry; bone marrow aspiration and biopsy

LYMPHOMA

Signs and symptoms (non-Hodgkin): constitutional symptoms (fatigue, fever, night sweats, weight loss), enlarged lymph nodes, chest pain, coughing, shortness of breath

Hodgkin lymphoma (less common): constitutional symptoms (fatigue, fever, night sweats, weight loss); enlarged lymph nodes; itching or pain on drinking alcohol, or increased sensitivity to alcohol

Investigations: blasts or cancer cells on peripheral blood smear; excess blasts or cancer cells on bone marrow examination

METASTATIC CANCER

Signs and symptoms: history of cancer; constitutional symptoms (weight loss, fever, night sweats)

Investigations: CBC with differential; platelet count; ESR; CT scan; tissue biopsy or fine needle aspiration biopsy for histology/cytology and immunophenotyping

FG

Drugs (e.g., hormone replacement therapy, anticoagulants)

Keys to patient encounter

Airway and hemodynamic status

Because the patient may be actively bleeding, check the patient's ABCs. Look in particular for hypotension and tachycardia. In unstable patients, establish large bore IV access and provide fluid resuscitation.

History

The differential diagnosis is extensive for this clinical presentation. Ask open-ended questions and listen for information that will help narrow the possibilities: What is the bleeding like? When did it start? When does it occur? What are your periods usually like? What medical conditions do you have? What medications do you take?

In a woman of childbearing age, ask whether she could be pregnant.

Physical exam

Pelvic:

- Note that pelvic exam is contraindicated in some circumstances (e.g., placenta previa).
- Look for enlarged or tender uterus and adnexa.

Investigations

β-HCG

CBC

Thyrotropin (TSH) in suspected thyroid disease

Urgent US in pregnant patients

Other specific investigations as indicated (see the differential diagnosis)

Management

Management depends on the specific diagnosis. Some patients will require referral to an obstetrician-gynecologist.

GYNECOLOGICAL PRESENTATIONS

Vaginal discharge, vulvar pruritus

Differential diagnosis

PHYSIOLOGIC DISCHARGE AND CERVICAL MUCOUS PRODUCTION

This discharge is caused by pregnancy, puerperium, lactation, premenstrual changes, ovulation, sexual excitement, OCs, and emotional stress.

GENITAL TRACT INFECTIONS (BACTERIAL VAGINOSIS, YEAST, SEXUALLY TRANSMITTED INFECTION)

Bacterial vaginosis

Signs and symptoms: often asymptomatic; foul vaginal odor; mild to moderate increase in vaginal discharge (homogenous, thin, gray, white, green); vulvar pruritus

Risk factors: unprotected sex with multiple partners or new partners; frequent douching; natural lack of *Lactobacillus*; recent antibiotic use

Investigations: vaginal pH $\geq$ 4.5; saline smear to detect clue cells

Yeast: vulvovaginal candidiasis

Signs and symptoms: thick, white, clumpy ("curd-like") vaginal discharge; vulvar pruritus, burning, soreness; thrush patches loosely adherent to the vulva; erythema and edema of the vestibule, labia majora, labia minora

Risk factors: diabetes; pregnancy; estrogen therapy; recent antibiotic use; contraceptive devices; immunosuppression

Investigations: normal vaginal pH (4–4.5); wet-mount test of discharge with potassium hydroxide preparation to detect yeast

Sexually transmitted infection

STIs include chlamydia and gonorrhea (very common), syphilis, HPV, HIV, HBV, HCV, and trichomonas.

Signs and symptoms (symptoms vary with the specific STI): often asymptomatic; vaginal or urethral discharge; ulcerative or nonulcerative genital disease; pelvic pain

Risk factors: unprotected sex with multiple or new partners; sex-trade work or sexual contact with sex workers; age 15 to 24; prior STIs

GENITAL TRACT INFLAMMATIONS (E.G., IRRITANTS)

Irritants

Signs and symptoms: vulvar pruritus; erythema

Risk factors: use of scented panty liners, pads, soaps, lotions, detergents, bubble baths; use of douches, spermicides, certain topical drugs (e.g., povidone-iodine)

Keys to patient encounter

Key concern

Distinguish STIs from other causes.

History

Establish the likely phase of the patient's menstrual cycle, and whether the patient may be pregnant.

Ask about symptoms. Examples of characteristic symptoms include:

Bacterial infection: foul odor and thin grey, white, or green discharge

Yeast infection: clumpy discharge with itching

STI: pelvic pain and/or genital ulcers

Ask about factors that make the symptoms better and worse, such as possible irritants.

Ask about risk factors for STI: unprotected sex with multiple partners or new partners; working in the sex trade; sexual contact with sex workers; age 15 to 24; and prior STIs.

Physical exam

Abdominal: Look for tenderness.

Pelvic:

- Perform a bimanual exam and a speculum exam for adnexal or uterine tenderness.
- Look for skin or mucosal abnormalities, and discharge.

Investigations

In practice, the diagnosis of bacterial vaginosis, yeast infection, and trichomonas is usually done together with swabs, rather than with pH and wet mount or potassium hydroxide (KOH) smears.

Yeast

Bacteria

IN PATIENTS WITH RISK FACTORS FOR STI

Gonorrhea

Chlamydia

HIV

HBV antibody

HCV antibody

Management

Positive gonorrhea and chlamydia tests require specific antibiotic treatment and reporting to public health authorities. Treat yeast infections with oral or intravaginal antifungals. Treat bacterial vaginosis with intravaginal antibiotics. In the case of chemical irritants, the treatment is to avoid the causative agent.

HAIR PRESENTATIONS

Hair presentations

Differential diagnosis

ALOPECIA

Scarring

Common causes include lichen planopilaris, chronic cutaneous lupus erythematosus, central centrifugal cicatricial alopecia, acne keloidalis nuchae, and dissecting cellulitis.

Signs and symptoms: onset during young adulthood (more common); absence of pores within the area of hair loss (sometimes magnification is needed to see this); history of skin disease, SLE, or autoimmune disease (possible)

Lichen planopilaris: itching scalp; lesions showing most inflammation at the center

Cutaneous lupus erythematosus: lesions showing most inflammation at the edges

Central centrifugal cicatricial alopecia, acne keloidalis nuchae, dissecting cellulitis: African descent

Investigations: microscopic examination of individual hairs for follicle damage; scalp biopsy

Nonscarring

ANDROGENIC ALOPECIA

This is a common form of alopecia.

Signs and symptoms: gradual-onset hair loss

Male-pattern hair loss: receding hairline, bald spots

Female-pattern hair loss: thinning hair over the crown of the head

ALOPECIA AREATA

This is a common form of alopecia.

Signs and symptoms: loss of hair in patches on the head or other parts of the body (e.g., beard); "exclamation point" hairs (short, broken-off hairs at the edge of bald patches); recovery within a year in mild cases; several episodes in a lifetime, with the first episode before age 30 (common); pitting of nails

Alopecia totalis (this is a type of alopecia areata): loss of all hair of the scalp; loss of eyebrows and eyelashes (often)

Risk factors: family history of alopecia areata

Cooccuring conditions: vitiligo; thyroiditis; pernicious anemia (due to vitamin B_{12} deficiency)

TELOGEN EFFLUVIUM (LOSS OF MATURE HAIR) DUE TO ACUTE ILLNESS OR SURGERY

Signs and symptoms: hair loss that occurs 3 to 4 months after an acute illness or surgery, and that decreases over 6 to 8 months (this is usually a temporary condition); diffuse hair loss

ANAGEN EFFLUVIUM (LOSS OF GROWING HAIR) DUE TO CHEMOTHERAPY

Chemotherapy drugs target fast-growing cells like cancer and hair. Hair regrowth starts 3 to 6 months after the cessation of chemotherapy. Regrowing hair may have a different texture or color at first.

Signs and symptoms: hair loss all over the body (e.g., the scalp, eyelashes, eyebrows, armpit hair, pubic hair) that begins 2 to 4 weeks after chemotherapy

TRICHOTILLOMANIA[1(p251)]

Signs and symptoms: visible hair loss from recurrent plucking or pulling (common sites are the head, eyebrows, eyelashes); repeated attempts to stop the behavior; symptoms with significant impact on day-to-day life

TINEA CAPITIS

This is a contagious fungal infection of the scalp and hair shafts.

Signs and symptoms: bald patches on the scalp that are itchy and scaly; contagious contacts (the infection is most common in toddlers and school children)

Investigations: potassium hydroxide wet mount of plucked hairs or scalp scrapings

HIRSUTISM

HIRSUTISM IN GENERAL

Signs and symptoms:

Women (more common than men): male-pattern hair growth of terminal body hair in androgen-stimulated areas (i.e., face, chest, areolae)

Men: excessive growth of terminal body hair in androgen-stimulated areas

Familial condition (no endocrine disorder)

Signs and symptoms: women of South Asian or Mediterranean descent (more common); symptom onset in puberty; normal rate of hair growth; **no** evidence of irregular menstruation or elevated serum testosterone

Androgen excess

ANDROGEN EXCESS IN GENERAL

Signs and symptoms: voice changes, increased libido, irregular menstruation, odorous perspiration, acne, clitoromegaly, increased muscle mass, temporal hair recession and balding, loss of normal female body shape

Investigations: elevated DHEA-S levels, elevated serum testosterone

POLYCYSTIC OVARY SYNDROME

Signs and symptoms: symptom onset after puberty, with increased rate of hair growth and male-pattern hair growth; irregular menstruation; infertility; obesity; acne

Investigations: elevated LH:FSH ratio (2:1 or 3:1) (usual); elevated testosterone; US to detect ovarian cysts; normal prolactin levels; normal thyroid function

OVARIAN TUMOR (ARRHENOBLASTOMA)

Signs and symptoms: abrupt-onset symptoms (often); hirsutism; virilization (e.g., clitoromegaly, increased muscle mass, temporal hair recession and balding, loss of normal female body shape); palpable ovarian mass

Investigations: suppressed LH and FSH levels; elevated androgen levels; CT scan or US of the pelvis

HYPERTRICHOSIS

HYPERTRICHOSIS IN GENERAL

Signs and symptoms (in men and women): excessive hair growth in nonandrogen-stimulated areas

Idiopathic

Signs and symptoms: diffuse increase in vellus hair growth

Investigations: normal serum androgen levels

Drugs (e.g., phenytoin, minoxidil)

Examples include phenytoin, minoxidil, cyclosporine hydrocortisone, and psoralens.

Systemic illness

HYPOTHYROIDISM

Signs and symptoms: history of hypothyroidism or symptoms of hypothyroidism (cold intolerance, decreased reflexes, dry skin, weight gain, impaired cognition)

Investigations: elevated thyrotropin (TSH)

ANOREXIA NERVOSA[1(pp338–339)]

Signs and symptoms: significantly low body weight; intense fear of gaining weight or persistent behavior that interferes with gaining weight; excessive focus on body weight or shape in self-evaluation, or persistent lack of recognition of current low body weight

Keys to patient encounter

Key concern

Determine the underlying cause of the condition and identify secondary causes requiring treatment.

History

HISTORY OF PRESENT ILLNESS

Ask when the patient's concerns about hair loss or growth started, and what the patient has noticed.

Examples of characteristic features include:

Androgenic alopecia: gradual-onset thinning with receding hairline (men) or thinning hair (women)

Alopecia areata: recent-onset patchy loss of head or beard hair

Tinea capitis: bald, itchy spots on the scalp

Ovarian tumor: sudden-onset male-pattern hair growth

In women, ask about menstrual irregularities and amenorrhea (these suggest androgen excess, including polycystic ovary syndrome).

Ask about a family history of hair loss (this is common in androgenic alopecia), and about ethnicity.

Ask about recent extreme stresses (surgery, severe illness, emotional crisis, pregnancy) that might precipitate telogen effluvium.

PAST MEDICAL HISTORY

Ask about skin disease, SLE, autoimmune disease, hypothyroidism, and psychiatric disorders.

MEDICATIONS

Ask about cortisone, penicillamine, psoralens, phenytoin, diazoxide, minoxidil, and cyclosporine.

H

Physical exam

Perform a full physical exam (including a pelvic exam in women) with particular attention to:

Dermatological:

- Identify the pattern of hair growth or loss.
- Note if it is localized or generalized.

Investigations

WOMEN

Thyrotropin (TSH) in hypertrichosis or hair loss

CBC in hair loss to assess for anemia

Vitamin D in hair loss to assess for low levels

HIRSUTE WOMEN

Tests for polycystic ovarian syndrome (see the differential diagnosis)

Tests for congenital adrenal hyperplasia

LOCALIZED HAIR LOSS (EITHER SEX)

Skin biopsy

Management

Treatment of hypertrichosis and hirsutism is directed at the underlying cause. Hyperandrogenic hirsutism may be treated with cyproterone acetate and spironolactone. Other options include bleaching agents, depilatory creams, shaving, waxing, and electrolysis.

Treatments for androgenic alopecia include hair transplantation, and topical minoxidil or oral finasteride. Note that medications for androgenic alopecia are only effective during the time the patient is taking the medication.

Reassure patients with telogen effluvium that spontaneous regrowth will occur over a period of 2 to 3 months.

In cases of scarring alopecia or where the diagnosis is uncertain, refer the patient to a dermatologist.

REFERENCE

1. American Psychiatric Association. Diagnostic and statistical manual of mental disorders. 5th ed. Arlington, VA: American Psychiatric Association; 2013. 991 p.

HEADACHE

Headache

Differential diagnosis

PRIMARY HEADACHE (E.G., MIGRAINE, CHRONIC DAILY HEADACHE WITH MEDICATION OVERUSE)

Migraine

Signs and symptoms: symptom onset in childhood or adolescence; known triggers for symptoms (e.g., light, weather changes, certain foods)

Prodrome: irritability, hyperactivity, depression, food craving

Aura: visual disturbances, vision loss, pins-and-needles sensations, aphasia, limb weakness

Attack: light-headedness; nausea, vomiting; light sensitivity; bilateral or unilateral pulsating or throbbing head pain

Chronic daily headache with medication overuse

Definition, chronic daily headache: headaches for ≥ 15 days a month for ≥ 3 months

Signs and symptoms: history of headaches; regular, daily, or clustered headaches, including headaches with migraine symptoms; routinely taking analgesics ≥ 2 days per week or ≥ 9 days per month

SECONDARY HEADACHE

Associated with vascular disorders (e.g., severe arterial hypertension)

SEVERE ARTERIAL HYPERTENSION

Signs and symptoms (hypertensive crisis): systolic BP ≥ 180 mmHg and/or diastolic BP ≥ 120 mmHg; family history of hypertension; renal conditions; diabetes; adrenal or thyroid conditions; vascular conditions; catecholamine excess; obstructive sleep apnea

Risk factors: lack of exercise, high-sodium diet, obesity

Associated with nonvascular disorders (e.g., intracranial infection)

INTRACRANIAL INFECTION

Signs and symptoms: triad of fever, neck stiffness, and altered mental status

History of infectious contacts (viral, bacterial, or fungal meningitis; or viral, bacterial, or fungal encephalitis); HIV or immunosuppression (this suggests abscesses, toxoplasmosis)

Investigations: MRI, CT scan; CSF analysis to detect abnormal cells or infection

Other (e.g., systemic viral infection, carbon monoxide exposure)

SYSTEMIC VIRAL INFECTION

Signs and symptoms: fever; malaise; myalgia or diffuse pain; respiratory symptoms; joint pain; dehydration on physical examination (skin turgor, sunken eyes, sunken fontanelle in babies); **no** focal neurological symptoms

Investigations: CBC, viral serology, systemic inflammatory markers, endotoxin testing

CARBON MONOXIDE EXPOSURE

Signs and symptoms: dull headache, weakness, dizziness, nausea, vomiting, shortness of breath, confusion, blurred vision, loss of consciousness

History of indoor chemical or charcoal heater use; indoor portable generator use

Investigations: elevated serum carboxyhemoglobin

Keys to patient encounter

Key concern

Differentiate benign from potentially serious causes.

History

Pay particular attention to evidence of red flags (see the pointer), which indicate the need for neuroimaging or urgent referral.

HISTORY OF PRESENT ILLNESS

CURRENT HEADACHE

Ask when the current headache started, how severe it is, and how it compares to previous headaches. Ask about recent head trauma, and medical and dental procedures.

Ask about associated symptoms. Examples of characteristic symptoms include:

Intracranial infection: neck stiffness with sudden-onset first or worst headache

Viral infection: fever and myalgia
Carbon monoxide exposure: nausea and shortness of breath

HEADACHE PATTERN

Ask how often the patient gets headaches, what age the headaches started, and whether they have recently increased in frequency or severity. Ask what triggers the patient has noticed.

Examples of characteristic features include:

Migraine: childhood-onset recurrent headaches with triggers and prodromal symptoms
Medication-overuse headache: recent-onset daily headaches

PAST MEDICAL HISTORY

Ask about hypertension, renal conditions, diabetes, adrenal conditions, thyroid conditions, vascular conditions, and obstructive sleep apnea (relevant to hypertensive crisis), or conditions associated with immunosuppression (relevant to intracranial infection).

MEDICATIONS

Ask about the use of analgesics, looking for overuse.

Physical exam

Vital signs: Look for hypertension and fever.
Neurological exam
Eyes: Examine the retinas for papilledema.

Investigations

Noncontrast CT neuroimaging in patients with red flags (see the pointer) or headaches associated with systemic illness
LP in patients with red flags if neuroimaging is normal, except if contraindicated (see the pointer)

POINTER

Red flags in acute headache

Sudden onset of headache
New onset of headaches after age 50
Increased frequency or severity of headaches
Focal neurologic symptoms
Papilledema
Headache subsequent to head trauma

H

Management

Treat tension headaches occurring fewer than 15 times per month with as-needed analgesics: acetylsalicylic acid, acetaminophen, or NSAIDs. Do not prescribe opioids. Patients with more frequent headaches may respond to daily TCAs, avoidance of triggers, and lifestyle modifications (adequate sleep, exercise, and limiting alcohol and caffeine).

Medication-overuse headaches are treated by the supervised withdrawal of the overused medication and lifestyle changes. Cluster headaches are treated acutely with 100% oxygen. Triptans are the mainstay of treatment for migraine headaches, and may also be used for cluster headaches. Preventive treatment for cluster headaches may include verapamil or prednisone.

Refer patients without a diagnosis, or who do not respond to management, to a neurologist or headache clinic.

POINTER

Contraindications for lumbar puncture

Cellulitis near the LP site
Increased intracranial pressure
Uncorrected coagulopathy
Acute spinal cord trauma

HEARING PRESENTATIONS

Hearing loss

Differential diagnosis

CONDUCTIVE HEARING LOSS

External ear pathology

CONGENITAL DISORDER (E.G., ATRESIA)

CONGENITAL AURAL ATRESIA

Causes include prenatal infections; prenatal environmental exposure to ototoxic agents, including aminoglycoside medications; and maternal drug abuse.

Signs and symptoms: absence of auricle and partial external auditory meatus; recurrent otitis media, mastoiditis, or cholesteatoma

Associated abnormalities: other ENT congenital abnormalities, including the following syndromes: Goldenhar, Treacher, Down, Nager, CHARGE

Risk factors: family history of congenital abnormalities

INFLAMMATION OR INFECTION (E.G., OTITIS EXTERNA)

OTITIS EXTERNA

The most common cause is bacterial infection (90% of cases).

Signs and symptoms: ear pain; ear pruritus (this can occur with chronic infection; it is more common with fungal infection); discharge; hearing loss; feeling of fullness; pain with jaw movement; erythema of the external ear; pain on traction of the pinna or pressure on the tragus (these typically do not cause pain in acute otitis media); normal tympanic membrane on otoscopy; pain on otoscopy

Fungal infection: white, flakey debris

Risk factors: water exposure ("swimmer's ear"); use of ear devices (e.g., headphones, hearing aids); trauma (e.g., Q-tip use); dermatitis

OBSTRUCTION OF CANAL (E.G., WAX, FOREIGN BODY)

Signs and symptoms: hearing loss; ear pain; tinnitus; vertigo; feeling of fullness; history of recent mechanical cleaning of the ears (e.g., Q-tip use); possible visible trauma; foreign body or cerumen impaction on otoscopy

Middle ear pathology

CONGENITAL DISORDER

Signs and symptoms: recurrent otitis interna; tympanic membrane abnormalities; inner ear ossicular or cochleosaccular abnormalities

Associated abnormalities: other ENT congenital abnormalities such as congenital rubella syndrome and VACTERL syndrome; vascular abnormalities (e.g., internal carotid artery aneurysms, jugular bulb abnormalities)

Investigations: CT scan, MRI; audiology assessment

INFECTION (E.G., OTITIS MEDIA)

OTITIS MEDIA

Signs and symptoms; ear pain; fever; hearing loss; tympanic membrane that is erythematous and may be opaque, white, yellow, or green (typically; this demonstrates pus behind the tympanic membrane); ear discharge (this indicates perforation of the tympanic membrane); loss of bony landmarks; middle ear effusion with bulging or reduced mobility of the tympanic membrane on pneumatic otoscopy

Infants and toddlers: ear tugging, irritability, poor feeding, vomiting, diarrhea

Risk factors: URTI; allergic rhinitis; chronic rhinosinusitis; attendance at a day care (for children); contact with infectious illness; exposure to secondhand smoke; age (the condition peaks age 6 to 24 months)

OSSICULAR PATHOLOGY (E.G., OTOSCLEROSIS)

This is diagnosed via investigations (not clinically).

Investigations: CT scan, MRI (findings: absence of part or all ossicular bones; intratympanic muscle changes; facial nerve aberrant course); abnormalities on audiology assessment

TRAUMA (E.G., TYMPANIC MEMBRANE PERFORATION)

TYMPANIC MEMBRANE PERFORATION

Signs and symptoms: ear pain; clear, pus-filled, or bloody discharge from the ear; hearing loss; tinnitus; dizziness

History of otitis media infection; barotrauma or head trauma; acoustic trauma; foreign object in the ear (e.g., cotton swab)

Investigations: culture of discharge; tympanometry; audiology assessment

TUMOR (E.G., GLOMUS, VESTIBULAR NEUROMA)

Signs and symptoms (in general): gradual hearing loss; tinnitus; problems with balance, vertigo; facial numbness, tingling, and weakness; changes in taste perception; difficulty swallowing; hoarseness; headaches; clumsiness; confusion; family history of neurofibromatosis type 2; personal history of vascular malformations and/or hemangiomas

Investigations: CT scan, MRI; biopsy; audiology assessment

SENSORY-NEURAL HEARING LOSS

Acquired disorder (e.g., presbycusis, noise-induced hearing loss)

PRESBYCUSIS

Signs and symptoms: gradual bilateral hearing loss; loss of ability to hear high-pitched sounds; loss of ability to discern sounds or voices in noisy areas; tinnitus; dizziness

Risk factors: older than 50 (most common); chronic noise exposure; family history of presbycusis; use of ototoxic medication (e.g., high-dose aspirin); genetic syndrome; prenatal infection (toxoplasmosis, rubella, herpes); history of meningitis, mumps, measles, scarlet fever; Ménière disease

Investigations: positive Rinne and Weber tests for sensory-neural hearing loss

NOISE-INDUCED HEARING LOSS

Signs and symptoms: unilateral or bilateral hearing loss that is gradual or sudden (depending on the cause); tinnitus

Sudden loss: history of exposure to a sudden, loud noise (e.g., explosion, gunshots, jet engine)

Gradual loss: history of chronic exposure to loud noise from an occupation (e.g., machinery noise in construction, factory work, farming) or recreation (e.g., listening to loud music; snowmobiling; woodworking)

Investigations: positive Rinne and Weber tests for sensory-neural hearing loss

Congenital disorder (e.g., Alport syndrome)

Signs and symptoms (in general): hearing loss at birth or in childhood (often bilateral); no startle response to loud noise; speech delay; family history of hearing loss; hematuria; renal failure

Investigations: genetic testing

Sudden sensorineural hearing loss

This is an emergency situation: the patient must be assessed without delay. Most cases are idiopathic but prompt treatment with steroids may help prevent permanent hearing loss.

Signs and symptoms: acute sensorineural hearing loss, nearly always unilateral, that occurs within a 72-hour period

Keys to patient encounter

Key concerns

Differentiate conductive from sensory-neural hearing loss.

Counsel patients about preventing further hearing loss.

Identify hearing loss in infants as early as possible to prevent developmental delay.

History

HISTORY OF PRESENT ILLNESS

Ask when the hearing loss began, which ear is affected, and what symptoms are associated with the hearing loss.

Stay alert to evidence of unilateral, unexplained sensory-neural hearing loss that has occurred within the last 72 hours, because this is a medical emergency.

Examples of characteristic features include:

Gradual hearing loss: infection or trauma

Sudden-onset hearing loss: sudden sensorineural hearing loss or tumor

Bilateral hearing loss: presbycusis or congenital disorder

Otitis externa: ear pain, redness, itchiness, and discharge

Otitis media: ear pain and discharge with fever

Tumor: hearing loss with neurologic symptoms and headache

Ask about trauma to the ear or head, and exposure to a sudden loud noise (e.g., an explosion).

MEDICATIONS

Ask about aminoglycosides and high-dose aspirin.

SOCIAL HISTORY

Ask about occupational and recreational exposure to noise. In cases of chronic noise exposure, ask whether the patient wears ear protection.

Physical exam

Ears:

- Perform an otoscope exam looking for wax, obstructions, tumor, infection, effusion, discharge, and tympanic perforation.
- Perform Rinne and Weber tests.

Cranial nerves

Investigations

Audiogram

CT scan of the head in suspected vestibular neuroma

Management

Treat reversible causes. Consider referral to an ENT specialist. Counsel the patient about preventing further hearing loss.

Sudden sensory-neural hearing loss (acute unexplained hearing loss, nearly always unilateral, that occurs over less than a 72-hour period) is a medical emergency. These cases may have viral or autoimmune causes. Some evidence supports administering prednisolone 1 mg/kg/day to a maximum of 60 mg/day for 7 to 14 days. In general, offer the patient steroid treatment and discuss the case with an ENT specialist.

HEARING PRESENTATIONS

Tinnitus

Differential diagnosis

TINNITUS IN GENERAL

This is commonly a sign of hearing loss or cochlear injury.

Signs and symptoms: intermittent or continuous ringing or other sounds (buzzing, clicking) without an external source; variable apparent location of sounds (1 or both ears; within or around the head; distant)

EXTERNAL OR MIDDLE EAR (E.G., OTITIS, WAX)

Otitis media

Signs and symptoms: ear pain; fever; hearing loss with possible discharge from the ear

Otoscopy: tympanic membrane that is erythematous (typically) or opaque, white, yellow, or green (this indicates pus behind the tympanic membrane); loss of bony landmarks

Risk factors: URTI; allergic rhinitis; chronic rhinosinusitis; crowded living conditions; contact with infected persons; exposure to secondhand smoke; family history of otitis media

Children: attending a day care; bottle feeding or pacifier use; age 6 to 24 months

Wax

Signs and symptoms: hearing loss; pain; tinnitus; vertigo; feeling of fullness; history of recent mechanical cleaning of ears (e.g., Q-tip use); cerumen impaction on otoscopy

COCHLEAR-VESTIBULAR END ORGAN (E.G., MEDICATIONS, OTOSCLEROSIS, ENVIRONMENTAL EXPOSURE)

Medications

Common ototoxic medications include antibiotics (some: e.g., gentamicin), ACE inhibitors, antimalarial drugs, bismuth, CCBs, cisplatin, COX-2 inhibitors, local anesthetics, TCAs, valproic acid, and aspirin (in large amounts: tinnitus stops when aspirin intake stops).

Otosclerosis

Signs (on imaging): missing ossicular bones (part or all); intratympanic muscle changes; facial nerve aberrant course

Environmental exposure

Noise exposure can lead to temporary tinnitus, but long-term exposure can lead to permanent tinnitus.

Common exposures include workplace saws, drills, and machines, and portable music devices.

COCHLEAR NERVE (E.G., ACOUSTIC NEUROMA)

Acoustic neuroma

Signs and symptoms: ear or mastoid pain; facial weakness; dizziness or vertigo

BRAINSTEM OR CORTEX (E.G., ISCHEMIA, INFECTION)

Signs and symptoms (in general): history of stroke, trauma, MS, encephalitis

Keys to patient encounter

Key concern

Acknowledge the distress caused by this usually benign condition.

History

HISTORY OF PRESENT ILLNESS

Ask about constant versus intermittent symptoms, and about hearing loss, fever, pain, and vertigo.

Ask how the tinnitus is affecting the patient's daily life and mental health.

PAST MEDICAL HISTORY

Ask about trauma, stroke, MS, and encephalitis.

MEDICATIONS

Ask about ototoxic medications.

SOCIAL HISTORY

Ask about occupational noise exposure and use of portable music devices.

Physical exam

Ears, head, neck:

- Perform an otoscopy looking for infection and impacted wax.
- Examine the head and neck looking for mastoid pain (this suggests infection), and muscle weakness (this suggests acoustic neuroma or stroke).

Investigations

Audiogram

CT scan of the head if neurological symptoms are present

Management

Management depends on the etiology. If impacted earwax is present, removal can decrease symptoms. If an ototoxic medication is being taken, it should be discontinued or substituted.

For cases caused by hearing loss or without known cause, the use of noise suppression may help. Options include white noise machines, hearing aids, and masking devices.

Counseling and the use of TCAs (e.g. amitriptyline, nortriptyline) or anxiolytics may be useful in some patients.

HEMATOLOGICAL PRESENTATIONS

Abnormalities of white blood cells

Differential diagnosis

LEUKOCYTOSIS

LEUKOCYTOSIS IN GENERAL

Leukocytosis usually indicates infection or a nonmalignant etiology.

Reactive (e.g., bacterial infection, infectious mononucleosis)

BACTERIAL INFECTION

Signs and symptoms: WBCs > 10 000/μL (10×10^9/L); fever

MONONUCLEOSIS

Signs and symptoms (classic triad): fever, pharyngitis, lymphadenopathy (usually posterior cervical)

Additional signs and symptoms: fatigue and malaise; headache; abdominal pain; nausea, vomiting; rash; splenomegaly; palatal exanthems or petechiae

Investigations: CBC, lymphocytosis (> 50%); peripheral blood smear to detect atypical lymphocytes; heterophile antibody test (e.g., Monospot); EBV-specific serology testing (definitive)

Neoplastic (e.g., leukemia)

LEUKEMIA

Signs and symptoms: fever; chills; persistent fatigue and weakness; frequent or severe infections; weight loss; pallor; swollen lymph nodes; enlarged liver or spleen; easy bleeding and bruising; recurrent nosebleeds; petechiae; excessive sweating; bone pain or tenderness

Investigations: CBC; peripheral blood smear; flow cytometry; bone marrow aspiration and biopsy

LEUKOPENIA

Increased destruction (e.g., bacterial infection, HIV)

BACTERIAL INFECTION

Examples of bacterial infections include typhoid fever, rickettsia, brucellosis, and dengue fever.

Signs and symptoms: acute neutropenia; fever (this indicates serious infection), shaking chills, hypothermia; increased respiratory and heart rate

Rickettsia: history of insect bites or contact (ticks, fleas); characteristic rash or petechiae; sudden-onset fever, severe headache, malaise

HIV

HIV develops into AIDS when the CD4 cell count is < 200 cells/µL (0.2×10^9/L) (reference range of CD4: 500–2000 cells/µL [$0.5–2 \times 10^9$/L]).

Signs and symptoms: flu-like symptoms in the first, acute phase; leukopenia in the second, latent, asymptomatic stage (200–499 CD4 cells/µL [$0.2–0.499 \times 10^9$/L]); lymphadenopathy

AIDS: recurrent, severe opportunistic infections or malignancies

Risk factors: unprotected sex; IV drug use

Investigations: positive HIV-1 p24 antigen in the blood followed by HIV antibody testing (positive ELISA result); PCR to determine HIV RNA level or viral load

Decreased production (e.g., marrow suppression)

This is commonly due to chemotherapy and can cause anemia, neutropenia, and thrombocytopenia.

Signs and symptoms:

Anemia: fatigue, pallor, dizziness, shortness of breath, tachycardia

Neutropenia: infections, fever, chills, diarrhea, cough, rash, mouth sores

Thrombocytopenia: bleeding, petechiae, easy bruising, hematuria, black stools

IHI

LEUKOCYTE DYSFUNCTION (E.G., HIV, CHRONIC GRANULOMATOUS DISEASE)

HIV—see above

Chronic granulomatous disease

This immunodeficiency produces recurrent or persistent bacterial and fungal infections, and granulomas.

Signs and symptoms: onset before age 2 (usual), but also during 20s; male (usual); failure to thrive (in infants), short stature (older patients); recurrent pyoderma (common) such as perianal, axillary, scalp abscesses; recurrent or persistent pneumonia, dermatitis, cutaneous disease, or infections; GI complications (diarrhea); abscesses (spleen, liver, gingival); septicemia

Investigations: nitroblue tetrazolium (NBT) dye test (this confirms that neutrophils, monocytes, macrophages, and eosinophils are not producing superoxide anions); peripheral blood leukocytosis (> 8500 neutrophils/μL [8.5×10^9/L]); anemia

Keys to patient encounter

Key concern

Differentiate life-threatening conditions that require immediate treatment (overwhelming sepsis, acute leukemia, febrile neutropenia) from nonurgent conditions.

History

HISTORY OF PRESENT ILLNESS

Review the patient's blood work, both recent and past.

Ask about symptoms of infection (fever, localized pain, redness) and malignancy (fever, weight loss, malaise). Ask about a recent history of infectious contacts and foreign travel.

PAST MEDICAL HISTORY

Ask about immunodeficiency (cancer, autoimmune disease, HIV, immunosuppressive therapy).

Physical exam

Vital signs: Look for fever and hypotension (note that hypotension is a key finding in sepsis).

General inspection: Look for sites of infection.
Lymph nodes: Check for lymphadenopathy.
Respiratory: Look for evidence of pneumonia.
Abdominal: Look for enlarged liver and spleen.

Investigations

Suspected infection: cultures of infection sites
Suspected sepsis: urgent blood cultures
Febrile neutropenia: urgent cultures (blood, urine, and, in some cases, CSF)

INTERPRETING RESULTS

Elevated neutrophils usually indicate infection. Elevated lymphocytes may be in response to viral infection or may be neoplastic. If blasts are present, or if lymphocytosis (more than 5000 monoclonal lymphocytes per μL [more than 5×10^9/L]) persists for several months, consider leukemia: order cell surface markers and consider a bone marrow biopsy.

Consider mononucleosis in younger individuals with elevated WBCs and atypical lymphocytes.

Management

Sepsis and febrile neutropenia require urgent management. Admit these patients to hospital (to ICU in the case of sepsis) and start empiric antibiotic treatment.

Other cases may require further testing or referral to specialists (e.g., a hematologist). These include:

- unexplained anemia
- erythrocytosis
- hemoglobinopathy
- persistent lymphocytosis (monoclonal lymphocytes greater than 5000/μL [5×10^9/L])
- neutropenia
- thrombocytosis or thrombocytopenia
- abnormal cells identified in peripheral blood smear

HEMATOLOGICAL PRESENTATIONS

Anemia

Differential diagnosis

NORMOCYTIC ANEMIA

Red blood cell loss

OBVIOUS (E.G., TRAUMA, METRO- OR MENORRHAGIA)

OCCULT BLOOD LOSS

Signs and symptoms: abdominal pain; black or tarry stools; blood in vomit; fatigue; dizziness

History of PUD; liver disease; abnormal coagulation or bleeding disorder; GI bleeding; alcoholism

Investigations: endoscopy; colonoscopy; CBC; peripheral blood smear; CT scan

Decreased red blood cell production

MARROW PRODUCTION (E.G., STEM CELL DISORDER, BONE MARROW REPLACEMENT)

STEM CELL DISORDER

Signs and symptoms: fatigue; tachycardia or tachypnea; bone pain; headaches; frequent infections; mucosal or joint bleeding

Investigations: CBC; peripheral blood smear; bone marrow biopsy; flow cytometry; chromosomal analysis; genetic testing to detect *JAK2* or *BCR-ABL* mutation

Increased red blood cell destruction (e.g., sickle cell anemia, immune-mediated conditions, mechanical conditions)

SICKLE CELL DISEASE

Signs and symptoms: family history of sickle cell disease; painful swelling of the hands and feet

Investigations: CBC to detect anemia, sickle cells; positive sickle cell screen; abnormalities on peripheral blood smear; abnormalities on hemoglobin electrophoresis

IMMUNE-MEDIATED CONDITIONS

Signs and symptoms: fatigue, weakness, fever, hepatosplenomegaly, jaundice, dark urine

> History of recent transfusion; recent infections (EBV, hepatitis, *Streptococcus*, *E. coli*); autoimmune disorders (SLE, Wiskott-Aldrich syndrome); new medications (e.g., antibiotics); leukemia or lymphoma; HELLP syndrome

Investigations: direct and indirect antiglobulin tests (DAT, IAT), CBC, peripheral blood smear, kidney function tests

MECHANICAL CONDITIONS

Signs and symptoms: fatigue, dizziness, tachycardia, tachypnea

> History of heart valve replacement; recent rapid transfusion or blood warmer use; arteriovenous malformations; genetic conditions or syndromes

Investigations: CT scan, MRI, US, ECG

Anemia of chronic disease

Signs and symptoms: fatigue, dizziness, tachycardia, tachypnea

> History of chronic systemic disease: autoimmune disorders, CKD, chronic infections, cancer

Investigations: normal to high serum ferritin, low iron, low reticulocyte count, low hemoglobin

MICROCYTIC ANEMIA (E.G., IRON DEFICIENCY, HEMOGLOBINOPATHIES)

Iron deficiency

Signs and symptoms: fatigue, dizziness, tachycardia, tachypnea, enlarged tongue

> History of menorrhagia, dietary restriction (e.g., anorexia, starvation, poverty), pregnancy, melena

Investigations: low serum ferritin, low iron, low reticulocyte count, low hemoglobin, colonoscopy

Hemoglobinopathies

Causes include sickle cell disease (see above), thalassemia, and chronic blood transfusions.

THALASSEMIA

Signs and symptoms: fatigue, dizziness, tachycardia, tachypnea

Risk factors: family history thalassemia; African, Middle Eastern, or South Asian descent

Investigations: abnormalities on CBC; low serum ferritin; low iron; low reticulocyte count; low hemoglobin; abnormalities on hemoglobin electrophoresis; abnormalities on hemoglobin HPLC

MACROCYTIC ANEMIA (E.G., VITAMIN B_{12} OR FOLATE DEFICIENCY, ALCOHOL USE)

Signs and symptoms (in general): fatigue; dizziness; tachycardia; tachypnea; ataxia; burning or prickling sensations

History of chemotherapy medication use; folate or vitamin B_{12} deficiency (pernicious anemia); alcoholism; poor diet

Investigations: abnormalities on CBC; abnormalities on peripheral blood smear; low vitamin B_{12} and folate levels; Schilling test to detect low vitamin B_{12} absorption

Keys to patient encounter

Key concerns

Pay particular attention to:

- red cell morphology
- common causes of anemia in specific populations
- risk factors for serious underlying conditions

History

HISTORY OF PRESENT ILLNESS

Review the patient's blood work, both recent and past.

Ask about malignancy and chronic disease. Ask about a family history of anemia and clarify the ethnic background of the patient (hemoglobinopathies are prevalent in patients of African, Middle Eastern, or South Asian descent).

Physical exam

Vital signs: Look for hypotension and tachycardia.

General inspection:

- Examine the skin for pallor, purpura, petechiae, and jaundice.
- Examine the sclera for icterus.

Cardiovascular: Look for a systolic ejection (flow) murmur at the left sternal border.

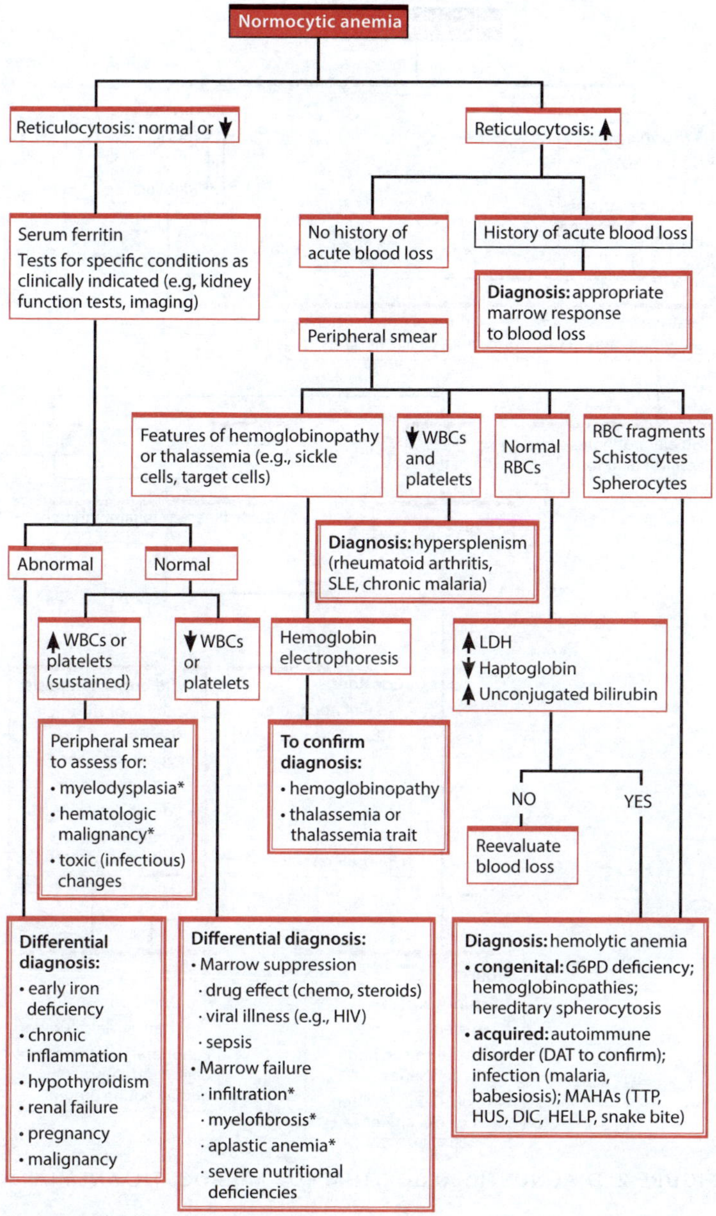

*Requires bone marrow biopsy or special tests to confirm.

FIGURE 1. DIAGNOSTIC ALGORITHM FOR NORMOCYTIC ANEMIA

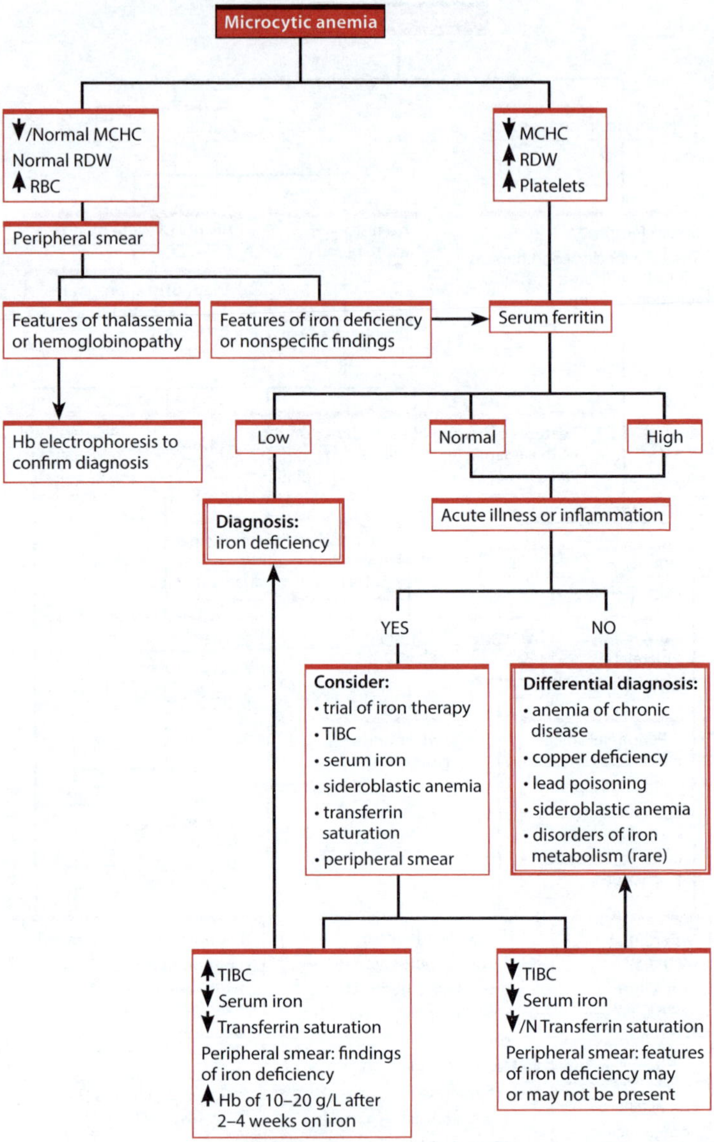

FIGURE 2. DIAGNOSTIC ALGORITHM FOR MICROCYTIC ANEMIA

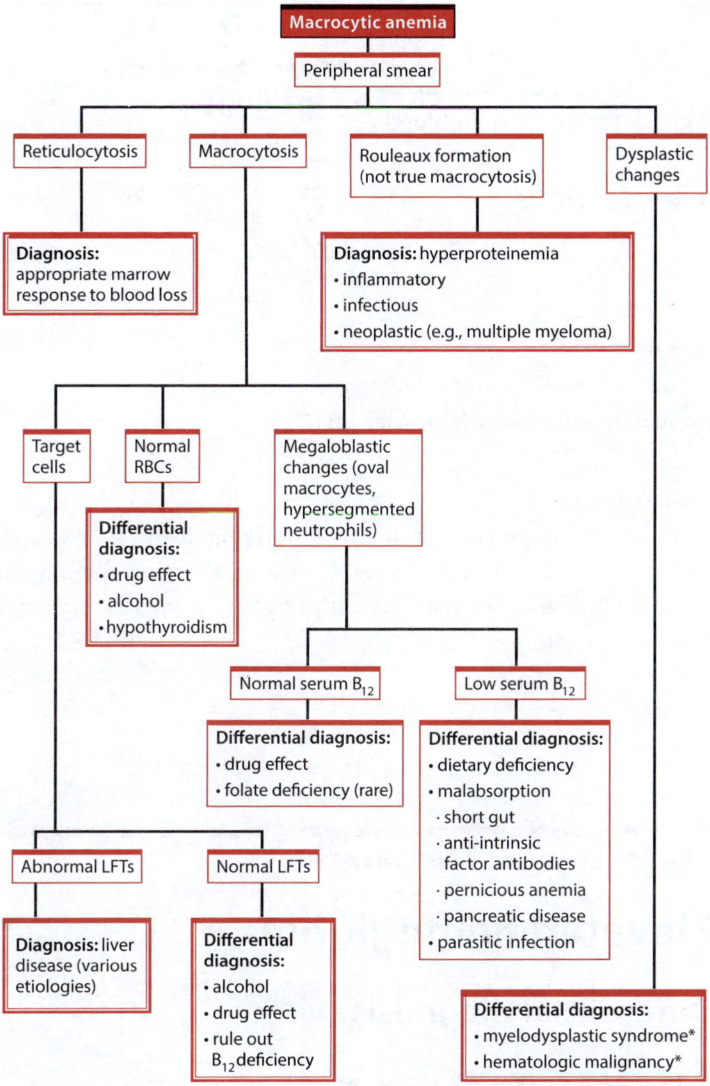

*Requires bone marrow biopsy or special tests to confirm.

FIGURE 3. DIAGNOSTIC ALGORITHM FOR MACROCYTIC ANEMIA

Abdominal: Look for hepatosplenomegaly.

DRE: Look for masses and check for fecal occult blood.

POINTER

Keys to anemia etiology

History (including family history) may give clues to the cause of anemia. However, red cell indices and findings on peripheral blood smear are key to making a diagnosis.

Investigations

CBC with peripheral blood smear

Serum ferritin

Serum iron

Serum vitamin B_{12} and folate in macrocytosis

Bone marrow biopsy (consider this)

Management

Optimize the management of any underlying disorders and correct any nutritional deficiencies. Consider referring the patient to a hematologist. For patients with refractory anemia, consider blood transfusion.

HEMATOLOGICAL PRESENTATIONS

Elevated hemoglobin

Differential diagnosis

INCREASED RED CELL MASS

Polycythemia vera: low or normal erythropoietin (EPO)

Signs and symptoms: possibly asymptomatic, pruritus (this is worse after warm baths), burning sensations in distal extremities, fatigue, dizziness, headache, gouty nodules, hepatomegaly, splenomegaly

Investigations:

Blood tests: elevated findings (platelets, hemoglobin, hematocrit, RBCs, WBCs); low EPO

Bone marrow biopsy: increased cellularity, panmyelosis (erythroid, granulocytic, megakaryocytic lines)

Secondary erythrocytosis: elevated EPO

APPROPRIATE EPO ELEVATION (E.G., HYPOXEMIA)

HYPOXEMIA

Causes include living in high altitudes, lung disease (e.g., COPD), smoking, and heart disease (e.g., CHD, arteriovenous malformations).

Signs and symptoms: cyanosis

INAPPROPRIATE EPO ELEVATION (E.G., EPO-EXCRETING TUMOR, RENAL ARTERY STENOSIS)

RENAL TUMOR

Signs and symptoms: possible palpable abdominal mass

Investigations: CT scan, US

RENAL ARTERY STENOSIS

Signs and symptoms: hypertension, renal artery bruit

Investigations: CT scan, US

RELATIVE POLYCYTHEMIA

Dehydration

Causes of dehydration include vomiting, diarrhea, sweating, and burns.

Signs and symptoms: low JVP, low BP, decreased skin turgor, dry mouth, sunken eyes, tachycardia

Investigations: elevated creatinine

Medications

Examples include darbepoetin, thiazide diuretics, and androgen therapy (i.e., testosterone or anabolic steroids).

Keys to patient encounter

History

Review the patient's blood work, which is how elevated hemoglobin is diagnosed.

The primary goal is to distinguish primary from secondary erythrocytosis. Ask about secondary causes of elevated hemoglobin including heart disease, respiratory disease, smoking, CHD, and causes of dehydration.

Physical exam

Cardiovascular

Respiratory

Abdominal:

- Look for an enlarged liver and/or spleen.
- Listen for renal artery bruits.

Investigations

The ULN for hemoglobin is 12–15 g/dL (120–150 g/L) for women and 14–17 g/dL (140–170 g/L) for men.

Creatinine in suspected dehydration

Blood tests for the *JAK2 V617F* mutation if common secondary causes have been ruled out, and especially if there are elevations in other blood cells (platelets and neutrophils)

- This is present in 97% of patients with polycythemia vera.

Bone marrow biopsy in suspected polycythemia vera, or in cases of unknown cause

Management

Manage any secondary causes identified. Refer patients with polycythemia vera to a hematologist. Reduce or discontinue contributing medications. Complications of polycythemia vera (stroke, blood clots) are managed with regular phlebotomy and low-dose acetylsalicylic acid. Hematologists may also treat polycythemia vera with chemotherapy.

HYPOTHERMIA

Hypothermia

Degrees of hypothermia

MIld hypothermia: 32°C to 35°C; vigorous shivering, cold white skin

Moderate hypothermia: 28°C to < 32°C; mental status changes (amnesia, confusion, apathy); slurred speech, hyporeflexia; loss of fine motor coordination; reduced shivering

Severe hypothermia: < 28°C; no shivering; cold edematous skin; areflexia; oliguria; fixed, dilated pupils; hypotension; pulmonary edema; bradycardia

Keys to patient encounter

Key concern

Recognize the degree of hypothermia and provide urgent care.

Steps in emergency management

Hypothermia is always an emergency situation.

- Obtain IV access.
- Provide supplemental oxygen.
- Attach a cardiac monitor.

History

Perform a history and physical exam at the same time. Ask accompanying caregivers for information on the setting and circumstances of any environmental exposure. Ask about possible contributing factors including drug or alcohol use, trauma, hypothyroidism, and dementia.

Ask about symptoms such as confusion, dizziness, chills, dyspnea, mood changes, irritability, poor judgment, and lassitude.

Physical exam

Vital signs

Core body temperature

Investigations

Check for possible underlying disorders (e.g., metabolic and neurologic disorders).

Finger-stick glucose
CBC
Electrolytes (see *Notes on labs and assessments*)
BUN
Creatinine
ECG
X-ray or CT scan in suspected trauma

IN MODERATE TO SEVERELY HYPOTHERMIC PATIENTS

INR/PTT

Fibrinogen (disseminated intravascular coagulation)

Serum lactate

CK

Troponin

Thyrotropin (TSH)

Cortisol

Toxicology screen

Lipase

Magnesium

Management

URGENT TREATMENT

Prevent further heat loss by removing wet clothing and replacing it with dry clothing or insulation. Admit the patient to ICU for continuous monitoring.

Mild hypothermia: Provide passive external rewarming and oral glucose. Provide active external rewarming if the patient does not respond to passive measures.

Moderate hypothermia: Provide active external rewarming with a heated air unit or warm water immersion (44°C to 45°C). Note that warm water immersion must be used with great caution.

Severe hypothermia: Provide active internal rewarming with warmed humidified air and warm IV fluids (40°C to 42°C). Consider lavage of the stomach, bladder, colon, peritoneum, and pleura with warm fluids. Consider extracorporeal warming methods, including hemodialysis and continuous arteriovenous rewarming. Consider cardiopulmonary bypass and ECMO in patients in cardiac arrest.

OTHER MANAGEMENT

Treat any underlying conditions.

POINTER

Rewarm arrested hypothermic patients

Remember the rule of thumb that a patient is not dead until they are warm and dead. This means that in arrested patients, rewarming is necessary before stopping resuscitation, especially in a child.

INCONTINENCE

Fecal incontinence

Differential diagnosis

PELVIC FLOOR INTACT

Neurologic conditions

Causes include diabetes, MS, ALS, spinal cord injury, acute brain injury, stroke, spina bifida, peripheral neuropathy, Parkinson disease, Huntington disease, Alzheimer disease, and dementia.

Overflow (e.g., impaction)

Causes include physical inactivity, malnutrition (especially lack of fiber), not drinking enough water, medications (opioids, sedatives, iron supplements), GI disorders (e.g., irritable bowel syndrome), neurological disorders, diabetes, autoimmune diseases (amyloidosis, celiac disease, SLE, scleroderma), hypothyroidism, spinal cord injury, and pelvic or colorectal surgery.

Signs and symptoms: chronic constipation; abdominal pain, bloating; leaking of liquid stool; nausea, vomiting; headache; weight loss; loss of appetite; necrosis and ulcers of rectal tissue

> Severe: rapid heart rate, hyperventilation, dehydration, fever, confusion, agitation

PELVIC FLOOR AFFECTED

Acquired condition (e.g., traumatic birth)

The most common cause is obstetric anal sphincter injury.

It is underreported: it could occur in up to 25% of women following vaginal birth.

Signs and symptoms: history of forceps delivery and/or third and fourth degree perineal tears

Congenital

HIRSCHSPRUNG DISEASE

This is caused by nerves in the colon that do not fully develop.

The condition is usually diagnosed in neonates (rarely in adults).

Risk factors: family history of Hirschsprung disease; other congenital conditions (e.g., Down syndrome, CHD)

Key concern

Incontinence may be multifactorial (e.g., patients may have a disease that affects mobility or cognition, which leads to incontinence in cases of fecal urgency or diarrhea; or they may have a defect in the pelvic floor that is overwhelmed by diarrhea).

History

HISTORY OF PRESENT ILLNESS

Ask when the incontinence started, what makes it better and worse, and what symptoms area associated with it. Listen for:

Recent-onset versus chronic incontinence: Recent onset could signal a new problem contributing to an underlying problem.

Incontinence made better or worse with diet or exercise: This suggests overflow incontinence.

GI symptoms: These suggest overflow incontinence, or a GI infection contributing to an underlying problem.

Ask about the patient's mobility.

PAST MEDICAL HISTORY

Ask about ulcerative colitis, Crohn disease, diabetes, neurological disorders, and chronic constipation. Ask about a history of radiation therapy to the pelvis.

In women, ask about a history of traumatic childbirth involving forceps or episiotomy.

Physical exam

DRE:

- Evaluate sphincter strength.
- Look for rectal abnormalities and stool in the rectum.
- Ask the patient to bear down and observe for rectal prolapse.

Investigations

Anal manometry

Colonoscopy or sigmoidoscopy

MRI to assess the anatomy of the anal sphincter (consider this)

Management

Kegel exercises, biofeedback, and maintenance of a regular defecation schedule may help reduce incontinence. Manage constipation by increasing exercise, fiber, and fluids; consider bulk laxatives (methylcellulose or psyllium). For diarrhea, consider treatment with loperamide hydrochloride, or diphenoxylate hydrochloride and atropine sulfate. Consider referring the patient to a gastroenterologist. Refer patients with rectal prolapse or damaged anal sphincters to a surgeon.

Pediatric urinary incontinence (enuresis)

Differential diagnosis

PRIMARY ENURESIS (E.G., FAMILY HISTORY)

This is bedwetting that occurs during sleep in children 5 years or older.

It is the most common type of enuresis.

Signs and symptoms: family history of nocturnal enuresis

Common contributing factors: nocturnal polyuria, detrusor overactivity, disturbed sleep

SECONDARY ENURESIS (E.G., URINARY TRACT INFECTION, VESICOURETERAL REFLUX)

Urinary tract infection

Signs and symptoms: frequent urination; painful urination; pelvic pain and/or flank pain; fever; tenderness over the bladder

Investigations: urinalysis, urine culture

Vesicoureteral reflux

The most common form (primary vesicoureteral reflux) resolves spontaneously as the child grows.

Signs and symptoms:

- Prenatal: fetal hydronephrosis on prenatal US
- Postnatal: recent UTI (this has a higher risk of vesicoureteral reflux if accompanied by fever)

Risk factors: family history, male (prenatal vesicoureteral reflux), female (postnatal vesicoureteral reflux), Caucasian

Investigations: contrast voiding cystourethrogram or radionuclide cystogram

Keys to patient encounter

Key concern

Determine whether a physical abnormality is causing incontinence in a child aged 5 years or older.

History

HISTORY OF PRESENT ILLNESS

Ask when the enuresis started. A key question is whether the child has never had nighttime bladder control (which indicates primary nocturnal enuresis) or has lost nighttime bladder control (which indicates secondary nocturnal enuresis).

Ask about coexisting symptoms, and listen for evidence consistent with UTI (e.g., fever, painful urination).

Ask about new or significant social stressors.

FAMILY HISTORY

Ask about a family history of enuresis.

Physical exam

Abdominal: Look for tenderness and masses.

GU: Look for rashes and physical abnormalities.

Investigations

In patients with a reassuring history and physical exam, investigations may not be necessary.

Urinalysis and urine culture to rule out UTI (consider this)

Management

Maintenance of the child's self-esteem is paramount. For primary nocturnal enuresis, educate and reassure the parents. Treatment should only be considered when enuresis poses a significant problem for the child. Behavioral modifications include avoiding caffeine-containing foods and excessive fluids before bedtime, having the child urinate before bedtime, and waking the child at night to urinate. Treatment with alarm devices may be useful, especially in older children. Desmopressin acetate may also be useful, especially on an as-needed basis for sleepovers and camps.

INCONTINENCE

Urinary incontinence in adults

Differential diagnosis

TRANSIENT CONDITION

Polyuria

Signs and symptoms: history of uncontrolled diabetes mellitus (this is the most common cause), primary polydipsia, central diabetes insipidus (DI), and/or nephrogenic DI

Investigations: water restriction test; plasma sodium; urine osmolality (except in suspected nephrogenic DI)

Urine output > 3 L/day in adults

Urine osmolality < 250 mOsm/kg (250 mmol/kg)

Drugs, alcohol

Examples include alcohol, caffeine, and loop diuretics (these increase urine production); antidepressants, antihistamines, and CCBs (these interfere with bladder contraction, which can lead to overflow incontinence); and antipsychotics and sedatives (these slow mobility and increase the urge to urinate).

NEUROLOGIC CONDITION (E.G., CAUDA EQUINA SYNDROME)

Cauda equina syndrome

This occurs when the spinal cord is compressed in the lumbar spine. Common causes include herniated disk, spinal stenosis, infection, and trauma.

Signs and symptoms: leg pain, numbness, weakness; urinary symptoms (incontinence, retention, frequent urination); fecal incontinence; loss of rectal tone; abnormal bulbocavernosus and anal wink reflexes; erectile dysfunction; decreased muscle tone and deep tendon reflexes in the legs; saddle anesthesia (loss of sensation in the inner thighs, back of the legs, around the rectum)

Investigations: x-ray, CT scan, MRI, myelography

ANATOMIC CONDITION

Stress incontinence

Signs and symptoms: female, aged 45 or older (more common); no bladder contractions during episodes of incontinence; incontinence during coughing, sneezing, running, heavy lifting, laughing, standing up, exercise, sexual intercourse

Risk factors: childbirth, especially vaginal deliveries; obesity; illnesses that cause sneezing or coughing; smoking (coughing); use of alcohol or caffeine; hormonal deficiency or HRT; hysterectomy; prostatectomy

Urgency incontinence (e.g., cystitis)

CYSTITIS

Signs and symptoms: bladder contractions during episodes; increased frequency of urination; painful urination; pelvic pain and/or flank pain; fever; tenderness over the bladder

Investigations: urinalysis, urine culture

Overflow incontinence (e.g., prostate enlargement, multiple sclerosis)

ENLARGED PROSTATE

Signs and symptoms: older male; urinary frequency, urgency, hesitancy, intermittency; nocturia; dribbling, incomplete bladder emptying; bladder distention (sometimes); nontender, enlarged prostate with rubbery consistency and lack of median furrow

Investigations: transrectal US of the prostate; PSA blood test

MULTIPLE SCLEROSIS

Signs and symptoms: variable depending on lesion location

- Spinal cord: sensory or motor dysfunction; Lhermitte sign (paresthesias radiating down the extremities or trunk with neck flexion); bowel, bladder or erectile dysfunction
- Brainstem: double vision; swallowing, speech difficulties; vertigo; pseudobulbar palsy
- Cerebrum: cognitive impairment; depression; upper motor neuron signs; unilateral motor or sensory deficits
- Cerebellum: problems with balance and coordination; vertigo
- Other symptoms: tonic spasms; fatigue; pain; exercise intolerance; temperature sensitivity; painful unilateral loss of visual acuity

Risk factors: younger than 50, female

Investigations: brain and spinal cord MRI, including advanced MRI techniques, with established occurrence of multiple episodes; CSF analysis

Keys to patient encounter

Key concern

Address the 2 most common causes: stress and urgency.

History

HISTORY OF PRESENT ILLNESS

Ask the patient about the circumstances associated with incontinence, looking for evidence to separate stress from urge incontinence, and to identify comorbid conditions (e.g., neurologic symptoms in cauda equina). Consider asking the patient to complete a voiding diary at home.

PAST MEDICAL HISTORY

Ask about diabetes, disorders in the lumbar spine, MS, and multiple vaginal deliveries.

SURGICAL HISTORY

Ask about hysterectomy, prostatectomy, and surgeries on the lumbar spine.

MEDICATIONS

Ask about antidepressants, antihistamines, CCBs, and HRT.

SOCIAL HISTORY
Ask about alcohol and caffeine.

Physical exam

Neurological

Pelvic

DRE:

- Check for masses and impacted feces.
- In men, check the prostate.

GU:

- *Cough stress test:*
  - Ask the patient to stand with a full bladder.
  - Ask the patient to cough and observe for leakage of urine.
- *Cotton swab test:* This assesses for bladder hypermobility.
  - Insert an anesthetic-lubricated swab into either the urethra or vagina (the vagina is better tolerated).
  - Ask the patient to perform the Valsalva maneuver.
  - Hypermobility (weak pelvic floor and urethral connective tissue) is demonstrated by a deviation of > 30° from horizontal during straining or a change in angle of > 30° during straining.

Investigations

Serum creatinine

Fasting glucose or HbA_{1c}

PSA

Urinalysis and culture to look for infection and hematuria

Urine cytology if hematuria is present

US to measure postvoid residual urine (normal is < 50 mL), and evaluate for hydronephrosis, hydroureter, and urinary tract stones

Urodynamic testing in patients with an unclear etiology (consider this)

Management

Several behavioral techniques can be useful for incontinence, including bladder training (delaying urination when the urge is felt), double voiding (urinating, then going again a few minutes later), scheduling toilet trips every 2 to 4 hours, weight loss, Kegel exercises, and reduced fluid intake. If these are ineffective, consider medications (anticholinergics, mirabegron, alpha-blockers, or topical estrogen for women). Consider referral to an incontinence program, or to a urologist (men) or gynecologist (women) for surgical options.

INFERTILITY

Infertility

Differential diagnosis

FEMALE

Ovulatory dysfunction (e.g., hypogonadotropic hypogonadism, polycystic ovary syndrome)

HYPOGONADOTROPIC HYPOGONADISM

Signs and symptoms: abnormal puberty; low libido and sexual function; absence or delay of normal Tanner stage for age

History of primary congenital syndrome (e.g., Kallmann syndrome, gonadotropin-releasing hormone sensitivity); secondary acquired syndrome (e.g., tumor; trauma; use of medications such as opioids, gonadotropin-releasing hormone analogs, gonadal analogs, glucocorticoids)

Investigations: decreased FSH; decreased LH; decreased estrogen; thyrotropin (TSH) (elevated in prolactinoma); prolactin (elevated in prolactinoma); decreased serum progesterone 1 week before expected onset of menstruation

POLYCYSTIC OVARY SYNDROME

Signs and symptoms: symptom onset after puberty, with increased rate of hair growth and male-pattern hair growth; irregular menstruation; infertility; obesity; acne

Investigations: LH:FSH ratio (elevated: 2:1 or 3:1) (usual); elevated testosterone; US to detect ovarian cysts; normal prolactin levels; normal thyroid function

Tubal and peritoneal abnormalities (e.g., pelvic inflammatory disease)

PELVIC INFLAMMATORY DISEASE

Signs and symptoms: lower abdominal and pelvic pain; pain during intercourse; fever; urinary symptoms; vaginal discharge; irregular menstruation; pelvic tenderness and pain associated with 1 or both adnexa

History of gonorrhea, chlamydia, or risk factors for them (multiple partners, unprotected sex); IUD; childbirth; gynecologic procedure

Investigations: cultures for gonorrhea and chlamydia; US (this has normal findings); hysterosalpingography to detect tubal abnormalities

Uterine and cervical factors (e.g., fibroids)

FIBROID (LEIOMYOMA)

Signs and symptoms: commonly asymptomatic; premenopausal (usual); heavy or prolonged menstrual bleeding; pelvic, abdominal pressure; painful intercourse; urinary symptoms (incontinence; frequent urination; difficulty emptying the bladder); constipation; pelvic mass or enlarged, irregular uterus on bimanual palpation

Risk factors: family history of leiomyoma; African descent

Investigations: US to detect mass ≥ 1 cm in diameter

MALE

Testicular dysfunction (e.g., hypogonadotropic hypogonadism, viral orchitis)

Signs and symptoms (in general): loss of libido, fever, testicular pain

History of medications (e.g., chemotherapy, anabolic steroids), chromosomal abnormality (e.g., Klinefelter syndrome), trauma, mumps, malaria, neoplasm, radiation, testicular surgery

Investigations: semen analysis (decreased quantity or quality of semen); abnormal FSH (elevated in primary hypogonadism, decreased in secondary hypogonadism); decreased serum testosterone; pelvic US to detect mass

Keys to patient encounter

Key concerns

Diagnose the cause and complications of infertility.

Explain therapeutic options.

History

Infertility is usually described as inability to conceive after 1 year of regular intercourse without contraception (6 months for women older than 35 years).

Ask female patients if they have ever become pregnant and male patients if they have ever fathered a child. Ask about the frequency of sex and its timing in terms of the menstrual cycle.

Ask women about their menstrual cycles: how often menstruation occurs and how regular it is. Ask about a history of endometriosis, pelvic infections, and ectopic pregnancies.

Ask men about a history of chemotherapy or radiation, testicular surgery or trauma, anabolic steroid use, chromosomal abnormalities, mumps, and malaria.

Physical exam

Men: Look for testicular abnormalities.

Women: Perform a pelvic exam, looking for masses and tenderness.

Investigations

MEN

Semen analysis

WOMEN

Serum progesterone at cycle day 21 (or 7 days before expected menstruation if the cycle is not 28 days) to confirm ovulation

Serum prolactin

Thyrotropin (TSH)

FOR ANATOMIC ABNORMALITIES OF THE REPRODUCTIVE TRACT

Hysterosalpingography in previously healthy women

Hysteroscopy or laparoscopy in women with a history of endometriosis, pelvic infections, or ectopic pregnancy

POINTER

Steps before conception

Remember to counsel all women contemplating pregnancy on the preconceptual use of folic acid and the need for up-to-date immunizations.

Management

Sperm abnormalities may be treated with gonadotropin therapy, intrauterine insemination, or in vitro fertilization.

Anovulation may be treated with aromatase inhibitors. In cases of polycystic ovary syndrome or obesity, the first line of treatment is weight loss (with or without metformin in polycystic ovary syndrome). Consider referral to a fertility clinic or to a gynecologist for treatment of female reproductive tract obstruction.

JAUNDICE

Jaundice

Differential diagnosis

UNCONJUGATED HYPERBILIRUBINEMIA (PREHEPATIC)

Overproduction (e.g., hemolysis)

HEMOLYTIC ANEMIA

Signs and symptoms: fatigue, shortness of breath, decreased exercise tolerance, dark urine

Severe: jaundice

Investigations: peripheral blood smear to detect schistocytes, spherocytes, and/or bite cells; blood tests (hemoglobin, WBCs, platelet count, RBCs, MCV, hematocrit, bilirubin, lactate dehydrogenase, haptoglobin, reticulocyte indices)

Decreased hepatic uptake (e.g., congestive heart failure)

CONGESTIVE HEART FAILURE

Signs and symptoms: history of heart disease (or risk factors for heart disease: diabetes, hypertension, hyperlipidemia, and smoking) or hepatic vein thrombosis (Budd-Chiari syndrome); severe shortness of breath; elevated JVP; edema in the abdomen and legs; pink phlegm; heart murmurs and extra cardiac sounds

Investigations: chest x-ray to detect pulmonary edema; NT-proBNP level; echocardiogram to distinguish forms of HF; cardiac stress testing, either with exercise or pharmacological agent

Decreased bilirubin conjugation (e.g., Gilbert syndrome)

GILBERT SYNDROME

This inherited disorder does not impair health and requires no treatment.

Signs and symptoms: usually asymptomatic, jaundice

> Triggers for jaundice in Gilbert syndrome: current illness (e.g., flu, cold) or menstruation; recent fasting; certain medications (e.g., acetaminophen, irinotecan)

Risk factors: family history of Gilbert syndrome (to inherit the disorder, both parents must carry the gene)

Investigations: elevated unconjugated bilirubin, normal CBC

CONJUGATED HYPERBILIRUBINEMIA (HEPATIC)

Intrahepatic cholestasis (e.g., drugs, cirrhosis)

DRUGS

These include antibiotics (e.g., penicillin, tetracycline, amoxicillin-clavulanate, macrolide), anabolic steroids, estrogen (e.g., estradiol), chlorpromazine, cimetidine, imipramine, prochlorperazine, terbinafine, and tolbutamide.

INFECTIONS

These include HBV, HBC, HIV, and EBV.

CIRRHOSIS

Signs and symptoms: jaundice; easy bruising, bleeding; itching; ascites; spiderlike blood vessels on the skin; systemic symptoms (anorexia, weight loss, weakness, fatigue)

History of chronic alcohol abuse; chronic HBV or HCV, or risk factors for them (unprotected sex, IV drug abuse, blood transfusions, tattoos, body piercings, imprisonment, workplace exposure to body fluids); hemochromatosis; nonalcoholic fatty liver disease

Investigations: liver function tests

Extrahepatic cholestasis (e.g., cholelithiasis)

CHOLELITHIASIS (GALLSTONES)

Symptoms: right upper quadrant abdominal pain, under the ribs; pain that prevents normal or deep breathing; Murphy sign (while palpating near the gallbladder, severe pain on taking a breath); vomiting

Pain characteristics: 15 minutes to 24 hours in duration; radiating to the right upper back or shoulder blade; no relief with moving or changing position; onset at night, on waking, or after eating

Symptoms of bile duct blocked by gallstone: jaundice, dark urine, light-colored stools, fever, chills

Risk factors: high BMI or obesity (see *Notes on labs and assessments*); high-fat diet; diabetes; older than 60; estrogen medications; family history of gallstones; female

Investigations: US, abdominal x-ray, CT scan, hepatobiliary scan, MRCP, ERCP

Hepatocellular injury (e.g., sepsis, hypoperfusion)

SEPSIS

Definition: infection with systemic inflammatory response, dysfunction of ≥ 1 organ system

Signs and symptoms: fever or hypothermia; tachycardia; tachypnea; infection (most common: pneumonia, abdominal infection, kidney infection, bacteremia)

Severe: oliguria; mental status changes; shortness of breath; extreme hypotension, unresponsive to fluid replacement (this indicates septic shock)

Risk factors: very young or very old; compromised immune system; wounds, burns; catheterization, intubation

Investigations: CBC with differential; cultures (blood, CSF, urine) to detect causative organism; ABG to detect acidosis; elevated creatinine; chest x-ray to detect pulmonary edema

HYPOPERFUSION (ISCHEMIC HEPATITIS)

Signs and symptoms: weakness, fatigue, mental confusion, low urine production, jaundice, loss of liver function (rare and transient)

Investigations: AST, ALT (both > 1000 U/L [16.7 µkat/L]); ALP; GGT; bilirubin (direct, total, indirect); albumin; PT/INR

Other (e.g., infiltrative states, fatty liver)

INFILTRATIVE STATES

Examples of causes include hepatocellular carcinoma, sarcoidosis, pancreatic cancer, cholangiocarcinoma, and lymphoma.

Signs and symptoms: nausea, abdominal pain, anorexia, malaise, fever, chills, jaundice, dark urine, light stools, pruritus

- Malignancy: recent weight loss

Investigations: liver function tests, MRI, biopsy

- AST, ALT: normal or mildly elevated (30–40 U/L [0.5–0.67 µkat/L], < 300 U/L [5 µkat/L]); AST:ALT ratio < 1
- ALP: > 4 times ULN
- Conjugated hyperbilirubinemia: direct bilirubin fraction > 20%

NONALCOHOLIC FATTY LIVER DISEASE

This is the most common form of chronic liver disease.

Signs and symptoms: usually asymptomatic, fatigue, right upper quadrant abdominal pain, enlarged liver, muscle weakness

- More severe: jaundice, gynecomastia, enlarged spleen, red palms

Risk factors: high cholesterol; high serum triglycerides; obesity; type 2 diabetes; metabolic syndrome; polycystic ovary syndrome; hypothyroidism; hypopituitarism; recent weight gain or loss

Investigations: blood tests (CBC, liver enzymes, lipid profile); abdominal US, CT scan, MRI; transient elastography (FibroScan)

Keys to patient encounter

Key objective

Identify life-threatening conditions.

History

HISTORY OF PRESENT ILLNESS

Ask when the jaundice started and what other symptoms the patient has. Ask specifically about systemic symptoms that may indicate the presence of malignancy or infection (fever, weight loss, fatigue, night sweats). Ask about risk factors for infectious hepatitis (unprotected sex, IV drug abuse, blood transfusions, tattoos, body piercings, imprisonment, workplace exposure to body fluids), and about possible occupational exposures to toxic substances.

PAST MEDICAL HISTORY

Ask about a history of gall bladder disease.

MEDICATIONS AND DRUGS

Ask about hepatotoxic drugs and alcohol abuse.

Physical exam

Vital signs: Look for fever.

General inspection: Examine the skin for jaundice and the sclera for icterus.

Cardiovascular:

- Auscultate the heart for murmurs.
- Check the extremities for edema (edema suggests CHF).

Respiratory: Auscultate the lungs for rales.

Abdominal: Look for masses and tenderness.

Investigations

Total and direct bilirubin to distinguish conjugated (direct) from unconjugated (indirect) hyperbilirubinemia

- A direct bilirubin level of ≥ 0.58 mg/dL (10 μmol/L), with an elevated total bilirubin level, indicates conjugated hyperbilirubinemia.

CBC (this is relevant for hemolysis)

AST

ALT

HCV antibody

HB_sAg

Anti-HB_cAb

HIV

Heterophile antibody (Monospot test)

Lipase to rule out pancreatic disease and/or obstruction

IN SUSPECTED BILIARY OBSTRUCTION

ALP

GGT

IF A DIAGNOSIS IS NOT MADE

Consider more specialized studies:

Liver US to exclude biliary obstruction and to look for fatty liver, tumor, and cirrhosis

- In cases of tumor, cirrhosis, or biliary atresia, refer the patient for liver biopsy.

Blood alcohol

Acetaminophen

Iron studies

Antimitochondrial antibody

Ceruloplasmin

ANA

Management

Management depends on the specific diagnosis. Remove any offending medications or drugs. In mechanical obstruction or tumor, refer the patient to a surgeon. In hemolysis, refer the patient to a hematologist. If indicated, consider referral to a hepatologist for diagnosis and treatment.

JAUNDICE

Neonatal jaundice

Differential diagnosis

UNCONJUGATED HYPERBILIRUBINEMIA

Increased bilirubin production

HEMOLYTIC CAUSE

This is sometimes diagnosed and treated before birth.

Signs and symptoms: jaundice that develops quickly after birth; Rh-negative mother and Rh-positive baby

Investigations: direct antibody test of cord blood (Coombs test) and blood type if the mother is Rh-negative; serum bilirubin; transcutaneous bilirubin; bilirubin:albumin (B:A) ratio; total and conjugated bilirubin

Decreased bilirubin conjugation

METABOLIC OR GENETIC CAUSE (E.G., GILBERT SYNDROME, HYPOTHYROIDISM)

GILBERT SYNDROME

This inherited disorder does not impair health and requires no treatment.

Signs and symptoms: usually asymptomatic, jaundice

> Triggers for jaundice in Gilbert syndrome: current illness (e.g., flu, cold), recent fasting, certain medications (e.g., acetaminophen, irinotecan)

Risk factors: family history of Gilbert syndrome (to inherit the disorder, both parents must carry the gene)

Investigations: elevated unconjugated bilirubin, normal CBC

HYPOTHYROIDISM

Signs and symptoms: history of hypothyroidism or symptoms of hypothyroidism (decreased reflexes, dry skin)

Investigations: elevated thyrotropin (TSH)

PHYSIOLOGIC CAUSE (E.G., BREAST MILK JAUNDICE)

JAUNDICE ASSOCIATED WITH BREASTFEEDING

Two types of neonatal jaundice are associated with breastfeeding: breastfeeding jaundice and breast milk jaundice.

Breastfeeding jaundice is very common, and develops during the period after birth when breastfeeding is becoming established. It is due to inadequate milk intake (because the mother's milk is not established, or the baby's latch is not established), which leads to jaundice through dehydration and delayed passage of meconium.

Breast milk jaundice generally occurs later (e.g., second week of life) and persists longer (e.g., 3 to 6 weeks). It is generally a diagnosis of exclusion.

Gastrointestinal (e.g., sequestered blood)

Examples of causes include anal fissure (most common); esophageal, gastric, or duodenal erosions; and stress gastritis.

Signs and symptoms: blood in the stool (bright red, dark red, black); blood in vomit; maternal use of acetylsalicylic acid, cephalothin, phenobarbital during pregnancy; prematurity; history of neonatal distress, mechanical ventilation

CONJUGATED HYPERBILIRUBINEMIA

Decreased bilirubin uptake

INFECTION (E.G., SEPSIS, NEONATAL HEPATITIS)

NEONATAL SEPSIS

Definition: infection with systemic inflammatory response, dysfunction of ≥ 1 organ system

Infection usually occurs by vertical transmission. Examples include group B streptococci, *E. coli*, *S. aureus*, *L. monocytogenes*, *S. viridans*, *H. influenzae*, CMV, RSV, human metapneumovirus, parainfluenza virus, human coronavirus, HSV, HIV, *C. albicans*, *C. parapsilosis*, and *Aspergillus*.

Signs and symptoms: fever, tachycardia, tachypnea, poor muscle tone, poor feeding, vomiting, jaundice, abdominal distention, poor perfusion

> Severe: oliguria; mental status changes; shortness of breath; extreme hypotension, unresponsive to fluid replacement (this indicates septic shock)

Risk factors: compromised immune system; wounds, burns; catheterization, intubation

> Maternal factors: chorioamnionitis (intrauterine onset of infection); intrapartum maternal temperature ≥ 38° C; < 37 weeks gestation; membrane rupture > 18 hours before delivery

Investigations: CBC with differential (elevated neutrophils is a common finding); CRP; blood culture; cultures of other fluids (CSF, urine)

NEONATAL HEPATITIS

Note that neonates are generally asymptomatic: symptoms generally appear 1 to 2 months after birth.

Signs and symptoms: maternal history of viral hepatitis, CMV, rubella; jaundice; enlarged liver and spleen; poor weight gain and growth

CHOLESTASIS (E.G., TOTAL PARENTERAL NUTRITION)

PARENTERAL NUTRITION–ASSOCIATED CHOLESTASIS

This is usually associated with long-term parenteral nutrition. It is chronic and irreversible, and leads to liver failure.

Signs and symptoms: poor feeding; vomiting; diarrhea; lethargy, hypotonia; symptoms of advanced liver failure (e.g., tarry or bloody stools; bleeding from the umbilical stump; bruising or purpura); hepatomegaly, possible splenomegaly, or ascites

Investigations: elevated direct/conjugated bilirubin (either > 20% of total serum bilirubin or at minimum > 1 mg/dL [17.1 μmol/L]); abdominal US; liver biopsy

Other tests for liver enzymes and liver function: AST, ALT, ALP, PT/INR, PTT, albumin, glucose, ammonia

METABOLIC CAUSE

GALACTOSEMIA, HEREDITARY FRUCTOSE INTOLERANCE, GLYCOGEN STORAGE DISEASES

Signs and symptoms: hypoglycemia, lethargy, vomiting, failure to thrive, diarrhea, jaundice, renal insufficiency

NIEMANN-PICK DISEASE, GAUCHER DISEASE, TYROSINEMIA

Signs and symptoms: hepatomegaly, splenomegaly, CNS dysfunction

Gaucher disease: bruising, anemia, low platelet count

α_1-ANTITRYPSIN DEFICIENCY

Signs and symptoms: liver symptoms with asthma-like symptoms (shortness of breath, wheezing, rhonchi, rales)

Investigations: newborn screening (enzyme function tests, DNA analysis); enzyme tests from blood or liver biopsy

GENETIC CAUSE

DUBIN-JOHNSON AND ROTOR SYNDROMES

These are generally benign disorders showing mild, nonitching jaundice with elevated conjugated bilirubin.

Obstructive cause (e.g., biliary atresia)

BILIARY ATRESIA

This is a rare disease of the bile ducts that occurs in infants.

Signs and symptoms: jaundice that develops 2 to 3 weeks after birth; dark urine; light stools; full term baby; low birth weight (often)

Associated disorders (10% to 15% of cases): cardiac anomalies (murmurs), polysplenia, blood vessel abnormalities (inferior vena cava, preduodenal portal vein), intestinal abnormalities (situs inversus or malrotation)

Investigations: blood tests for liver function, liver biopsy

Keys to patient encounter

Key objective

Pay particular attention to jaundice within the first 3 days of birth or that has rapid onset.

History

HISTORY OF PRESENT ILLNESS

Ask how often the baby has a wet diaper, what the baby's stools are like, and if the baby is breastfed and how often.

Evidence of dehydration suggests infrequent feeding. Tarry or bloody stools suggest a GI cause.

Ask about risk factors for neonatal jaundice (see the pointer).

PAST MEDICAL HISTORY

Ask about complications during pregnancy and delivery. Listen for evidence of neonatal distress and risk factors for infection (e.g., premature birth, intrapartum maternal fever, early membrane rupture in labor). Ask about the infant's birth weight.

FAMILY HISTORY

Ask about Gilbert syndrome, Dubin-Johnson syndrome, and Rotor syndrome.

POINTER

Risk factors for neonatal hyperbilirubinemia

- Jaundice < 24 hours after delivery or while still in hospital
- ABO incompatibility and positive Coombs test
- Glucose-6-phosphate dehydrogenase (G6PD) deficiency
- Premature delivery (< 36 weeks gestation)
- History of sibling jaundice or phototherapy
- Significant neonatal bruising
- Exclusively breastfed
- East Asian descent

JKL

Physical exam

Weight: Compare current weight to birth weight (a loss of more than 10% of birth weight suggests inadequate milk intake).

General inspection: Look for jaundice, scleral icterus, and bruising.

Investigations

Total serum bilirubin or transcutaneous bilirubin should be plotted on a nomogram against the infant's age in hours. This will indicate the need for treatment, further investigations, or further testing.

IN RAPIDLY RISING BILIRUBIN OR INFANTS RECEIVING PHOTOTHERAPY

Total and direct serum bilirubin to help distinguish between conjugated (direct) and unconjugated (indirect) hyperbilirubinemia

- Direct bilirubin is considered elevated when it exceeds 20% of total bilirubin.

Infants with elevated direct bilirubin: urinalysis and urine culture

Infants receiving phototherapy: blood type and Coombs test

INFANTS WITH PROLONGED JAUNDICE (WEEKS)

Review the neonatal tests for hypothyroidism and galactosemia.

Management

Admit all neonates to hospital who require treatment according to the nomogram. The nomogram will indicate the need for phototherapy or exchange transfusion. In neonates with mild jaundice not requiring phototherapy, increasing the frequency of feedings will help lower the bilirubin level. Provide IV fluids if the infant is dehydrated. Retest bilirubin levels according to advice given in the nomogram.

All newborns should have frequent clinical assessments for jaundice in the first 24 hours after birth, and a follow-up assessment within 48 hours after birth. Infants with risk factors for hyperbilirubinemia should have their total serum bilirubin (or transcutaneous bilirubin) measured 24 to 72 hours after discharge.

POINTER

Considerations in neonatal jaundice

Breastfed neonates are less likely to develop jaundice if fed 8 to 12 times per 24 hours, as opposed to less frequently.

It is unconjugated (indirect) bilirubin that is toxic to the CNS.

KIDNEY PRESENTATIONS

Acute kidney injury (anuria or oliguria)

Differential diagnosis

ACUTE KIDNEY INJURY IN GENERAL

Definition: rising serum creatinine over a short period of time

Investigations: increase in serum creatinine by ≥ 0.29 mg/dL (26 μmol/L) within 48 hours, or ≥ 1.5 times baseline; or urine volume < 0.5 mL/kg/hour for 6 hours

PRERENAL CAUSE

PRERENAL CAUSE IN GENERAL

Signs and symptoms: thirst; reduced fluid intake; blood or fluid loss (from vomiting, diarrhea, bleeding, severe burns)

Renal hypoperfusion (e.g., hepatorenal syndrome)

RENAL HYPOPERFUSION IN GENERAL

Predisposing conditions for localized renal hypoperfusion include renal artery obstruction due to expanding AAA; hypercalcemia; renal artery stenosis or occlusion; and use of NSAIDs, cox-2 inhibitors, ARBs, norepinephrine, radio-contrast agents, amphotericin B, and calcineurin inhibitors. **ACE inhibitors are contraindicated for patients with bilateral renal artery stenosis.**

HEPATORENAL SYNDROME

Signs and symptoms: renal dysfunction (progressive or rapid) in the context of cirrhosis with ascites; arterial hypotension; circulatory dysfunction; signs of liver disease (jaundice, edema, ascites); history of bacterial peritonitis, cirrhosis, hepatitis, alcohol use

Investigations: BUN:creatinine ratio > 20:1; blood tests (electrolytes, WBCs, CRP, culture); urine tests (proteinuria, microhematuria, sodium, osmolality, culture)

Systemic hypoperfusion (e.g., shock, hypovolemia)

CIRCULATORY SHOCK

Signs and symptoms: persistent hypotension; tachycardia; acute ischemia; HF; chest trauma; cold cyanotic extremities; poor organ perfusion; history of HF, CAD, infarction, angina

Investigations: blood tests (cardiac troponin; ABG; lactate)

HYPOVOLEMIA

Signs and symptoms: weakness; lethargy; change in thirst or drinking pattern; dry mucous membranes; sunken eyes; slow capillary refill; hypotension; resting tachycardia; orthostatic changes

History of acute or chronic illness (GI illness, cirrhosis, nephrotic syndrome, HF, prolonged fever, blood loss); use of diuretics, laxatives, ADH antagonists, lithium, narcotics, alcohol; medical procedures including surgery, nasogastric suction, enemas, tube feeding

Investigations: ECG; chest x-ray; BUN:creatinine ratio > 20:1; decreased urinary sodium (unless on diuretics); blood tests (electrolytes, osmolality, glucose, calcium); nonactive urine sediment

RENAL CAUSE

RENAL CAUSE IN GENERAL

Signs and symptoms: fatigue; weight loss; fever; muscle and joint pain; cough with blood

Tubulointerstitial condition (e.g., acute tubular necrosis, interstitial nephritis)

ACUTE TUBULAR NECROSIS

Causes include ischemic injury (e.g., prolonged kidney hypoperfusion) and toxic injury (e.g., from calcineurin inhibitors, radio-contrast agents, or antibiotics such as aminoglycoside and amphotericin B).

Investigations: BUN:creatinine ratio 10:1–20:1; signs of tubular necrosis (urinary sediment with muddy brown casts, renal tubular epithelial cells, granular casts); urine osmolality < 350–400 mOsm/kg (350–400 mmol/kg); urine sodium > 40 mEq/L (40 mmol/L); blood electrolytes

ACUTE INTERSTITIAL NEPHRITIS

Signs and symptoms: fever; rash; arthralgia; use of diuretics, antibiotics, analgesics (usual); history of autoimmune disorders

Investigations: urine eosinophils (their presence is suggestive); urinalysis (normal findings for RBCs, proteinuria, and red cell casts); blood tests (normal creatinine; normal complement level); renal biopsy (definitive)

Glomerular condition (e.g., glomerulonephritis, thrombotic thrombocytopenic purpura, or hemolytic uremic syndrome)

INFECTION-RELATED GLOMERULONEPHRITIS AND MEMBRANOPROLIFERATIVE GLOMERULONEPHRITIS

The common cause for infections is *Streptococcus* in the upper respiratory tract or skin. Contributing factors include alpha-interferon treatment, HBV, HCV, HIV, and hematologic abnormalities.

Signs and symptoms: hypertension; edema, oliguria, or anuria (infection related); frothy urine; gross hematuria

THROMBOTIC THROMBOCYTOPENIC PURPURA

Signs and symptoms: neurologic symptoms (headache, seizures, coma, sensory-motor deficits, TIAs); skin symptoms (purpura, jaundice, pallor); use of associated medications (quinine, ticlopidine, mitomycin C, cyclosporine A); microangiopathic hemolytic anemia; thrombocytopenia; decreased *ADAMTS13* activity

HEMOLYTIC UREMIC SYNDROME

This commonly follows infection from Shiga toxin–producing *E. coli*.

Signs and symptoms: GI symptoms (abdominal pain, bloody diarrhea); anemia (fatigue, weakness, pallor); neurologic symptoms (irritability, confusion, seizures); peripheral edema (this is a sign of renal failure); thrombocytopenia

Investigations: blood tests (BUN, creatinine, electrolytes, peripheral smear); urinalysis (to detect proteinuria and RBCs); elevated PT/INR

POSTRENAL CAUSE OR OBSTRUCTION (E.G., PROSTATIC HYPERTROPHY, CERVICAL CANCER, CALCULI)

Predisposing conditions for ureteral or urethral obstruction include nephrolithiasis; benign prostatic hyperplasia or hypertrophy; and prostate or cervical cancer.

Signs and symptoms (in general): palpable bladder, enlarged prostate (prostatic hypertrophy), pelvic mass (cervical cancer), history of kidney stones

Investigations: renal US to detect obstruction; noncontrast CT scan to see calculi; PSA or Pap test for prostate or cervical conditions

Keys to patient encounter

Key concern

Identify patients who need urgent intervention.

History

HISTORY OF PRESENT ILLNESS

Start with questions that target prerenal, renal, and postrenal causes. This will help structure the interview and narrow the possible diagnosis.

Prerenal causes: Ask about increased thirst, and recent sources of fluid loss (e.g., vomiting, diarrhea, bleeding, severe burns). Ask about a history of bilateral renal artery stenosis.

Renal causes: Ask about a pattern of fatigue, weight loss, and fever.

Postrenal causes: Ask about a history of kidney stones, prostate trouble, and cervical cancer.

Ask about the patient's symptoms and listen for evidence consistent with the likely cause (e.g., cyanosis and heart disease, or jaundice and liver disease, in prerenal causes; rash and autoimmune disorders, or hematuria and *Streptococcus* infection, or neurologic symptoms and *E. coli* in renal causes).

MEDICATIONS

Ask about medications relevant to the likely cause (e.g., ACE inhibitors in the context of bilateral renal artery stenosis in prerenal causes; calcineurin inhibitors and antibiotics in renal causes).

Physical exam

Vital signs: Look for shock and hypovolemia.

Abdominal: Look for masses and a palpable bladder.

Investigations

Urinalysis

Urine sediment analysis

Serum creatinine

Serum and urine electrolytes

Renal US and CT scan to assess for renal or bladder obstruction

Management

Assess the need for urgent intervention, which could include dialysis, fluid resuscitation, or urinary catheterization. Institute dialysis in patients with a GFR < 15 mL/minute, and with 1 or more of the following:

- symptoms or signs of uremia (progressive fatigue; anorexia; nausea, vomiting; muscle atrophy; tremors; mental function changes; shallow breathing; metabolic acidosis)
- inability to control hydration status or BP
- inability to maintain nutritional status

Refer the patient to a nephrologist.

KIDNEY PRESENTATIONS

Chronic kidney injury

Differential diagnosis

PRERENAL CAUSES (E.G., HYPERTENSION)

Hypertension

Signs and symptoms: systolic BP ≥ 140 mmHg and/or diastolic BP ≥ 90 mmHg

History of renal conditions, diabetes, adrenal or thyroid conditions, vascular conditions, catecholamine excess, obstructive sleep apnea, family history of hypertension

Risk factors: lack of exercise; high-sodium diet; obesity

RENAL CAUSE

Glomerular condition (e.g., IgA nephropathy, diabetic nephropathy)

GLOMERULAR CONDITION IN GENERAL

Signs and symptoms: hematuria (gross or microscopic, often following UTI); proteinuria; dysmorphic RBCs in urine

IgA NEPHROPATHY

Signs and symptoms: often asymptomatic; low-grade fever; loin pain; hypertension; edema

Investigations: renal biopsy

DIABETIC NEPHROPATHY

Signs and symptoms: usually asymptomatic; hypertension; edema

Investigations: elevated albumin:creatinine ratio in urine (i.e., albuminuria)

Tubulointerstitial condition (e.g., drug toxicity)

DRUG TOXICITY

ANALGESIC NEPHROPATHY

There is conflicting evidence on the risk of CKD from analgesic use (NSAIDs, acetylsalicylic acid, lithium).

Signs and symptoms: headache; anemia (fatigue, pallor, dizziness, shortness of breath, tachycardia); hypertension; pyuria; proteinuria; possible renal papillary necrosis and chronic interstitial nephritis (on CT scan) due to capillary sclerosis

DECREASED GLOMERULAR FILTRATION RATE

Chemotherapy can cause kidney disease. Examples of chemotherapeutic drugs include cisplatin, ifosfamide, methoxyamine, pemetrexed, and bisphosphonates.

Signs and symptoms: features of uremia (progressive fatigue; anorexia; nausea, vomiting; muscle atrophy; tremors; mental function changes; shallow breathing; metabolic acidosis)

Investigations: GFR < 60 mL/min; BUN; creatinine; elevated cystatin C; proteinuria; albuminuria; urine sediment abnormalities

OTHER

Kidney injury (acute or chronic) can be caused by use of ACE inhibitors, ARBs, diuretics, and NSAIDs in combination (the first 3 drugs are often used in combination to treat hypertension and HF); antimicrobials including aminoglycosides, sulfa-based antibiotics, vancomycin, ciprofloxacin; and herbal supplements.

Ischemic condition

RENAL ARTERY STENOSIS

The common cause is atherosclerosis.

Signs and symptoms: usually asymptomatic; sudden-onset hypertension; bruits from arteries in the kidneys

Risk factors: older than 55; hypertension; hyperlipidemia; diabetes; obesity; family history of heart disease; smoking; lack of exercise

Investigations: blood tests (GFR, BUN, electrolytes); urinalysis (protein, blood, pH); renal US with Doppler

Congenital condition (e.g., dysplasia, polycystic kidney disease)

MULTICYSTIC DYSPLASTIC KIDNEY

This is usually detected on prenatal US.

Signs and symptoms: palpable mass in abdomen

AUTOSOMAL DOMINANT POLYCYSTIC KIDNEY DISEASE

This is the most common inherited cause of kidney disease.

It may not be detected in patients younger than 30.

Signs and symptoms: family history of polycystic kidney disease; hypertension with pain (abdomen, flank, lower back); hematuria; UTIs

Investigations: renal US; genetic testing; serum creatinine and GFR to assess disease; urine tests (hematuria, micro or gross; culture to detect UTI or cyst infection)

AUTOSOMAL RECESSIVE POLYCYSTIC KIDNEY DISEASE

This is usually detected on prenatal US.

Signs and symptoms: enlarged kidney (neonates, infants); bilateral flank or abdominal masses; tachypnea; grunting, respiratory distress; impaired renal function

POSTRENAL CAUSE (E.G., OBSTRUCTIVE UROPATHY)

Obstructive uropathy

Signs and symptoms: flank pain; fever; nausea, vomiting; weight gain; edema; frequent urge to urinate; difficulty voiding or abnormal urine stream; reduced urine volume; hematuria

Investigations: US or CT scan of the pelvis, abdomen; IV pyelogram; voiding cystourethrogram; renal nuclear scan

Keys to patient encounter

The differential diagnosis for this clinical presentation is large and complex. Keep in mind that the most common conditions associated with chronic kidney injury are diabetes and hypertension.

History

HISTORY OF PRESENT ILLNESS

Ask about urinary problems (e.g., UTIs, hematuria); and symptoms of uremia (e.g., progressive fatigue; tremors; mental function changes).

PAST MEDICAL HISTORY

Ask about diabetes, hypertension, kidney disease, and heart disease.

MEDICATIONS

Ask about chemotherapy, analgesics, ACE inhibitors, and antimicrobials.

FAMILY HISTORY

Ask about kidney problems.

Physical exam

Vital signs: Look for hypertension and fever (fever suggests IgA nephropathy or obstructive uropathy).

Abdominal: Look for masses.

Investigations

Serum creatinine

Serum electrolytes

Serum glucose

Urinalysis

Serum protein electrophoresis

Kidney biopsy as indicated (some causes require this for diagnosis)

Management

Manage immediately life-threatening metabolic abnormalities (fluids, electrolytes, acidosis). Institute immediate measures to prevent further loss of renal function (BP control, steroids for autoimmune disorders). Refer the patient to a nephrologist.

Institute dialysis in patients with a GFR < 15 mL/minute, and with 1 or more of the following:

- symptoms or signs of uremia (progressive fatigue; anorexia; nausea, vomiting; muscle atrophy; tremors; mental function changes; shallow breathing; metabolic acidosis)
- inability to control hydration status or BP
- inability to maintain nutritional status

KIDNEY PRESENTATIONS

Proteinuria

Differential diagnosis

ORTHOSTATIC PROTEINURIA

This is generally found incidentally on urinalysis for another condition (as a positive urine dipstick for protein).

Signs and symptoms: asymptomatic (generally); child or adolescent (it is uncommon in adults older than 30); elevated protein excretion while in upright position (daytime proteinuria), but normal in supine or recumbent position

Investigations:

Protein:creatinine ratio in urine samples collected in recumbent and upright positions in the daytime and nighttime; elevated ratio in upright sample; normal ratio in recumbent sample

Urinary protein excretion rate in daytime and nighttime collections: normal rate in daytime collection (> 4 mg/m^2 per hour for children over an 8-hour period); normal rate in nighttime collection (< 4 mg/m^2 per hour)

TUBULOINTERSTITIAL PROTEINURIA (INTERSTITIAL NEPHRITIS)

Interstitial nephritis

Signs and symptoms: fever; rash; arthralgia; use of diuretics, antibiotics, analgesics

Investigations: urine eosinophils (this is suggestive); renal biopsy (definitive)

GLOMERULAR PROTEINURIA

Active urine sediment

PRIMARY (E.G., IgA NEPHROPATHY, MEMBRANOPROLIFERATIVE GLOMERULONEPHRITIS)

IgA NEPHROPATHY

Signs and symptoms: recurrent macroscopic hematuria (brown-colored urine) or persistent microscopic hematuria (this is found incidentally on routine exam)

Risk factors: age 20 to 40 (peak incidence); male (more common); Caucasian, Asian, Indigenous descent (highest incidence); URTI; cirrhosis; liver disease; celiac disease; HIV; family history of IgA nephropathy

Investigations: kidney biopsy with immunofluorescence or immunoperoxidase studies for IgA deposits

MEMBRANOPROLIFERATIVE GLOMERULONEPHRITIS

Signs and symptoms: asymptomatic (generally); nephrotic syndrome, or recurrent gross hematuria, or hypertension; proteinuria and hematuria on routine urinalysis; normal or elevated creatinine on blood work

> Nephrotic syndrome: progressive lower extremity edema (ankles and feet); swelling around the eyes; weight gain (from water retention); foamy urine

Risk factors: child, young adult (if idiopathic); Caucasian descent; history HBV, HCV, cancer, autoimmune disease

Investigations: renal biopsy; immunofluorescence microscopy; hypocomplementemia

SECONDARY (E.G., SYSTEMIC LUPUS ERYTHEMATOSUS, POSTINFECTION)

SYSTEMIC LUPUS ERYTHEMATOSUS

Signs and symptoms: personal or family history of SLE; malar rash; arthritis; cytopenias

Investigations: elevated ANA titer; elevated dsDNA

POSTSTREPTOCOCCAL GLOMERULONEPHRITIS

Signs and symptoms: child 5 to 12 years, or adult older than 60 (increased risk); asymptomatic (often); gross hematuria (brown or cloudy urine); proteinuria; edema; hypertension; acute kidney injury; recent skin or throat infection due to nephritogenic strains of group A β-hemolytic streptococcus

Investigations: elevated serum creatinine; positive throat or skin culture for recent infection; decreased total complement activity in the first 2 weeks of disease (C3, CH50); elevated antibody titres for extracellular streptococcal products (positive for ASO, AHase, ASKase, anti-NAD, anti-DNase B)

Nonactive urine sediment

PRIMARY (E.G., MINIMAL CHANGE, FOCAL SEGMENTAL GLOMERULOSCLEROSIS)

MINIMAL CHANGE DISEASE

This is a major cause of nephrotic syndrome in children (mostly younger than 6) and adults (the average age of onset is 40).

Signs and symptoms: facial edema that is preceded by URTI, allergic reaction to a bee sting, use of NSAIDs, or cancer; malaise; fatigue; weight gain; hypovolemia; hypertension (often in adults, less commonly in children), thromboembolism, or infection; wet retina; dependent and subungual edema; muscle wasting; thinning of the skin; growth failure in children if prolonged proteinuria

Investigations: profound proteinuria; random albumin to creatinine ratio > 5; slightly elevated plasma creatinine

FOCAL SEGMENTAL GLOMERULOSCLEROSIS

Signs and symptoms: asymptomatic proteinuria (usual)

> If symptomatic: nephrotic syndrome (progressive lower extremity edema; swelling around the eyes; weight gain from water retention; foamy urine)
>
> Severe symptoms: severe hypertension; massive proteinuria; poor response to corticosteroids

Investigations: histology

SECONDARY (E.G., DIABETES, AMYLOID)

DIABETES MELLITUS

Signs and symptoms: personal or family history of diabetes; history of diabetic complications and/or inadequate monitoring; polydipsia, polyuria, and/or weight loss

> In the context of proteinuria: heavy proteinuria (protein excretion > 3.5 g in a 24-hour urine collection) with or without nephrotic syndrome

AMYLOIDOSIS

Signs and symptoms: male, older than 50 (higher incidence); asymptomatic until advanced; enlarged tongue (this causes swallowing difficulty, shortness of breath); skin symptoms (thickening; easy bruising; purpura around the eyes); numbness, tingling, pain in the extremities; diarrhea or constipation; feeling full quickly on eating, with weight loss; variable additional symptoms depending on the organ or system affected

> Renal amyloidosis: nephrotic syndrome, heavy proteinuria
>
> Cardiac amyloidosis: shortness of breath; cardiac arrhythmia; diastolic and systolic HF symptoms (edema of the ankles and feet; fatigue; weakness; nausea)
>
> Liver amyloidosis: enlarged liver; elevated serum ALT; elevated ALP
>
> GI amyloidosis: decreased appetite; diarrhea; nausea; abdominal pain; weight loss

Investigations: detection of monoclonal paraprotein in serum or urine (primary amyloidosis)

Keys to patient encounter

Key concern

Proteinuria is a predictor of CKD. The diagnosis of proteinuria is based largely on lab tests and subsequent ancillary testing; once discovered, the key concern is the patient's risk of CKD.

History

Ask about a personal or family history of kidney problems, and conditions associated with kidney problems (diabetes, hypertension).

Physical exam

Except to assess BP, physical exam will not likely contribute useful information.

Vital signs: Look for hypertension.

Investigations

Qualitative measure of the proteinuria: albumin:creatinine ratio, random or 24-hour collection

IF THE DIAGNOSIS REMAINS UNCERTAIN

Blood glucose for diabetes

Serum protein electrophoresis for amyloidosis and multiple myeloma

Management

The goals of management are to treat any underlying causes (hypertension and diabetes). In hypertension, consider treatment with an ACE inhibitor.

LANGUAGE AND SPEECH DISORDERS

Language and speech disorders

Differential diagnosis

LANGUAGE DISORDER

Delayed and developmental language impairment in children (e.g., hearing impairment, autism spectrum disorder, neglect, abuse)

DELAYED AND DEVELOPMENTAL LANGUAGE IMPAIRMENT IN GENERAL (PEDIATRIC)

Signs and symptoms: differences in language development compared to other children of the same age; problems with social interactions with other children

HEARING IMPAIRMENT

Signs and symptoms: problems identifying the sources of sounds; complications during gestation (e.g., toxin exposure such as alcohol) and/or delivery; blocked (from impacted wax or mass) or nonmobile (from chronic effusion) tympanic membranes

Investigations: hearing test

AUTISM SPECTRUM DISORDER[1(pp50–51)]

Signs and symptoms: deficits in social interaction and communication; repetitive, stereotyped behaviors (motor and/or vocal); restricted interests; sensory problems; presence of symptoms in all contexts (e.g., home, school); presence of symptoms from early childhood

NEGLECT

Neglect involves failure to provide all or some basic physical, emotional, educational, and medical needs. Examples include rejecting a child and not giving love; not feeding a child; not dressing a child in proper clothing; not giving needed medical or dental care; and abandonment by leaving a child alone for a long time.

Signs and symptoms: not attending school regularly; poor hygiene, dental care; malnutrition; reports by the child suggesting lack of physical and/or emotional care at home

ABUSE

Signs and symptoms: disclosed abuse (victims do not always disclose abuse); resistance by the parent or caregiver to having the patient interviewed alone (usual)

Physical abuse: inconsistency between an injury and the explanation for the injury and/or the developmental stage of the child; facial contusions; marks on the neck or limbs; burn marks; ligature marks on the wrists or ankles; bite marks; lash marks; bruises or broken bones unexplainable by usual activities

Sexual abuse: behavior and knowledge that is inappropriate for the child's age; pregnancy or STI; blood in the child's underwear; trouble walking or sitting, or complaints of genital pain; sexual abuse of other children by victim

Psychological abuse: problems in school; eating disorders leading to weight loss or poor weight gain; emotional issues (anxiety, low self-esteem); depression; extreme behavior (e.g., acting out to seek attention); trouble sleeping

No evidence of medical conditions that could mimic abuse (e.g., malabsorption; developmental delay due to complications during gestation or delivery; genetic or metabolic disorders)

Risk factors: history of substance abuse by the parents or caregivers; unstable living situation of the parents or caregivers

Degenerative, vascular, or other central nervous system disorders (e.g., stroke)

Signs and symptoms (in general): older age (more common); personal or family history of cardiovascular or cerebrovascular disease; obesity; smoking; diabetes; hypertension; dyslipidemia; lack of physical activity; poor diet

Head injury

Signs and symptoms: history of trauma or assault (high-risk mechanisms include pedestrian-vehicle accidents; accidents where people are ejected from vehicles; and falls from heights ≥ 1 metre, or down ≥ 5 stairs); motor or sensory deficits on neurological exam

Investigations: CT scan of the head

SPEECH DISORDER

Articulation disorder (e.g., dysarthria)

DYSARTHRIA

Causes include trauma, neurological injury, stroke, cerebral palsy, muscular dystrophy, ALS, and MS.

Signs and symptoms: drooling and/or difficulty swallowing; incomprehensible speech; limited movement of the tongue, lip, or jaw on speaking; abnormalities in voice rate, quality, pitch, nasality, or rhythm; motor or sensory deficits on neurological exam

Fluency (e.g., stuttering, Parkinson disease)

FLUENCY IN GENERAL

Signs and symptoms: involuntary repetition of sounds (initial consonants usually); prolongation of sounds or syllables; involuntary silent pauses

STUTTERING

Signs and symptoms: childhood onset

PARKINSON DISEASE

Signs and symptoms (mnemonic **TRAP**): **t**remor at rest; **r**igidity of the lower limbs; **a**kinesia, bradykinesia; **p**ostural instability

Other symptoms: cognitive impairment; dementia; shuffling gait with stooped posture and loss of arm swing; micrographia; hypophonia; masklike facies; "pill rolling"; lack of blinking; orthostatic hypotension

History of use of antipsychotics, antiemetics; toxin ingestion (e.g., carbon monoxide, cyanide); head trauma; vascular disease; other neurodegenerative disease (e.g., Lewy body dementia, Huntington disease); brain tumor, hydrocephalus; metabolic conditions (e.g., hypoparathyroidism, Wilson disease, chronic liver failure); infections that spread to the brain (HIV/AIDS, syphilis, prion disease, toxoplasmosis, encephalitis lethargica, progressive multifocal leukoencephalopathy)

Speech apparatus lesions (e.g., cleft palate, head and neck neoplasm)

CLEFT PALATE

This is usually diagnosed at birth. When it affects only the muscles of the palate (submucous cleft palate), it may not be detected until later.

Signs and symptoms (submucous cleft palate): difficulty swallowing, hypernasal voice resonance, auditory issues, frequent ear infections

HEAD AND NECK CANCER

Signs and symptoms: symptoms for > 3 weeks; persistent unilateral throat discomfort

Lesion in the oral cavity: persistent red and/or white patches on the oral mucosa; ulceration and/or swelling of the oropharynx or mucosa; persistent mass; tongue pain; tongue deviation; hoarseness; unexplained tooth mobility and/or looseness; earache; difficulty swallowing; bleeding in the oral cavity; stridor; facial pain or numbness

Lesion in the nasopharynx: neck lump; bloody nasal discharge; nasal blockage; unilateral hearing loss; ringing in the ear; recurrent otitis media; headache; facial pain or numbness; double vision; persistent cough

Investigations: endoscopic visualization; fine needle aspiration or core biopsy of mass

Keys to patient encounter

Key concern

Differentiate language disorders from speech disorders:

Language disorder: impaired comprehension and/or use of the form, content, or function of language (difficulty understanding speech or sharing thoughts)

Speech disorder: impaired articulation, fluency, voice (difficulty producing speech sounds correctly)

History

IN A CHILD

Ask about the child's speech and language milestones (see the pointer). Ask whether the family can understand what the child says. Ask about a family history of ADHD and autism spectrum disorder. Ask about a history of head injury.

IN AN ADULT

Ask when the speech issues started. Ask about a history of head trauma, brain tumor, Lyme disease, facial paralysis, poorly fitting dentures, head injury, stroke, and neurodegenerative diseases (e.g., MS, MD, Parkinson disease). Ask about alcohol consumption.

Physical exam

Observe the patient speaking.

Ears, nose, and throat (including otoscopy)

Full neurological exam

POINTER

Simplified speech and language milestones

12 months: babbles and uses gestures

15 months: says a few words and correctly points to objects or pictures

18 months: understands simple commands and has more than 20 words

24 months: has 50 to 100 words, joins 2 words together

36 months: has more than 300 words, asks questions, makes simple, grammatically correct sentences

4 years: able to tell a simple story

Investigations

Hearing test

CT or MRI scan of the head in the presence of trauma or neurologic symptoms

Management

Refer pediatric patients for speech therapy. Consider referral to an ENT surgeon or neurologist, as appropriate.

REFERENCE

1. American Psychiatric Association. Diagnostic and statistical manual of mental disorders. 5th ed. Arlington, VA: American Psychiatric Association; 2013. 59–60. 991 p.

LIPIDS (ABNORMAL SERUM LIPIDS)

Lipids (abnormal serum lipids)

Differential diagnosis

HYPERCHOLESTEROLEMIA

Primary (familial)

Signs and symptoms: extreme hypercholesterolemia (LDL) without secondary causes; corneal arcus at younger than 45; xanthomas in the tendons of the feet, hands, elbows, knees (the Achilles tendon is the most common site), and around the eyes (xanthelasma)

Family history: elevated LDL; early onset (younger than 50) CAD (especially premature MI)

Personal history: premature CAD, cardiovascular disease

Secondary

ENDOCRINE DISORDER (E.G., DIABETES MELLITUS, HYPOTHYROIDISM)

DIABETES

Signs and symptoms: personal or family history of diabetes; history of diabetic complications and/or inadequate monitoring; polydipsia, polyuria, and/or weight loss

Investigations: fasting glucose or HbA_{1c}

HYPOTHYROIDISM

Signs and symptoms: history of hypothyroidism or symptoms of hypothyroidism (cold intolerance, decreased reflexes, dry skin, weight gain, impaired cognition)

Investigations: elevated thyrotropin (TSH)

CHOLESTATIC LIVER DISEASE

Signs and symptoms: abdominal pain; nausea, vomiting; jaundice; itchiness; palpable, tender liver and/or gallbladder; history of liver disease, gallstones, cancer; current pregnancy

Investigations: abnormal liver enzyme tests, elevated bilirubin, abdominal US

NEPHROTIC SYNDROME OR CHRONIC KIDNEY INJURY

NEPHROTIC SYNDROME

Signs and symptoms: progressive lower extremity edema (ankles and feet); swelling around the eyes; weight gain (from water retention); foamy urine

Risk factors: conditions that damage the kidneys (e.g., diabetes, SLE, amyloidosis); use of NSAIDs, antibiotics; history of HIV, HBV, HCV, malaria

Investigations: urine (proteinuria, spot urine protein:creatinine ratio, lipuria); hyponatremia with low fractional sodium excretion; low serum albumin; high total cholesterol (hyperlipidemia); elevated BUN

CHRONIC KIDNEY INJURY

Signs and symptoms: history of kidney disease, chronic renal failure, and/or current renal dialysis; bilateral lower limb swelling; shortness of breath; paroxysmal nocturnal dyspnea; orthopnea

Risk factors: diabetes, diabetic complications, and/or inadequate monitoring; hypertension; smoking

OTHER

OBESITY

Signs and symptoms: BMI ≥ 30.0 (see *Notes on labs and assessments*)

DRUGS (E.G., STEROIDS)

Examples of steroids include corticosteroids, anabolic steroids, and progestins.

Glucocorticoids and estrogens elevate triglycerides and raise HDL.

Oral anabolic steroids reduce HDL.

Injectable testosterone does not affect the LDL:HDL ratio.

Progestins have different effects on HDL, LDL, and triglycerides.

HYPERTRIGLYCERIDEMIA

Primary (familial)

Signs and symptoms: family history of hypertriglyceridemia; personal or family history of CAD; pancreatitis; elevated BP; xanthomas

> Xanthomas: palmar (yellow creases on the palms); tuberous (red/orange, shiny nodules on the elbows and knees); or eruptive (small yellow papules on the back, chest, proximal extremities)

Secondary

OBESITY—SEE ABOVE

DIABETES MELLITUS—SEE ABOVE

NEPHROTIC SYNDROME OR CHRONIC KIDNEY INJURY—SEE ABOVE

DRUGS

Examples of drugs associated with hypertriglyceridemia include OCs, beta-blockers, and thiazide-type diuretics.

ALCOHOL

LOW HIGH-DENSITY LIPOPROTEIN

Primary

Signs and symptoms: personal or family history of premature atherosclerosis, CAD, stroke

Secondary

OBESITY—SEE ABOVE

DRUGS

Examples of drugs associated with low HDL include progesterone, anabolic steroids, and beta-blockers.

METABOLIC SYNDROME

Signs and symptoms: obesity, elevated BP, elevated serum glucose, dyslipidemia

> Diagnostic criteria (at least 3): increased waist circumference ($\geq$ 102 cm for men and $\geq$ 88 cm for women);
> systolic BP $\geq$ 130 mmHg, diastolic BP $\geq$ 85 mmHg; fasting

glucose ≥ 110 mg/dL (6.1 mmol/L); triglycerides ≥ 150 mg/dL (1.7 mmol/L); HDL (men) < 40 mg/dL (1.0 mmol/L); HDL (women) < 50 mg/dL (1.3 mmol/L)

Keys to patient encounter

Key concern

Identify patients who will benefit from serum cholesterol reduction, as well as primary and secondary prevention.

History

PAST MEDICAL HISTORY

Ask about heart disease, diabetes, kidney disease, and stroke.

FAMILY HISTORY

Ask about high cholesterol, premature heart disease, and stroke.

SOCIAL HISTORY

Ask about the patient's diet and exercise routines.

Physical exam

Vital signs

Height and weight:

- Calculate the patient's BMI (see *Notes on labs and assessments*).
- Measure the patient's waist circumference.

General inspection: Examine the eyes for corneal arcus and the skin for xanthomas.

Cardiovascular

Respiratory

Investigations

Lipids (see *Notes on labs and assessments*)

Creatinine

HbA_{1c}

Thyrotropin (TSH)

Liver function (see *Notes on labs and assessments*)

Albumin

Urinalysis

Management

Calculate the patient's risk of cardiovascular disease with the Framingham Risk Score (FRS).

For all patients, recommend lifestyle changes (diet, exercise, weight reduction). Discuss the risks and benefits of lipid-lowering drugs.

Prescribe lipid-lowering drugs in the following cases:

- high FRS (higher than 20%) or intermediate FRS (10% to 19%) with LDL ≥ 135 mg/dL (3.5 mmol/L) or non-HDL ≥ 166 mg/dL (4.3 mmol/L)
- men aged 50 or older, and women aged 60 or older, with 1 additional risk factor (low HDL, smoking, hypertension, impaired fasting glucose, large waist circumference)
- presence of clinical atherosclerosis (ACS, stable angina, stroke, TIA, peripheral arterial disease), AAA, diabetes mellitus (in patients 40 years or older, or 30 years or older with diabetes for at least 15 years; or with microvascular complications), CKD, LDL ≥ 193 mg/dL (5.0 mmol/L)

LIVER FUNCTION (ABNORMAL LIVER FUNCTION TESTS)

Liver function (abnormal liver function tests)

Differential diagnosis

HEPATOCELLULAR CAUSE

Acute condition (e.g., infection, medication)

Infectious causes include HAV, HBV, HEV, CMV, HSV, EBV, and yellow fever.

Medication causes include acetaminophen (most common), antibiotics, NSAIDs, antiepileptics, statins, antihypertensives, and antivirals (also herbs and supplements: kava kava, Herbalife, Hydroxycut).

Signs and symptoms: viral-like illness; right upper quadrant abdominal pain; jaundice; intracranial hypertension; progression to encephalopathy over weeks

Viral hepatitis: skin lesions, enlarged liver

Intracranial hypertension: posturing, peripheral reflex changes, systemic hypertension, bradycardia

Encephalopathy: behavioral change, disorientation, drowsiness, confusion, incoherent speech, coma, unresponsiveness to pain

Investigations: blood tests (electrolytes, phosphate, glucose); liver enzyme and function tests (PT/INR, AST, ALT, ALP, GGT, bilirubin, albumin); toxicology screen; viral hepatitis serologies

Chronic condition (e.g., infection, medication)

CHRONIC LIVER DISEASE IN GENERAL

Patients with compensated cirrhosis may be asymptomatic.

Common causes include viral hepatitis, nonalcoholic fatty liver disease, and alcohol abuse. Medication-induced chronic liver disease is less common.

Signs and symptoms: jaundice; abdominal pain, swelling; swelling in the legs and ankles; systemic symptoms (anorexia, weight loss, weakness, fatigue); itching; easy bruising

Investigations: CBC (decreased platelets); liver enzyme and function tests (e.g., PT/INR, PTT, AST, ALT, bilirubin total, direct and indirect); liver biopsy; Doppler US; CT scan; MRI; transient elastography

CHRONIC HBV OR HCV INFECTION

HCV is often asymptomatic.

Risk factors: autoimmune conditions, unprotected sex, IV drug abuse, blood transfusions, tattoos, body piercings, imprisonment, workplace exposure to body fluids

NONALCOHOLIC FATTY LIVER DISEASE

This is the most common form of chronic liver disease.

Signs and symptoms: usually asymptomatic, fatigue, right upper quadrant abdominal pain, enlarged liver, muscle weakness

More severe: jaundice, gynecomastia, enlarged spleen, red palms

Risk factors: high cholesterol; high serum triglycerides; obesity; type 2 diabetes; metabolic syndrome; polycystic ovary syndrome; hypothyroidism; hypopituitarism; recent weight gain or loss

CHOLESTATIC CAUSE

Intrahepatic condition (e.g., pregnancy)

PREGNANCY

Signs and symptoms: amenorrhea; sexual activity, especially without contraception or with inconsistent use of contraception; nausea, vomiting (common early sign); breast enlargement and tenderness; increased frequency of urination without pain or difficulty; fatigue

Investigations: blood or urine β-HCG

Extrahepatic condition (e.g., gallstones)

GALLSTONES

Symptoms: right upper quadrant abdominal pain, under the ribs; pain that prevents normal or deep breathing; Murphy sign (while palpating near the gallbladder, severe pain on taking a breath); vomiting

> Pain characteristics: 15 minutes to 24 hours in duration; radiating to the right upper back or shoulder blade area; no relief with movement or changing position; onset at night, on waking, or after eating
>
> Symptoms of bile duct blocked by gallstone: jaundice, dark urine, light-colored stools, fever, chills

Risk factors: high BMI or obesity (see *Notes on labs and assessments*); high-fat diet; diabetes; older than 60; estrogen medications; family history of gallstones; female

Investigations: US, abdominal x-ray, CT scan, hepatobiliary scan, MRCP, ERCP

CONGENITAL ABNORMALITIES (E.G., GILBERT SYNDROME)

Gilbert syndrome

This inherited disorder does not impair health and requires no treatment.

Signs and symptoms: usually asymptomatic, jaundice

> Triggers for jaundice in Gilbert syndrome: current illness (e.g., flu, cold) or menstruation; recent fasting; certain medications (e.g., acetaminophen, cancer drug irinotecan)

Risk factors: family history of Gilbert syndrome (to inherit the disorder, both parents must carry the gene)

Investigations: elevated unconjugated bilirubin, normal CBC

OTHER (E.G., CELIAC DISEASE)

Celiac disease

Signs and symptoms: family history of celiac disease, or signs and symptoms of celiac disease (chronic abdominal pain, rashes)

Investigations: positive serum anti-tTG (with IgA level); duodenal biopsy to detect villous blunting

Keys to patient encounter

Note that abnormal liver function may be discovered incidentally, as part of the workup for systemic disease, abdominal pain, or jaundice.

Key concern

Identify underlying liver disorder or systemic disease.

History

HISTORY OF PRESENT ILLNESS

Ask how the abnormal liver function was discovered and what symptoms the patient has. Listen for incidental discovery associated with a specific workup, and symptoms associated with particular entities. Examples of characteristic symptoms include:

Pregnancy: missed menstrual periods

Gallstones: sudden-onset abdominal pain that is worse with deep breaths

Celiac disease: rash and chronic abdominal pain

FAMILY HISTORY

Ask about a family history of liver disease.

SOCIAL HISTORY

Ask about alcohol and drug use. Ask about risk factors for viral hepatitis (unprotected sex, IV drug abuse, blood transfusions, tattoos, body piercings, imprisonment, workplace exposure to body fluids) and about immunizations for HAV and HBV.

Physical exam

Vital signs: Look for fever.

General inspection:

- Examine the skin and sclera for jaundice.
- Check for stigmata of chronic liver disease (e.g., palmar erythema, spider angioma, gynecomastia).

Abdominal: Look for an enlarged and/or tender liver and spleen, and for ascites.

Lymph nodes: Check for lymphadenopathy (posterior cervical in infectious mononucleosis).

Investigations

CBC

Liver function (see *Notes on labs and assessments*)

Creatinine

Serology for infectious causes

US or CT scan of the abdomen

Other specific tests depending on the likely entity

Management

Treat the underlying condition. Identify complications from the presence of liver disease (e.g., bleeding, ascites). Consider referring the patient to a hepatologist or general surgeon.

LUMPS AND MASSES

Abdominal or pelvic mass

Differential diagnosis

ORGANOMEGALY

Hepatomegaly

Signs and symptoms: palpable, enlarged liver; signs of CHF (severe shortness of breath; elevated JVP; edema in the abdomen and legs;

pink phlegm; heart murmurs and extra cardiac sounds); signs of infection or malignancy (fever, enlarged lymph nodes)

History of CHF; hepatic vein thrombosis (Budd-Chiari syndrome); myeloproliferative disorders; hepatitis, or risk factors for HBV or HCV infection (unprotected sex, IV drug abuse, blood transfusions, tattoos, body piercings, workplace exposure to body fluids); lipid storage disease (e.g., Gaucher disease)

Investigations: abnormal serum liver function tests (this indicates liver disease)

Splenomegaly

Signs and symptoms: palpable, enlarged spleen

History of viral infection (especially mononucleosis), myeloproliferative disorders, lymphoma, liver disease, hemolytic anemia

Investigations: abnormal serum liver function tests (this indicates liver disease); blood tests to detect hemoglobinopathy, hemolytic anemia; heterophile antibody test to detect mononucleosis; abnormal differential and blood smear in the case of hematologic malignancy

Enlarged kidneys (e.g., cysts, hydronephrosis)

Signs and symptoms: palpable, enlarged kidneys

History of oliguria, hypertension; personal or family history of polycystic kidney disease, renal stones

Investigations: elevated creatinine (this indicates renal impairment)

NEOPLASM (BENIGN OR MALIGNANT)

Lymphoma or sarcoma

Signs and symptoms (in general): constitutional symptoms (weight loss, fever, night sweats), enlarged lymph nodes, palpable abdominal mass

Investigations: peripheral blood smear to detect blasts or cancer cells; bone marrow examination to detect excess blasts or cancer cells

Gastrointestinal tumor (e.g., gastric, colon, pancreas, hepatoma, gastrointestinal stromal tumor)

Signs and symptoms (in general): weight loss, abdominal pain, blood in the stool, change in bowel habits, family history of GI cancer, palpable abdominal mass

Investigations: elevated CEA, elevated CA 19-9

Gynecologic tumor (e.g., ovarian, uterine)—see below

Renal or adrenal neoplasm

Signs and symptoms (in general): flank pain, constitutional symptoms (weight loss, night sweats), blood in the urine, hypertension (this suggests renal tumor), palpable abdominal mass

Neuroblastoma

Neuroblastoma usually affects children younger than 5 years.

Signs and symptoms: abdominal pain; swollen legs; palpable, painless mass

GYNECOLOGIC

Ovary (e.g., benign or malignant mass)

Signs and symptoms (in general): pelvic pain; pain on intercourse; menstrual irregularities; change in bowel or bladder habits; family or personal history of gynecological or breast cancer

> Malignant ovarian masses: constitutional symptoms (fever, weight loss, night sweats)

Investigations (for malignancy); elevated CA 125

Fallopian tube (e.g., ectopic pregnancy)

ECTOPIC PREGNANCY

Signs and symptoms: symptoms of pregnancy and/or positive pregnancy test; pelvic pain; vaginal bleeding; painful intercourse; shoulder pain; palpable tubal mass; pelvic tenderness and pain associated with 1 or both adnexa

> Severe symptom: syncope

Risk factors: previous ectopic pregnancy, PID, pregnancy during IUD use

Investigations (pathognomonic): β-HCG above discriminatory zone (> 1500–2000 mIU/mL [1500–2000 IU/L]) **with** transvaginal US findings of a lack of intrauterine gestational sac, complex (mixed solid and cystic) masses in the adnexa, and free fluid in the cul-de-sac

Uterus (e.g., leiomyoma, pregnancy)

LEIOMYOMA

This is the most common pelvic tumor in women.

Signs and symptoms: commonly asymptomatic; premenopausal (usual); heavy or prolonged menstrual bleeding; pelvic, abdominal

JKL

pressure; pain on intercourse; urinary symptoms (incontinence; frequent urination; difficulty emptying the bladder); constipation; pelvic mass or enlarged, irregular uterus on bimanual palpation

Risk factors: family history of leiomyoma; African descent

Investigations: US to detect mass ≥ 1 cm in diameter

PREGNANCY

Signs and symptoms: amenorrhea, especially during childbearing years (some experience spotting); sexual activity, especially without contraception or with inconsistent use of contraception; nausea, vomiting (common early sign); breast enlargement and tenderness; increased frequency of urination without other urinary symptoms; fatigue

Investigations: blood or urine β-HCG

BLADDER OR PROSTATE CONDITIONS (E.G., URINARY RETENTION, CANCER)

Signs and symptoms (in general): change in urinary habits (reduced urination in prostate conditions; blood in the urine; reduced and/or frequent urination in bladder conditions; new-onset nocturia in adults); palpable bladder mass, or enlarged or irregular prostate on palpation

Investigations: urine cytology; CT scan or cytoscopy to detect bladder mass

OTHER

Pancreatic pseudocyst

Signs and symptoms: history of pancreatitis (usual), fever, abdominal tenderness, palpable abdominal mass

Abdominal aortic aneurysm

Signs and symptoms: back pain; abdominal pain; syncope; palpable pulsatile midabdominal mass

Risk factors: history of smoking; family history of AAA; previous aneurysms; hypertension

Abdominal wall masses

Signs and symptoms: abdominal pain; change in bowel or bladder habits; renal obstruction; constitutional symptoms (weight loss, fever, fatigue, night sweats)

Keys to patient encounter

Key concern

Recognize features of a mass that indicate the need for immediate intervention.

History

CHARACTERISTICS OF THE MASS

Localize and characterize the mass. Ask where the mass is, and when and how the patient discovered it. Ask whether the mass has grown.

Ask whether the patient could be pregnant.

ASSOCIATED SYMPTOMS

Ask about pain; constitutional symptoms (these suggest malignancy: fever, weight loss, night sweats, fatigue); urinary symptoms (these suggest gynecological, bladder, or prostate conditions); nausea; vomiting; constipation; diarrhea; and changes in menstruation.

PAST MEDICAL HISTORY

Ask about abdominal or pelvic surgeries.

MEDICATIONS

Ask in particular about narcotics, opiates, and anticholinergic medications (these may cause urinary retention or constipation).

Physical exam

Vital signs: Look for hypotension and fever.

Abdominal: Palpate the mass. Check for AAA.

DRE: Look for masses and blood.

Pelvic: Look for ovarian or uterine masses.

Investigations

CBC

β-HGC in women of childbearing age

Tumor markers
Creatinine
Electrolytes (see *Notes on labs and assessments*)
Liver function (see *Notes on labs and assessments*)
Urinalysis
Abdominal US
Abdominal CT scan with contrast to assess for bowel or pelvic pathology, and organomegaly
KUB x-ray to look for constipation, obstruction, and free intraperitoneal air
Colonoscopy in suspected bowel mass

Management

Stabilize any patient with a life-threatening cause (e.g., ruptured AAA). Treat the specific entity identified. Most patients with a mass require referral to a general surgeon, urologist, or gynecologist. Discontinue any contributing medications.

LUMPS AND MASSES

Lymphadenopathy

Differential diagnosis

LOCALIZED

Reactive condition (e.g., tonsillitis)

TONSILLITIS

Signs and symptoms: sore throat; difficulty swallowing; fever; scratchy voice; bad breath; stiff neck; intense erythema of tonsils and pharynx; swollen tonsils that may be coated in pus; swollen, tender regional lymph nodes

Investigations: throat swab

Neoplastic (e.g., metastatic cancer)

METASTATIC CANCER

Signs and symptoms: history of cancer; constitutional symptoms (weight loss, fever, night sweats)

Investigations: CBC with differential; platelet count; ESR; CT scan; tissue biopsy or fine needle aspiration biopsy for histology/cytology and immunophenotyping

DIFFUSE

DIFFUSE LYMPHADENOPATHY IN GENERAL

Signs and symptoms: swollen lymph nodes in multiple locations, fever, fatigue, nausea, vomiting, loss of appetite, headaches, joint pain, sore throat

Infection (e.g., viral)

Signs and symptoms:

> Mononucleosis: classic triad of fever, pharyngitis, lymphadenopathy (usually posterior cervical); fatigue and malaise; headache; abdominal pain; nausea, vomiting; rash; splenomegaly; palatal exanthems or petechiae
>
> Hepatitis: viral-like illness; abdominal pain; jaundice; palpable, tender liver; history of HAV, HBV, or HCV, or risk factors for them (autoimmune conditions, unprotected sex, IV drug abuse, blood transfusions, tattoos, body piercings, imprisonment, workplace exposure to body fluids)
>
> HCV: often asymptomatic
>
> HIV: flu-like symptoms in the first, acute phase; leukopenia in the second, latent, asymptomatic stage (200–499 CD4 cells/μL [$0.2–0.499 \times 10^9$/L]); lymphadenopathy
>
> CMV: muscle aches, rash
>
> Dengue: pain behind the eyes; rash that appears 2 to 5 days after fever onset

Investigations: blood antigen or antibody tests; urinalysis; throat culture (in suspected strep throat)

Inflammatory condition (e.g., sarcoidosis)

SARCOIDOSIS

Signs and symptoms: lymphadenopathy (a mass in the middle of the mediastinum is the most common lesion), fever, fatigue, weight loss, lung symptoms (dry cough, shortness of breath, wheezing, chest pain)

Risk factors: age 20 to 40, African descent, family history of sarcoidosis

Investigations: chest x-ray to detect enlarged hilar and mediastinal lymph nodes; biopsy to detect granulomas

Neoplastic condition (e.g., lymphoma)

LYMPHOMA

Signs and symptoms (non-Hodgkin): constitutional symptoms (fatigue, fever, night sweats, weight loss), enlarged lymph nodes, chest pain, coughing, shortness of breath

Hodgkin lymphoma (less common): constitutional symptoms (fatigue, fever, night sweats, weight loss); enlarged lymph nodes; itching or pain on drinking alcohol, or increased sensitivity to alcohol

Investigations: blasts or cancer cells on peripheral blood smear; excess blasts or cancer cells on bone marrow examination

Keys to patient encounter

Key concern

Determine the need for biopsy.

History

HISTORY OF PRESENT ILLNESS

Ask how long the patient has had swollen lymph nodes and what other symptoms the patient has. Listen for recent swelling versus long-standing, more insidious swelling (long-standing swelling suggests a noninfectious condition); and for constitutional symptoms (fever, weight loss, fatigue, and/or night sweats), which also suggest a noninfectious condition.

PAST MEDICAL HISTORY

Ask about cancer and sarcoidosis.

FAMILY HISTORY

Ask about cancer and sarcoidosis.

Physical exam

General inspection: Look for rash.

Lymph nodes:

- Examine the submandibular, axillary, inguinal, and supraclavicular regions.
- Examine any enlarged nodes noted by the patient.
- If you identify localized lymphadenopathy, look for an adjacent precipitating lesion (e.g., local infection).
- Ask the patient if identified enlarged lymph nodes are tender (nontender nodes are more likely in malignant conditions).

Head and neck: In the case of cervical lymphadenopathy, perform a full exam of the head and neck, including the oral cavity, looking for infections and tumors.

Breast: In the case of axillary lymphadenopathy, perform a breast exam.

Abdominal: Examine the spleen for enlargement.

Investigations

CBC

Lymph node biopsy in cases of generalized lymphadenopathy, or where lymphadenopathy has been present for more than 3 to 4 weeks

Tests for infection as indicated in the differential diagnosis

CT scan or MRI of the affected area(s) to look for internal masses and additional lymphadenopathy

Management

GENERALIZED LYMPHADENOPATHY

This usually represents systemic disease. Order specific tests as indicated by the differential diagnosis. If no diagnosis is made based on these tests, a node should be biopsied.

LOCALIZED LYMPHADENOPATHY

Order a biopsy of nodes in patients with constitutional symptoms (weight loss, fever, fatigue) and/or risk factors for malignancy.

POINTER

Size: abnormal lymph nodes

As a general rule, lymph nodes > 1 cm in diameter are considered abnormal.

JKL

In patients with unexplained lymphadenopathy that is localized, and an otherwise reassuring clinical picture, biopsy may be delayed by 3 to 4 weeks to see if the lymphadenopathy resolves on its own.

Mediastinal mass

Differential diagnosis

ANTERIOR

Tumor (e.g., thymoma, lymphoma)

THYMOMA

This is the most common neoplasm of the thymus in adults, and the most common anterior mediastinal mass.

It is usually found incidentally during imaging.

It is benign unless it invades through the capsule.

Signs and symptoms: age 40 to 60 (more common); asymptomatic (usual); thoracic symptoms in large tumors (chest pain, shortness of breath, cough, phrenic nerve palsy); paraneoplastic syndrome (myasthenia gravis is the most common: weakness of voluntary skeletal muscles, fatigue, double vision, drooping eyelids, difficulty swallowing)

> Metastasized thymoma: pleural or pericardial effusion, thoracic symptoms

Investigations: CT scan or MRI of mass; resection of mass

LYMPHOMA

Signs and symptoms (non-Hodgkin): constitutional symptoms (fatigue, fever, night sweats, weight loss), enlarged lymph nodes, chest pain, coughing, shortness of breath

> Hodgkin lymphoma (less common): constitutional symptoms (fatigue, fever, night sweats, weight loss); enlarged lymph nodes; itching or pain on drinking alcohol, or increased sensitivity to alcohol

Investigations: blasts or cancer cells on peripheral blood smear; excess blasts or cancer cells on bone marrow examination

Other (e.g., aneurysm)

ANEURYSM

Examples include thoracic aortic aneurysm in the chest cavity and AAA.

Signs and symptoms: pain in the chest or abdomen; back pain

Investigations: echocardiogram or transesophageal US (in thoracic aneurysm) or abdominal US (in abdominal aneurysm); chest x-ray to detect masses; CT scan for detailed images; MRI to characterize for size and location

MIDDLE

Tumor (e.g., bronchogenic cancer)

BRONCHOGENIC CANCER (LUNG CANCER)

Signs and symptoms: asymptomatic (usual in early disease); changes in a chronic cough; hemoptysis; shortness of breath; wheezing; hoarseness; weight loss; bone pain; headache

Risk factors: smoking or secondhand-smoke exposure; family history of lung cancer

Investigations: x-ray, CT scan to detect masses and lesions; biopsy

Other (e.g., sarcoidosis)

SARCOIDOSIS

This involves growth of tiny granulomas, most commonly in the lungs, lymph nodes, and skin.

It is usually detected incidentally through x-ray for another reason.

Signs and symptoms: lymphadenopathy (a mass in the middle of the mediastinum is the most common lesion), fever, fatigue, weight loss, lung symptoms (dry cough, shortness of breath, wheezing, chest pain)

Risk factors: age 20 to 40, African descent, family history of sarcoidosis

Investigations: chest x-ray to detect enlarged hilar and mediastinal lymph nodes; biopsy to detect granulomas

POSTERIOR

Tumor (e.g., esophageal cancer)

ESOPHAGEAL CANCER

Signs and symptoms: asymptomatic (often in early disease); pain with swallowing; heartburn-like pain; hoarse cough; nausea, vomiting (sometimes with blood)

Risk factors: smoking, alcohol use, family history

Other (e.g., hiatal hernia)

HIATAL HERNIA

Signs and symptoms: asymptomatic (sometimes); symptoms of GERD (burning chest pain radiating into the throat with bitter taste in mouth; pain that is worse with lying down and certain foods, better with standing up or antacids; acid damage to teeth)

Larger hernias: syncope (swallow syncope syndrome); shortness of breath; edema; reduced exercise tolerance with HF

Investigations: esophageal x-ray (barium swallow); upper GI endoscopy; manometry; ECG (if cardiac involvement is suspected)

Keys to patient encounter

Key concern

Differentiate among causes based on compartment location.

History

Confirm the patient's mediastinal mass symptoms. Listen for cough, stridor, hemoptysis, shortness of breath, chest pain, difficulty swallowing, and vocal hoarseness.

Physical exam

Vital signs: Look for hypotension, which may be present due to tamponade or cardiac compression.

General inspection: Examine the face and upper limbs for swelling (relevant to superior vena cava syndrome).

Eyes: Look for Horner syndrome (unilateral decreased pupil size and drooping eyelid).

Respiratory: Auscultate the lungs for stridor.

Investigations

CT scan or MRI of the chest

Other specific tests as indicated in the differential diagnosis

Management

Refer the patient to a thoracic surgeon for tissue biopsy and further management.

LUMPS AND MASSES

Musculoskeletal lump or mass

Differential diagnosis

NEOPLASTIC CONDITIONS

Soft tissue

BENIGN (E.G., LIPOMA)

LIPOMA

This is a subcutaneous lesion made of adipose tissue.

Signs and symptoms: age 40 to 60 years (more common); family history of lipoma (often); smooth, soft, movable, painless, mass; usually small (< 5 cm in diameter); slow growing; located on the upper extremities, neck, trunk, axillae (common)

Investigations: US; MRI

MALIGNANT (E.G., LEIOMYOSARCOMA)

LEIOMYOSARCOMA

This is a smooth muscle tumor.

Symptoms: postmenopausal bleeding; vaginal discharge; pelvic pain (in uterine leiomyosarcoma); abdominal pain; bloating

Common locations: uterus, stomach, small intestine, retroperitoneum

Investigations: biopsy to detect microscopic features (tumor cell necrosis, atypia, high mitotic activity)

Bone

BENIGN (E.G., CYST)

CYST

This is a fluid-filled hole inside a bone.

It can clinically or radiologically mimic solitary bone tumor.

Signs and symptoms: child, young adult (more common); generally asymptomatic; pain; swelling

Investigations: x-ray

MALIGNANT (E.G., EWING SARCOMA)

EWING SARCOMA

This is a rare cancer. It can occur in any bone.

Signs and symptoms: child, young adult (typically); pain and swelling at the site of the tumor

Common location: in and around the bone

Investigations: bone scan, x-ray, or CT scan to locate the primary tumor and detect possible metastasis; biopsy

NONNEOPLASTIC

Infection (e.g., osteomyelitis)

OSTEOMYELITIS

Signs and symptoms: fever; lethargy; irritability; site-specific pain; bone instability and tenderness; erythema; swelling; delayed wound healing; exposed bone (highly specific for osteomyelitis)

Children: acute osteomyelitis (more common) in the long bones of the legs and upper arms (more common)

Adults: chronic osteomyelitis (more common) in the vertebrae (more common); motor and/or sensory dysfunction in the limbs

Risk factors: diabetes mellitus; peripheral vascular disease; trauma; IV drugs or catheters

Investigations: CBC to detect inflammation markers; bone biopsy (definitive)

Trauma (e.g., hematoma)

HEMATOMA

Hematomas may reduce the mobility of an affected limb and present with symptoms similar to fracture.

Signs and symptoms: history of trauma; painful lump or mass that is initially firm, and purple/blue in color (later: spongy, flattening, and yellow/brown)

Investigations (the diagnosis is usually clinical): blood tests (CBC, hemoglobin, hematocrit, PT/INR)

Inflammatory condition (e.g., rheumatoid nodules, tendonitis)

RHEUMATOID ARTHRITIS

This is a chronic, systemic, inflammatory disease that involves synovial joints.

Signs and symptoms: symmetrical symptoms; pain, stiffness (morning stiffness); swelling in multiple joints that improves with movement; symptoms that progress from the periphery to proximal joints; decreased grip strength; fatigue; fever; weight loss; impaired ADLs; joint deformities and locomotor disability (in later disease);

rheumatoid nodules in the fingers, knuckles, elbows, forearms, knees, backs of heels (in about 25% of cases)

Common locations: metacarpophalangeal and proximal interphalangeal joints of the fingers; interphalangeal joints of the thumbs and wrists; metatarsophalangeal joints of the toes

Other locations: synovial joints of the upper and lower limbs (elbows, shoulders, ankles, knees)

Investigations: blood tests (to detect autoantibodies of rheumatoid factors and/or anti–citrullinated peptide or protein antibodies; anemia; thrombocytosis; elevated ESR; elevated CRP); tests of synovial fluid (leukocyte count of 1500–25 000/μL [1.5–25 × 10^9/L]) with predominance of polymorphonuclear cells); x-rays of the hands and feet to detect narrowing joint spaces, and erosions of bone and cartilage

TENDINITIS

Signs and symptoms: history of chronic repetitive low-grade trauma or overuse (common); history of sports injury (common); pain on palpation of the affected tendon; pain with tendon loading

Achilles tendon: heel pain (this is common in runners)

Biceps: anterior shoulder pain in the bicipital groove that is worse on flexing the shoulder or supination of the forearm

Lateral epicondylitis ("tennis elbow"): pain of the lateral elbow that is worse on grasping and twisting

Medial epicondylitis ("golfer's elbow"): pain of the medial elbow

Patellar ("jumper's knee"): male (more common); history of sports involving jumping and running (common); pain on standing up from sitting, and climbing stairs or hills

Rotator cuff, shoulder: dull, aching shoulder pain that is difficult to localize and radiates into the upper arm; painful range of motion

Keys to patient encounter

Key concern

Distinguish benign from malignant disease.

History

HISTORY OF PRESENT ILLNESS

Ask how the patient discovered the mass, how it has changed, and what other symptoms the patient has.

Examples of characteristic symptoms include:

Leiomyosarcoma: pelvic or abdominal pain

Tendinitis: worsening pain with use

RA: morning stiffness

Osteomyelitis and RA: systemic symptoms

PAST MEDICAL HISTORY

Ask about radiation therapy for cancer, or other exposure to radiation.

FAMILY HISTORY

Ask about sarcoma and genetic disorders that predispose to sarcoma (neurofibromatosis, Gardner syndrome, retinoblastoma, Li-Fraumeni syndrome).

Physical exam

The main goal is to determine the need for imaging and biopsy.

Mass:

- Examine the mass (or surrounding area if it was discovered by radiology) to assess size, firmness, and tenderness.
- Look for skin changes and enlarged regional lymph nodes.

Investigations

Imaging as indicated (see the differential diagnosis)

Tissue biopsy especially for a mass of large size and/or a firm, painless mass (have a low threshold of suspicion)

Management

In malignant masses, refer the patient to a surgeon or oncologist.

POINTER

Biopsy and masses

Remember that a tissue specimen for histology is often necessary for diagnosis: "tissue is the issue."

LUMPS AND MASSES

Neck mass, goiter, thyroid disease

Differential diagnosis

BENIGN

Congenital condition (e.g., thyroglossal duct cyst)

THYROGLOSSAL DUCT CYST

This is the most common form of congenital cyst in the neck.

Bacterial infection is a common complication.

Signs and symptoms: child aged 2 to 10 years (most common); midline upper cystic neck mass that is at or below the hyoid bone; cyst that moves up when swallowing or when patient sticks out their tongue; possible cyst tenderness; ectopic thyroid glands (usual); history of recent URTI (often)

Investigations: CT scan to confirm size, extent, and location of cyst

Inflammatory condition (e.g., reactive lymph nodes)

REACTIVE LYMPH NODES

Signs and symptoms: history of infections, immune system disorders (e.g., SLE, RA), other inflammatory conditions; nodes that may initially appear as simple palpable enlargements, with possible progression to red, painful, and tender lumps on the neck

Investigations: blood tests to detect infection response and any thyroid condition

Neoplasm (e.g., lipomas)

LIPOMA

This is a subcutaneous lesion made of adipose tissue.

Signs and symptoms: age 40 to 60 (more common); family history of lipoma (often); smooth, soft, movable, painless mass; mass that is small (< 5 cm in diameter, usually), slow growing, and commonly located on the upper extremities, neck, trunk, axillae

Investigations: US, MRI

Goiter

Goiter involves abnormal growth of the thyroid gland, and may be associated with normal, decreased, or increased thyroid hormone production.

Signs and symptoms: diffuse or nodular neck enlargement; compressive symptoms in large goiters (hoarse voice, difficulty swallowing, dyspnea)

Investigations: thyrotropin (TSH), thyroid US

MALIGNANT

MALIGNANT NECK MASSES IN GENERAL

Signs and symptoms of malignancy: nodes that are fixed, large, firm; voice changes; difficulty swallowing; shortness of breath; hemoptysis; high thyrotropin (TSH); systemic symptoms (e.g., pulmonary symptoms, neurologic symptoms)

Thyroid cancer

Signs and symptoms: female (more common); asymptomatic early in disease (symptoms are present once the tumor is large enough); palpable lump on the anterior neck due to swollen lymph nodes or thyroid nodule; voice change; difficulty speaking; increased hoarseness; difficulty swallowing; shortness of breath; pain in the neck and throat

> Papillary carcinoma (slowest growing): most common type of thyroid cancer; well differentiated; patient age commonly 30 to 50
>
> Follicular thyroid cancer: well differentiated; patient age commonly older than 50
>
> Medullary thyroid cancer: elevated calcitonin in blood
>
> Anaplastic thyroid cancer (fastest growing, rare): undifferentiated; highly aggressive and metastatic; patient age commonly older than 60

Risk factors: exposure to radiation; family history of thyroid cancer or goiters; abnormal amount of iodine in diet

Nonthyroid head and neck cancers

Signs and symptoms: symptoms for > 3 weeks; persistent unilateral throat discomfort

> Lesion in oral cavity: persistent red and/or white patches on the oral mucosa; ulceration and/or swelling of the oropharynx or mucosa; persistent mass; tongue pain; tongue deviation; hoarseness; unexplained tooth mobility and/or looseness; earache; difficulty swallowing; bleeding in the oral cavity; stridor; facial pain or numbness
>
> Lesion in nasopharynx: neck lump; bloody nasal discharge; nasal blockage; unilateral hearing loss; ringing in the ear;

recurrent otitis media; headache; facial pain or numbness; double vision; persistent cough

Investigations: endoscopy; fine needle aspiration or core biopsy of mass

Lymphoma

Signs and symptoms: neck or thyroid nodules or lesions that are asymptomatic (often); firm, painless, fixed, persistent, or rapidly enlarging lesions that are "rubbery"; constitutional symptoms (fatigue, weight loss, night sweats)

Non-Hodgkin lymphoma: constitutional symptoms (fatigue, fever, night sweats, weight loss), enlarged lymph nodes, chest pain, coughing, shortness of breath

Hodgkin lymphoma (less common): constitutional symptoms (fatigue, fever, night sweats, weight loss); enlarged lymph nodes; itching or pain on drinking alcohol, or increased sensitivity to alcohol

Investigations: CBC with differential, platelet count; CT scan; excisional biopsy for immunophenotyping; fine needle aspiration biopsy for cytologic classification, cytogenetics

Keys to patient encounter

Key concern

Exclude malignancy.

History

Ask about the patient's symptoms. Listen for evidence of thyroid dysfunction (e.g., weight gain, cold intolerance, impaired cognition in hypothyroidism; weight loss, tremor, diarrhea in hyperthyroidism), and difficulty swallowing and/or constitutional symptoms (these suggest malignancy). Ask about risk factors for malignancy (smoking, family history, radiation exposure).

Physical exam

Vital signs: Look for signs of thyroid dysfunction (tachycardia in hyperthyroidism, diastolic hypertension in hypothyroidism).

Head and neck:

- Palpate the thyroid and assess for goiter or nodules.
- Look for enlarged lymph nodes.

Investigations

US or CT scan if malignancy is possible

Thyrotropin (TSH) in suspected thyroid disorder or mass

Management

Management depends on the entity identified. Consider referral to an ENT surgeon and/or endocrinologist.

MOVEMENT DISORDERS

Ataxia

Differential diagnosis

CEREBELLAR ATAXIA

CEREBELLAR ATAXIA IN GENERAL

Signs and symptoms: imbalance; head and trunk swaying; impaired ability to control movement in the limbs; vertigo with nausea and vomiting; positive Romberg test; rapid eye movements that occur in irregular episodes, especially nystagmus; dysdiadochokinesia; intention tremor; scanning speech

Tumors

Tumors cause symptoms due to hemorrhage, or compression of the cerebellum and associated structures.

Signs and symptoms: history of cerebellar primary tumors (this is more common in children; examples include meningioma, astrocytoma, hemangioblastoma) or metastatic cancer (this is more common in adults; examples include breast cancer, small cell lung cancer, ovarian cancer, Hodgkin lymphoma)

Investigations: head imaging to detect cerebellar mass

Vascular conditions

Signs and symptoms: history of vascular conditions such as stroke, cerebellar arterial dissection, vasculitis, hemorrhage (burst aneurysm, arteriovenous malformation), hypertension, repeat subarachnoid bleeding

Hereditary conditions

Signs and symptoms: chronic symptoms; family history of hereditary spinocerebellar ataxia, Friedrich ataxia, telangiectasia, mitochondrial disorders, fragile X syndrome, Tay-Sachs disease, Niemann-Pick disease

Multiple sclerosis

Signs and symptoms: variable depending on lesion location

> Spinal cord: sensory or motor dysfunction; Lhermitte sign (paresthesias radiating down the extremities or trunk with neck flexion); bowel, bladder or erectile dysfunction
>
> Brainstem: double vision; swallowing, speech difficulties; vertigo; pseudobulbar palsy
>
> Cerebrum: cognitive impairment; depression; upper motor neuron signs; unilateral motor or sensory deficits
>
> Cerebellum: problems with balance and coordination; vertigo
>
> Other symptoms: tonic spasms; fatigue; pain; exercise intolerance; temperature sensitivity; painful unilateral loss of visual acuity

Risk factors: younger than 50, female

Investigations: brain and spinal cord MRI, including advanced MRI techniques, with established occurrence of multiple episodes; CSF analysis

Drugs

Examples include sedatives, anticonvulsants, benzodiazepines, amiodarone, metronidazole, chemotherapeutic drugs (fluorouracil), solvents, and lithium.

Alcohol

Signs and symptoms: history of alcohol abuse (this is associated with Wernicke encephalopathy); difficulty balancing; ataxia that affects the legs and gait, not the arms

> Wernicke encephalopathy: ataxia, confusion, ophthalmoplegia

Investigations: elevated liver enzymes (AST:ALT ratio > 2; elevated GGT)

SENSORY ATAXIA

Vestibular condition

ACOUSTIC NEUROMA

Signs and symptoms: unilateral hearing loss; unilateral tinnitus; vertigo; feeling as if the body is tilted; veering towards the side of the affected ear; facial weakness

Investigations: CT scan or MRI of the head

Proprioceptive condition

Signs and symptoms: clumsiness; high stepping gait with stamping; history of diabetes, spinal myelopathy, brain lesion

Investigations: MRI of spinal cord and head

Visual condition

Signs and symptoms: decreased visual acuity, depth perception, and/or contrast sensitivity

OTHER (E.G., PARKINSON DISEASE)

Parkinson disease

Signs and symptoms (mnemonic **TRAP**): **t**remor at rest; **r**igidity of the lower limbs; **a**kinesia, bradykinesia; **p**ostural instability

Other symptoms: cognitive impairment; dementia; shuffling gait with stooped posture and loss of arm swing; micrographia; hypophonia; masklike facies; "pill rolling"; lack of blinking; orthostatic hypotension

History of use of antipsychotics, antiemetics; toxin ingestion (e.g., carbon monoxide, cyanide); head trauma; vascular disease; other neurodegenerative disease (e.g., Lewy body dementia, Huntington disease); brain tumor, hydrocephalus; metabolic conditions (e.g., hypoparathyroidism, Wilson disease, chronic liver failure); infections that spread to the brain (HIV/AIDS, syphilis, prion disease, toxoplasmosis, encephalitis lethargica, progressive multifocal leukoencephalopathy)

Keys to patient encounter

Key concerns

Distinguish ataxia from other abnormalities.

Establish the localization and cause.

History

The most important information to obtain from the history is the age at onset of the movement disorder, the tempo of disease (acute onset, gradual onset, progressive), and the presence or absence of a family history of the same condition.

HISTORY OF PRESENT ILLNESS

Ask when the movement disorder began and how it has progressed.

Ask about vertigo, tinnitus, and hearing loss (this suggests a peripheral vestibular problem), and headache, nausea, and vomiting (this suggests increased intracranial pressure).

PAST MEDICAL HISTORY

Ask about a history of neurological problems, including motor weakness and sensory loss (this suggests MS). Ask about stroke and cancer.

FAMILY HISTORY

If there is a family history of relevant hereditary conditions, try to determine the pattern of inheritance (autosomal recessive, autosomal dominant, X-linked).

MEDICATIONS

Ask about medications that may have movement side effects (neuroleptics).

SOCIAL HISTORY

Ask about alcohol use and possible nutritional deficits.

Physical exam

The physical examination starts with an assessment of the patient's speech during the history, looking for scanning speech (variation in speech volume) and difficulty speaking.

Neurological:

- Pay particular attention to observing the patient's gait for ataxia, and assessing for broad-based stance and gait.
- Test tandem walking.
- Look for limb dysmetria by performing a finger-to-nose test on both sides.

Neck: Assess for stiffness.

Eyes:

- Look for nystagmus.
- Perform a funduscopic exam (this is relevant to increased intracranial pressure).

Investigations

Brain imaging (consider this for most patients)

- CT scan is the usual first choice.

- This is particularly important in detecting strokes, masses, lesions, and demyelination.
- Vascular lesions may require evaluation with angiography, CT angiogram, or MR angiogram.

LP in suspected infection, except when contraindicated (see the pointer)

POINTER

Contraindications for lumbar puncture

Cellulitis near the site for the lumbar puncture
Increased intracranial pressure
Uncorrected coagulopathy
Acute spinal cord trauma

Management

Consider referring the patient to a neurologist for assistance in diagnosis and management. Wernicke encephalopathy is treated with vitamin B_1 and usually shows rapid improvement.

MOVEMENT DISORDERS

Involuntary movement, tic disorders

Differential diagnosis

HYPERKINETIC MOVEMENT

Tics

PRIMARY

TOURETTE SYNDROME

Signs and symptoms: symptom onset during childhood or adolescence (symptoms are commonly present by age 12); presence of motor and vocal tics (not necessarily concurrently); presence of tics for ≥ 1 year

Motor tics (examples): eye blinking, facial grimacing, head jerking

Vocal tics (examples): grunting, repeating what others say, repeating particular words or phrases

Risk factors: male (3 to 4 times more common); family history of Tourette syndrome or other tic disorder (chronic motor or tic disorder, provisional tic disorder)

HUNTINGTON DISEASE

Signs and symptoms: family history of Huntington disease; abnormal eye movements; tics (uncontrolled movement in the fingers, feet, face, trunk); myoclonus; chorea (progressive chorea in late-onset Huntington disease; older than 50); psychiatric symptoms (depression; apathy; anxiety; obsessions, compulsions; irritability; psychosis; paranoid and acoustic hallucinations; hypersexuality); cognitive symptoms (impaired executive function; loss of mental flexibility, concentration, judgment, memory, awareness); motor symptoms (bradykinesia, dystonia, muscle weakness); profuse sweating from autonomic disturbance

Investigations: DNA analysis (PCR or Southern blot); neuroimaging (MRI, CT scan, SPECT, PET scan) for progression monitoring

SECONDARY

INFECTION (E.G., ENCEPHALITIS, CREUTZFELDT-JAKOB DISEASE)

ENCEPHALITIS

Signs and symptoms: seizures; fever; headache; nausea, vomiting; altered mental status, behavior, personality; abrupt-onset tic disorder; repetitive, uncontrollable muscle contractions; movements or sounds that occur intermittently and unpredictably outside of normal motor activity

CREUTZFELDT-JAKOB DISEASE

This is the most common form of prion disease (most commonly sporadic), but still rare.

Signs and symptoms: mental deterioration; dementia; myoclonus; personality changes; impaired memory, judgment, cognition, and/or vision; tics and myoclonus that are triggered on startling (common)

Brain atrophy (common): ventricular enlargement; deep gray structures (caudate, putamen, thalamus); **no** alteration of hippocampus

DRUGS (E.G., STIMULANTS, LEVODOPA)

Dystonia

DYSTONIA IN GENERAL

The diagnosis is primarily clinical.

PRIMARY (SPORADIC AND INHERITED)

Signs and symptoms: sustained involuntary muscle contractions, typically of antagonistic muscle groups in the same body part (the contractions resemble abnormal twisting, spasm, or tremor) and that are generalized, focal, or segmental (depending on body distribution); variable onset

Inherited: symptom onset in childhood; positive response to low-dose levodopa

Investigations: neurological testing of nerve and muscle function

DYSTONIA-PLUS SYNDROMES (E.G., MEDICATION)

MEDICATIONS

Dystonia-plus syndromes, in general, are nondegenerative neurochemical disorders associated with other neurological conditions.

Causative medications include antipsychotics (e.g., phenothiazines, thioxanthenes, butyrophenones) and antiemetics (e.g., metoclopramide, prochlorperazine).

Signs and symptoms: uncontrollable, sometimes painful muscle spasms; symptoms that develop after weeks (sometimes years) of medication use

Investigations: neurological testing of nerve and muscle function

Stereotypies (typically with mental retardation or autism)

Signs and symptoms: skin picking; mouth opening; facial grimacing; involuntary noises; head nodding or banging; body rocking (this may cause self-injury in severe cases); absence of movements during sleep and on distraction (e.g., calling the patient's name)

Triggers for movements: excitement, happiness, concentration, tiredness, anxiety

In autistic children: movements > 1 minute in duration that occur multiple times a day

Chorea, athetosis, ballism

CHOREA

This is found in many diseases, for example Huntington disease, chorea gravidarum, Sydenham chorea, Creutzfeldt-Jakob disease, drug-induced chorea, and metabolic and endocrine-related chorea.

Signs and symptoms: nonrepetitive, nonperiodic, involuntary jerking movements of the face, trunk, or limbs that are often enhanced during voluntary movement

Progressive chorea: increased movements with stress; absence of movements during sleep; movements that cause walking and balance problems

ATHETOSIS

Causes include brain lesions and cerebral palsy.

Signs and symptoms: slow, writhing, continuous movements in the fingers, hands, toes, feet (occasionally in the limbs, neck, tongue); unbalanced, involuntary movements; difficulty maintaining a symmetrical posture

BALLISM

This is a rare type of chorea.

Causes include stroke, TBI, and ALS.

Signs and symptoms: repetitive, but constantly varying, large amplitude involuntary movement of the proximal parts of the limbs; almost ceaseless activity, often complex and combined

Essential tremor

Essential tremor is the most common form of tremor.

Signs and symptoms (highly variable): tremors in the hands (usual), head (horizontal or vertical movement), voice; tremors on holding out the hands; tremors made worse with movement (usual) and better with alcohol

Risk factors: family history of tremor (autosomal dominant); older age

Myoclonus

This may indicate a nervous system disorder such as MS, Parkinson disease, dystonia, Alzheimer disease, Gaucher disease, Creutzfeldt-Jakob disease, serotonin toxicity, Huntington disease, epilepsy, or intracranial hypotension.

Signs and symptoms:

Positive myoclonus: sudden muscle contractions (twitches; jerks; seizures; hypnic jerk while falling asleep)

Negative myoclonus: brief lapses of contraction

Investigations: EMG, EEG

BRADYKINETIC MOVEMENT

Parkinson disease

Signs and symptoms (mnemonic **TRAP**): **t**remor at rest; **r**igidity of the lower limbs; **a**kinesia, bradykinesia; **p**ostural instability

Other symptoms: cognitive impairment; dementia; shuffling gait with stooped posture and loss of arm swing; micrographia; hypophonia; masklike facies; "pill rolling"; lack of blinking; orthostatic hypotension

History of use of antipsychotics, antiemetics; toxin ingestion (e.g., carbon monoxide, cyanide); head trauma; vascular disease; other neurodegenerative disease (e.g., Lewy body dementia, Huntington disease); brain tumor, hydrocephalus; metabolic conditions (e.g., hypoparathyroidism, Wilson disease, chronic liver failure); infections that spread to the brain (HIV/AIDS, syphilis, prion disease, toxoplasmosis, encephalitis lethargica, progressive multifocal leukoencephalopathy)

Wilson disease

This causes accumulation of copper in the body and can be fatal.

Signs and symptoms:

Neurologic: asymmetric tremor; dysphasia; ataxia; drooling; clumsiness; Fleischer rings in the cornea; masklike facies

Hepatic: liver dysfunction (cirrhosis, acute hepatitis, chronic active hepatitis), jaundice, abdominal pain

Musculoskeletal: osteopenia on radiological exam; joint inflammation that resembles premature osteoarthritis (this is symptomatic after age 20 and occurs in the spine, hips, knees, wrists)

Neuropsychiatric (not as common; usually coexistent with cirrhosis): personality changes, irritability, impaired cognition

Investigations: serum ceruloplasmin < 20 mg/dL (200 mg/L); urinary copper excretion rate > 100 mcg/day

Huntington disease—see above

TREMOR

Resting tremor (e.g., Parkinson disease, severe essential tremor)

PARKINSON DISEASE—SEE ABOVE

ESSENTIAL TREMOR—SEE ABOVE

Intention tremor (e.g., cerebellar disease, multiple sclerosis)

INTENTION TREMOR IN GENERAL

This is sometimes difficult to distinguish from cerebellar ataxia.

Signs and symptoms: large amplitude tremor whose severity typically increases on approaching a target (e.g., finger to nose, heel to shin)

CEREBELLAR DISEASE

Signs and symptoms: variable depending on etiology

Common symptoms: ataxia; other motor dysfunction (dysmetria, decomposition of movement, dysdiadochokinesia, nystagmus); speech dysfunction (difficulty speaking, scanning speech); hypotonia

MULTIPLE SCLEROSIS

Signs and symptoms: variable depending on lesion location

Spinal cord: sensory or motor dysfunction; Lhermitte sign (paresthesias radiating down the extremities or trunk with neck flexion); bowel, bladder or erectile dysfunction

Brainstem: double vision; swallowing, speech difficulties; vertigo; pseudobulbar palsy

Cerebrum: cognitive impairment; depression; upper motor neuron signs; unilateral motor or sensory deficits

Cerebellum: problems with balance and coordination; vertigo

Other symptoms: tonic spasms; fatigue; pain; exercise intolerance; temperature sensitivity; painful unilateral loss of visual acuity

Risk factors: younger than 50, female

Investigations: brain and spinal cord MRI, including advanced MRI techniques, with established occurrence of multiple episodes; CSF analysis

Postural/action tremor (e.g., enhanced physiologic tremor, essential tremor)

POSTURAL TREMOR IN GENERAL

Signs and symptoms: tremor on maintaining a position against gravity (e.g., holding the arms outstretched)

ENHANCED PHYSIOLOGIC TREMOR

Enhanced physiologic tremor is the most common type of postural or action tremor.

Signs and symptoms: tremor with stress, after strenuous exertion, and/or after ingesting substances (drugs, medications, chemicals); **no** neurologic symptoms

Substances: amphetamines, SSRIs, TCAs, nicotine, caffeine, corticosteroids, sodium valproate, mercury, lead, arsenic

ESSENTIAL TREMOR—SEE ABOVE

Keys to patient encounter

Key concern

Look for treatable symptoms and causes (e.g., in Parkinson disease, Wilson disease) and reversible causes (medication side effects).

MNO

History

MEDICATIONS

Ask about antiemetics and, in particular, antipsychotics.

FAMILY HISTORY

Ask about tics, tremors, dystonia, Huntington disease, autism, ALS, Parkinson disease, Wilson disease, and MS.

SOCIAL HISTORY

Ask about street drug use.

Physical exam

Movement: Carefully observe the clinical features of the movement disorder: Are the movements hyperkinetic or bradykinetic?

Neurological: Perform a full exam.

Investigations

CT scan or MRI of the brain

Genetic studies in suspected Huntington disease

Serum ceruloplasmin in suspected Wilson disease

Management

Consider referral to a neurologist. Parkinson disease is treated with levodopa. Wilson disease is treated with chelating agents (e.g., D-penicillamine, trientine).

Drug-induced movement disorders are most common with atypical and typical neuroleptics. The offending medication should be gradually withdrawn. Consult a psychiatrist for guidance on withdrawal and replacement with another agent.

MUSCULOSKELETAL PRESENTATIONS

Back pain and related symptoms

Differential diagnosis

MECHANICAL PROBLEM

Common back pain

Causes include muscle or ligament damage; bulging or ruptured disks; arthritis; skeletal irregularities; and osteoporosis.

Signs and symptoms: symptoms that last ≥ 6 weeks in the acute form (usual); muscle aches; shooting or stabbing pain; pain radiating down the leg; limited range of motion of the back; **no** bowel or bladder changes, fever, or history of trauma (e.g., a fall)

Acute, discogenic nerve root entrapment

Lumbar radiculopathy arises from a compressed nerve root in the lower back, which often results in inflammation of the nerve root. It is commonly called *sciatica*, because nerve roots comprising the sciatic nerve are often involved in this condition.

Causes include changes in the tissues surrounding the nerve root (typically); herniation of a spinal disc between vertebrae; bone spurs; and ossification of spinal ligaments.

Signs and symptoms: numbness, paresthesia, sharp pain in the back or legs; weakness or loss of reflexes in the legs; sciatic pain on straight leg raise

Investigations: nerve conduction studies, EMG, MRI

Spinal stenosis and/or cauda equina syndrome

SPINAL STENOSIS

This is narrowing of the intraspinal canal, commonly caused by osteoarthritis.

Signs and symptoms: lower back pain (usual); symptoms that develop over months to years; motor weakness; pain or claudication in the buttocks, thighs, calves when the patient is active (standing, walking, running, climbing stairs); **no** pain when sitting, lying down, squatting, or bending forward

Risk factors: older than 50; history of spinal surgery

Investigations: x-ray, CT scan, or MRI of the spine

CAUDA EQUINA SYNDROME

This occurs when the spinal cord is compressed in the lumbar spine.

Common causes include herniated disk, spinal stenosis, infection, and trauma.

Signs and symptoms: leg pain, numbness, weakness; urinary symptoms (incontinence, retention, frequent urination); fecal incontinence; loss of rectal tone; abnormal bulbocavernosus and anal wink reflexes; erectile dysfunction; decreased muscle tone and deep tendon reflexes in the legs; saddle anesthesia (loss of sensation in the inner thighs, back of the legs, around the rectum)

Investigations: x-ray; CT scan; MRI (this is preferred for suspected spinal cord compression); myelography

INFLAMMATORY ARTHRITIS

Ankylosing spondylitis

Signs and symptoms: unilateral or bilateral pain in the buttocks that spreads to the upper thighs, chest, hips, peripheral joints; back pain or stiffness that is worse on waking, lasts ≥ 30 minutes, and improves with activity; loss of mobility; anterior uveitis (unilateral eye symptoms including pain, photophobia, redness, watering, irregularly shaped pupil, slow-reacting pupil); diffuse swelling in the fingers, toes; large joint arthritis; stooped posture with cautious gait

Investigations: x-ray

Rheumatoid arthritis

This is a chronic, systemic, inflammatory disease that involves synovial joints.

Signs and symptoms: symmetrical symptoms; pain, stiffness (morning stiffness); swelling in multiple joints that improves with movement; symptoms that progress from the periphery to proximal joints; decreased grip strength; fatigue; fever; weight loss; impaired ADLs; joint deformities and locomotor disability (later disease); rheumatoid nodules in the fingers, knuckles, elbows, forearms, knees, backs of heels (in about 25% of patients)

> Commonly affected joints: metacarpophalangeal and proximal interphalangeal joints of the fingers; interphalangeal joints of the thumbs and wrists; metatarsophalangeal joints of the toes
>
> Other joints: synovial joints of the upper and lower limbs (elbows, shoulders, ankles, knees)

Investigations: blood tests (to detect autoantibodies of rheumatoid factors and/or anticitrullinated peptide/protein antibodies; anemia; thrombocytosis; elevated ESR; elevated CRP); tests of synovial joint fluid (leukocyte count of 1500–25 000/μL [1.5–25 × 10^9/L] with predominance of polymorphonuclear cells); x-rays of the hands and feet to detect narrowing joint spaces, and erosions of bone and cartilage

Psoriatic arthritis

Signs and symptoms: symptoms of psoriasis (chronic plaque psoriasis is the most common form); joint pain, stiffness, swelling; pain and stiffness in the morning or after inactivity (pain lasts > 30–45 minutes); symptoms that affect ≥ 5 joints with asymmetric distribution and distal interphalangeal joint involvement; finger and/or toe swelling (sausage-like dactylitis); inflammation at sites of tendon insertion; nail lesions

Chronic plaque psoriasis: symmetrically distributed cutaneous lesions that are erythematous, raised above normal skin, 1–10 cm in diameter, with clearly defined margins, and a thick, coarse, silvery scale; located on the scalp, elbows, knees, back (most common sites)

Investigations: x-ray

INFECTION

Factors that suggest infection include immunosuppression, IV drug use, unexplained fever, chronic steroid use, infection at another site, and progressive, disabling symptoms.

Investigations (infection detection): blood tests (glucose, WBCs, protein, culture); antigen and antibody tests (blood, urinalysis); imaging

FRACTURE

Signs of spinal fracture: history of trauma (e.g., a fall from a height; car accident; strenuous lifting, especially with osteoporosis); sudden-onset severe pain in the spine; point tenderness over vertebrae; structural spine deformity

Pain is made better by lying down or reclining.

Pain is made worse by prolonged sitting; activities where the arms are elevated or used away from the body (e.g., vacuuming); and bending forward.

Investigations: x-ray of the lumbar spine; CT scan to detect stress fractures; MRI to detect disk lesions

NEOPLASM

Spinal cord tumor

Tumors can be malignant or benign (e.g., osteoblastoma, neurofibroma).

Signs and symptoms: chronic pain for > 1 month that is unimproved by bed rest or therapy; focal spine pain that is tender on palpation; possible neurologic effects (weak or numb limbs; lack of coordination; bladder or bowel dysfunction); constitutional symptoms (weight loss, vomiting, fever, chills)

Risk factors: history of cancer (especially lung, prostate, breast, multiple myeloma)

Investigations: spinal x-ray, MRI, CSF analysis

Keys to patient encounter

Key concern

Identify patients who require urgent intervention.

History

Ask when the pain started, what the patient was doing when it started, and how constant the pain is. Ask about other symptoms the patient has. Listen for evidence of sudden onset and trauma (this suggests common back pain or fracture); chronic pain (this suggests neoplasm or an inflammatory condition); symptoms of infection (e.g., fever); and neurological symptoms (e.g., associated leg pain and/or incontinence in cauda equina syndrome). Determine the presence of red flags (see the pointer). Ask how the pain affects function, including work and recreation.

POINTER

Red flags in back pain

Back pain concurrent with any of the following findings suggests a serious cause (e.g., aortic aneurysm, cancer, GI bleed, or infection) with the possible need for urgent intervention:

- Abdominal aorta > 5 cm
- Lower extremity pulse deficit
- Acute, tearing midback pain
- Cancer, either diagnosed or suspected
- Duration of pain longer than 6 weeks
- Fever
- GI findings (e.g., localized abdominal tenderness)
- Infection risk factors
- Meningismus
- Neurologic deficits
- Severe nocturnal or disabling pain
- Unexplained pain after age 55
- Unexplained weight loss

Physical exam

Vital signs: Look for fever.

Gait and range of motion

Abdominal: Check for an enlarged aorta.

Neurological

Straight-leg-raise test: This assesses for herniated lower lumbar disc.

Lower extremity pulses: Check for pulse deficit.

Investigations

Imaging (X-ray, CT scan, or MRI) for patients whose pain has lasted more than 4 to 6 weeks despite conservative treatment, and for patients with red flags

IN SUSPECTED INFECTION OR FEVER

CBC

CRP

POINTER

Imaging for back pain without red flags

In patients without red flags, delay imaging for 4 to 6 weeks. The pain usually resolves, avoiding the need for imaging.

Management

In the absence of red flags, treat patients conservatively with acetaminophen, NSAIDs, muscle relaxants, heat, and/or physical therapy. Advise patients to stay active. Refer patients with neurological symptoms, fracture, infection, or malignancy to an orthopedic surgeon or neurosurgeon.

MUSCULOSKELETAL PRESENTATIONS

Limp in children

Differential diagnosis

CONGENITAL CONDITIONS

Lower limbs, spine

HIP DYSPLASIA

This generally develops around the time of birth and is screened for in well-baby exams.

Signs and symptoms (if undiagnosed in infancy): long-standing limp with no pain (usual); walking on the toes of the foot (this is especially true in older children); limited range of motion in the hips; 1 leg shorter than the other (often)

Investigations: bilateral hip x-ray to detect subluxation of 1 or both hips

COXA VARA

Signs and symptoms: waddling gait with no pain (usual); mild discrepancy in limb length

Investigations: bilateral hip x-ray to detect unilaterally prominent greater trochanter

SLIPPED CAPITAL FEMORAL EPIPHYSIS

This is the most common hip disorder in adolescents.

It requires accurate diagnosis and immediate treatment.

Symptoms: hip pain (sometimes groin, thigh, or knee pain) that becomes worse with physical activity; altered gait (limping; walking with a leg turned outward; waddling walk)

Risk factors: obesity, hypothyroidism, growth hormone deficiency, Down syndrome, prior radiation therapy

Investigations: x-ray (anteroposterior and lateral views of the bilateral hips)

> Anteroposterior view shows a blurry junction between the metaphysis and the growth plate.
>
> Both views show the line of Klein passing outside the epiphysis (instead of intersecting it) or passing just at its superior edge.

ACQUIRED CONDITIONS

Infection

SEPTIC ARTHRITIS

Signs and symptoms: fever (often); severe pain, usually in 1 joint

> History of recent joint injury and/or surgery; structural joint abnormality; recent or current infections (e.g., GU, pulmonary, skin); systemic disease (e.g., diabetes mellitus, liver disease, malignancy, CKD); use of immunosuppressants; **no** vaccine for *H. influenzae* type b (Hib)

Investigations: elevated WBCs; very high CRP; synovial fluid analysis (WBCs, Gram stain, culture)

VIRAL SYNOVITIS

Signs and symptoms: low-grade fever (usual); pain (this is not as severe as in septic arthritis), usually in 1 joint; history of recent viral illness (usual)

Investigations: x-ray, US of affected joint to detect effusion

Inflammation

JUVENILE IDIOPATHIC ARTHRITIS

Signs and symptoms: swollen, tender joints; skin rash; iritis

Investigations: normal WBCs; moderately high CRP; x-ray of affected joints to detect boney overgrowth, decreased joint space, decreased bone density

Tumor

Signs and symptoms: weakness in the lower limbs; possible palpable mass in the abdomen, pelvis, back

Malignant: constitutional symptoms (fever, weight loss, night sweats, fatigue)

Benign: often asymptomatic

Investigations: WBCs; CRP; x-ray, CT scan, MRI, and/or nuclear scan

OTHER

Growing pains

Signs and symptoms: bilateral leg pain; pain that occurs only at night; no pain or limp during the day

Pain amplification syndromes

Signs and symptoms: pain in several parts of the body (e.g., headache, abdominal pain); pain from light touching of the skin

History of sedentary lifestyle, inadequate sleep

Keys to patient encounter

Key concern

Rule out the most serious diagnoses, which are usually unilateral.

History

HISTORY OF PRESENT ILLNESS

Ask when the limp started and what other symptoms the patient has. Examples of characteristic symptoms include:

Hip dysplasia: long-standing limp with no pain

Infection: sudden-onset fever and unilateral severe pain

Malignant tumor: lower-limb weakness and constitutional symptoms

If the patient has pain, ask how constant it is. Listen for suggestive patterns of pain (e.g., pain only at night suggests growing pains; hip pain that becomes worse with physical activity suggests slipped epiphysis). Pay particular attention to severe unilateral pain with fever (red flags for septic arthritis: see the pointer).

Ask about possible trauma associated with the symptoms. Screen for possible child abuse.

Physical exam

Vital signs: Look for fever.

Gait: Observe the patient walking and running.

Legs, hips, and pelvis:

- Palpate for tenderness.
- Look for bruising, swelling, redness, and deformities.
- Assess the active and passive range of motion in each joint.

Specific tests:

Trendelenburg sign: Ask the patient to stand on the affected limb and lift the unaffected limb from the floor. A positive sign is when the pelvis drops down toward the unaffected side.

Galeazzi sign: In the supine position, the patient flexes their hips and knees, with knees together. Assess leg length discrepancy by noting if 1 knee is lower than the other.

Test for flexion, abduction, and external rotation (FABER test): With the patient supine, flex, abduct, and externally rotate the hip joint. A positive test is when pain occurs in the sacroiliac joint.

Pelvic compression test: With the patient supine, compress the iliac wings toward each other looking for pain in the sacroiliac joint.

Psoas sign: With the patient lying on their side, passively extend the hip. Pain indicates a positive test.

Investigations

CBC

CRP

Anteroposterior and lateral x-rays of both lower extremities

Hip US in suspected hip effusion

Bone scan if other imaging is negative

Joint aspirate for Gram stain, culture, and cell count in suspected septic arthritis

Blood and bone cultures in suspected osteomyelitis

POINTER

Red flags for septic arthritis

Severe, unilateral joint pain

Temperature > 38.5°C

Refusal to bear weight on the affected leg

ESR > 40 mm/hour or CRP > 2 mg/dL (20 mg/L)

WBCs > 12 000/μL (12×10^9/L)

Management

Management depends on the specific entity identified. Consider referring the patient to a pediatrician or orthopedic surgeon.

MUSCULOSKELETAL PRESENTATIONS

Neck pain

Differential diagnosis

MECHANICAL PROBLEM

Neck strain

Signs and symptoms: history of neck injury (a common cause is whiplash from an automobile accident or sports injury; pain may have delayed onset after injury); stiffness, numbness, tingling, weakness in the arms, face, scalp; loss of range of motion; pain that is worse with movement; headaches that start at the base of the skull; fatigue; dizziness

Other: shortness of breath, hoarse voice, difficulty swallowing, blurred vision, tinnitus, irritability

Investigations: CT scan, MRI

Spondylosis

Cervical spondylosis is difficult to distinguish from other causes of neck pain.

Signs and symptoms: older adult (often: aging is an important factor in disc degeneration); pain that originates in the lower cervical spine (common); pain and/or stiffness that is chronic or intermittent in the neck and shoulders; **no** associated neurologic signs (often)

> Other symptoms (less common): headache; suboccipital and arm pain; tingling and weakness

Acute, discogenic nerve root entrapment

Cervical radiculopathy arises from a compressed nerve root in the neck, which often results in inflammation of the nerve root.

Causes include changes in the tissues surrounding the nerve root (typically); herniation of a spinal disc between vertebrae; bone spurs; and ossification of spinal ligaments.

Signs and symptoms: numbness, paresthesia, sharp pain, or weakness in the shoulders and arms (nerves in the neck primarily control sensation in the arms and hands)

Investigations: nerve conduction studies, EMG, MRI

Spinal stenosis and/or cord compression

CERVICAL SPINAL STENOSIS (CHRONIC CORD COMPRESSION)

This is narrowing of the intraspinal canal, commonly caused by osteoarthritis.

Signs and symptoms: male, older than 55 (more common); symptoms that develop over months to years; numbness, weakness, or tingling in the limbs and extremities (tingling in the hand is the most common symptom); subtle loss of hand dexterity; positive Hoffman or Babinski sign; hyperreflexia; clonus

Investigations: x-ray, CT scan, or MRI of the cervical spine

ACUTE AND SUBACUTE CORD COMPRESSION

The usual cause is extramedullary lesions (in subacute compression; another common cause of subacute compression is herniated disk).

Signs and symptoms: localized neck pain with radicular pain

> Acute compression: symptoms that develop over minutes to hours; history of trauma (often)

> Subacute compression: symptoms that develop over days to weeks; history of cancer (metastatic cancer is a common cause)

Investigations: immediate MRI

INFLAMMATORY ARTHRITIS

Ankylosing spondylitis

Signs and symptoms: unilateral or bilateral pain in the buttocks that spreads to the upper thighs, chest, hips, peripheral joints; back pain or stiffness that is worse on waking, lasts ≥ 30 minutes, and improves with activity; loss of mobility; anterior uveitis (unilateral eye symptoms including pain, photophobia, redness, watering, irregularly shaped pupil, slow-reacting pupil); diffuse swelling in the fingers, toes; large joint arthritis; stooped posture with cautious gait

Investigations: x-ray

Rheumatoid arthritis

This is a chronic, systemic, inflammatory disease that involves synovial joints.

Signs and symptoms: symmetrical symptoms; pain, stiffness (morning stiffness); swelling in multiple joints that improves with movement; symptoms that progress from the periphery to proximal joints; decreased grip strength; fatigue; fever; weight loss; impaired ADLs; joint deformities and locomotor disability (later disease); rheumatoid nodules in the fingers, knuckles, elbows, forearms, knees, backs of heels (in about 25% of patients)

> Commonly affected joints: metacarpophalangeal and proximal interphalangeal joints of the fingers; interphalangeal joints of the thumbs and wrists; metatarsophalangeal joints of the toes
>
> Other joints: synovial joints of the upper and lower limbs (elbows, shoulders, ankles, knees)

Investigations: blood tests (to detect autoantibodies of rheumatoid factors and/or anticitrullinated peptide/protein antibodies; anemia; thrombocytosis; elevated ESR; elevated CRP); tests of synovial joint fluid (leukocyte count of 1500–25 000/μL [1.5–25 × 10^9/L] with predominance of polymorphonuclear cells); x-rays of the hands and feet to detect narrowing joint spaces, and erosions of bone and cartilage

Psoriatic arthritis

Signs and symptoms: symptoms of psoriasis (chronic plaque psoriasis is the most common form); joint pain, stiffness, swelling; pain and stiffness in the morning or after inactivity (pain lasts > 30–45 minutes); symptoms that affect ≥ 5 joints with asymmetric distribution and distal interphalangeal joint involvement; finger and/or toe swelling (sausage-like dactylitis); inflammation at sites of tendon insertion; nail lesions

> Chronic plaque psoriasis: symmetrically distributed cutaneous lesions that are erythematous, raised above normal skin, 1–10 cm in diameter, with clearly defined

margins, and a thick, coarse, silvery scale; located on the scalp, elbows, knees, back (most common sites)

Investigations: x-ray

INFECTION

INFECTION IN GENERAL

Factors that suggest infection include immunosuppression; IV drug use; unexplained fever; chronic steroid use; infection at another site; and progressive, disabling symptoms.

Infections particularly associated with neck pain include meningitis and retropharyngeal abscess. Other infections may also cause neck pain (e.g., strep throat, mononucleosis, TB, catscratch disease, HIV, CVM, toxoplasmosis).

Investigations (infection detection in general): CSF glucose, WBCs, protein, culture; throat culture; antigen and antibody tests (blood, urinalysis); imaging

Meningitis

Signs and symptoms: fever; stiff neck; headache; Kernig sign (flexing the patient's hip 90 degrees, then extending the knee, causes pain); Brudzinski neck sign (flexing the patient's neck causes flexion of the hips and knees)

Investigations: positive culture in CSF; meningeal inflammation (increased pleocytosis, low glucose in CSF); CSF absolute neutrophil count ≥ 1000/μL (1×10^9/L); CSF protein level ≥ 80 mg/dL (0.8 g/L); peripheral blood absolute neutrophil count ≥ 10 000/μL (10×10^9/L); CT, MRI

Retropharyngeal abscess

Signs and symptoms: pain on swallowing; fever; enlarged lymph nodes in the neck; noisy breathing; stridor (in children); severe neck pain (in adults)

Investigations: neck x-ray, CT scan

FRACTURE

Signs and symptoms: history of trauma; neck symptoms (pain, tenderness, tightness, inability to move, swelling, muscle spasms); numbness, pain, tingling at the base of the head; difficulty swallowing; loss of feeling or pinprick pain in the arms and legs; double vision; loss of consciousness

Investigations: C-spine x-ray, CT scan, MRI

Range of motion test: if the patient can rotate their neck 45 degrees left and right, imaging is not required (perform range of motion testing only in low-risk neck injury)

NEOPLASM

Spinal cord tumor

Tumors can be malignant or benign (e.g., osteoblastoma, neurofibroma).

Signs and symptoms: chronic pain for > 1 month that is unimproved by bed rest or therapy; focal spine pain that is tender on palpation; possible neurologic effects (weak or numb limbs; lack of coordination; bladder or bowel dysfunction); constitutional symptoms (weight loss, vomiting, fever, chills)

Risk factors: history of cancer (especially lung, prostate, breast, multiple myeloma)

Investigations: spinal x-ray, MRI, CSF analysis

Thyroid cancer

Signs and symptoms: female (more common); asymptomatic early in disease (symptoms are present once the tumor is large enough); palpable lump on the anterior neck, resulting from swollen lymph nodes; voice change; difficulty speaking; increased hoarseness; difficulty swallowing; shortness of breath; pain in the neck and throat

- Papillary carcinoma (slowest growing): most common type of thyroid cancer; well differentiated; patient aged 30 to 50 (common)
- Follicular thyroid cancer: well differentiated; patient older than 50 (common)
- Medullary thyroid cancer: elevated serum calcitonin
- Anaplastic thyroid cancer (fastest growing, rare): undifferentiated; highly aggressive and metastatic; patient older than 60 (common)

Risk factors: exposure to radiation; family history of thyroid cancer or goiters; residence in an iodine-deficient area of the world

Investigations: thyroid US

Head and neck cancer

Signs and symptoms: symptoms for > 3 weeks; persistent unilateral throat discomfort

- Lesion in oral cavity: persistent red and/or white patches on the oral mucosa; ulceration and/or swelling of the oropharynx or mucosa; persistent mass; tongue pain; tongue deviation; hoarseness; unexplained tooth mobility and/or looseness; earache; difficulty swallowing; bleeding in the oral cavity; stridor; facial pain or numbness
- Lesion in nasopharynx: neck lump; bloody nasal discharge; nasal blockage; unilateral hearing loss; ringing in the ear;

recurrent otitis media; headache; facial pain or numbness; double vision; persistent cough

Investigations: endoscopic visualization; fine needle aspiration or core biopsy of mass

PAIN FROM SOFT TISSUE STRUCTURES (E.G., THYROID, PHARYNX)

Thyroiditis

Causes of thyroiditis include suppurative thyroiditis, Hashimoto thyroiditis, fibrous thyroiditis, thyroid cancer (see above), and use of amiodarone and lithium.

Signs and symptoms: swollen, tender thyroid; neck pain that is worse on swallowing and that may radiate locally; difficulty swallowing; voice changes; fever

Investigations: blood tests to assess thyroid function (thyrotropin, T_3, T_4, anti-TPO antibodies); CBC with differential; thyroid US or CT scan; radioactive iodine uptake; endoscopic laryngoscopy

Pharyngitis

Signs and symptoms: history of URTI (usual); sore throat; fever; runny nose; cough; headache; hoarse voice

Keys to patient encounter

Key concern

Identify patients who require urgent intervention.

History

HISTORY OF PRESENT ILLNESS

Ask when the pain started, how constant it is, what makes it better and worse, and how severe it is (on a scale of 1 to 10). Ask what other symptoms the patient has.

Examples of characteristic features include:

Neck strain: pain that is worse with movement

Discogenic nerve root entrapment: pain, numbness, or weakness in the shoulders and hands

Cervical spinal stenosis: slow-developing tingling in the hand

Inflammatory arthritis: pain that improves with movement

Retropharyngeal abscess: severe pain, fever, and pain on swallowing

Thyroid, head, and neck cancer: difficulty swallowing

Ask how the pain affects function, including work and recreation.

PAST MEDICAL HISTORY

Ask about trauma and cancer.

Physical exam

Vital signs: Look for fever.

Neck: Assess for tenderness, masses, and range of motion.

Oropharynx: Look for a retropharyngeal abscess.

Neurological

Signs of meningitis: Assess for Kernig sign and Brudzinski neck sign.

Investigations

CBC and CRP in patients with fever

Imaging (x-ray, CT scan, or MRI depending on most likely diagnosis)

LP with culture and blood cultures in suspected meningitis

Management

Management depends on the diagnosis. Cases of fracture must be immobilized with emergent referral to a neurosurgeon. Cases of cord compression must be emergently referred to a neurosurgeon. Patients with meningitis require hospital admission and IV treatment with broad-spectrum antibiotics with or without steroids.

MUSCULOSKELETAL PRESENTATIONS

Nonarticular musculoskeletal pain

Differential diagnosis

GENERALIZED PAIN

Acute pain (e.g., viral infections)

VIRAL INFECTIONS

Myalgia without trauma is often due to viral infections (e.g., influenza).

Signs and symptoms: fever, headache, malaise, nonproductive cough

Investigations: blood culture and testing to detect infectious agents

Chronic pain (e.g., fibromyalgia, polymyalgia rheumatica)

FIBROMYALGIA

This is a diagnosis of exclusion.

Signs and symptoms: female (more common); chronic, widespread pain for ≥ 3 months; pain that is bilateral, and above and below the waist; aching pain; fatigue; long sleep; restless leg syndrome; sleep apnea; impaired concentration, memory; dizziness; cramping (e.g., menstrual, abdominal); morning stiffness; numbness, tingling in the extremities; tender points; urinary symptoms (difficult or painful urination; irregular urination); sensitivity to noise, light, temperature

Coexisting conditions (often): headaches, irritable bowel syndrome, interstitial cystitis

POLYMYALGIA RHEUMATICA

Signs and symptoms: older than 50 (always); female (more common); northern European descent (higher incidence); history of giant cell temporal arteritis (many patients have this, but it may not be active at the same time as polymyalgia rheumatica); symmetrical symptoms (usual); shoulder pain (more common), hip pain, neck pain; stiffness (morning stiffness usually lasts ≥ 30 minutes, with inability to abduct shoulders past 90 degrees); pain that is worse with movement; synovitis and bursitis (many patients have distal musculoskeletal manifestations)

Investigations: elevated ESR (≥ 50 mm/h); elevated serum CRP

LOCALIZED PAIN

Acute pain

TRAUMA

Trauma is the most common cause of nonarticular musculoskeletal pain.

Signs and symptoms: history of trauma; pain with active movement or stretches, or with movement in specific planes; pain localized to an extraarticular structure; superficial tenderness; limited range of motion

> Trauma to muscle: deep, penetrating, or dull pain (but not as intense as bone pain); possible muscle cramp or spasm
>
> Trauma to tendon or ligament: sharp pain that is worse on stretching or movement, and better with rest

Investigations: x-ray (this may show soft tissue calcifications)

INFECTION (E.G., OSTEOMYELITIS, NECROTIZING FASCIITIS)

OSTEOMYELITIS

Signs and symptoms: fever; lethargy; irritability; site-specific pain; bone instability and tenderness; erythema; swelling; delayed wound healing; exposed bone (highly specific for osteomyelitis)

> Children: acute osteomyelitis (more common) in the long bones of the legs and upper arms (more common)
>
> Adults: chronic osteomyelitis (more common) in vertebrae (more common); motor and/or sensory dysfunction in the limbs

Risk factors: diabetes; peripheral vascular disease; trauma; IV drugs or catheters

Investigations: CBC to detect inflammation markers; bone biopsy (definitive)

NECROTIZING FASCIITIS

This is an emergency requiring immediate surgery.

Signs and symptoms:

> Early symptoms: severe disproportionate pain (this precedes skin changes by 1 to 2 days); influenza-like symptoms; gastroenteritis-like symptoms
>
> In-course symptoms (day 3 or 4): erythema, swelling, blisters, bullae, ulcers, black-blue skin, loss of sensation, severe worsening pain, symptoms of systemic toxicity (fever, tachycardia, hypotension, delirium)

Risk factors: damage to skin from trauma, injury, lesions, skin infections, ulcers; immune-suppressing comorbidities (e.g., diabetes, cancer, alcohol abuse)

Investigations: biopsy

MNO

VASCULAR (E.G., COMPARTMENT SYNDROME, SICKLE CELL ANEMIA)

COMPARTMENT SYNDROME

Signs and symptoms: history of trauma or hemorrhagic event; symptoms in the limbs (usual: the lower leg is the most common site); palpable swelling; tenderness; escalating pain disproportionate to the injury; pain on passive stretch; paresthesia; paresis; pallor overlying compartment; absence of distal pulses

Investigations: limb intracompartment pressure measurement

SICKLE CELL ANEMIA

Signs and symptoms: family history of sickle cell disease; painful swelling of the hands and feet; jaundice (if concomitant liver disease)

Investigations: CBC to detect anemia, sickle cells; positive sickle cell screen

Chronic pain

MECHANICAL (E.G., TENDINOPATHY, BURSITIS)

TENDINOPATHY

Signs and symptoms: history of chronic repetitive low-grade trauma or overuse (common); history of sports injury (common); pain on palpation of the affected tendon; pain with tendon loading

Achilles tendon: heel pain (this is common in runners)

Biceps: anterior shoulder pain in the bicipital groove that is worse on flexing the shoulder or supination of the forearm

Lateral epicondylitis ("tennis elbow"): pain of the lateral elbow that is worse on grasping and twisting

Medial epicondylitis ("golfer's elbow"): pain of the medial elbow

Patellar ("jumper's knee"): male (more common); history of sports involving jumping and running (common); pain on standing up from sitting, and climbing stairs or hills

Rotator cuff, shoulder: dull, aching shoulder pain that is difficult to localize and radiates into the upper arm; painful range of motion; pain that is worse at night

BURSITIS

This is inflammation of the bursae, which are sacs that cushion bones and the structures surrounding joints.

The most common cause is repetitive pressure on bursae (e.g., kneeling, leaning on the elbows, sitting for long periods on hard surfaces).

Investigations: x-ray, US, or MRI to rule out other causes; blood tests or analysis of fluid from inflamed bursae to identify the cause

VASCULAR (E.G., INTERMITTENT CLAUDICATION)

INTERMITTENT CLAUDICATION

Signs and symptoms: muscle pain, cramps, numbness, fatigue; calf-muscle symptoms (usual); symptoms worse with muscle use, better with rest; acute limb ischemia (paresthesia, paralysis, pallor, pulselessness, urgent pain); positive Buerger test (redness on returning a limb to a dependent position)

Severe: cyanosis, hair loss, shiny skin, decreased temperature, bradycardia

Investigations: MRA; duplex US

NEOPLASTIC

Signs and symptoms: history of cancer

Types of pain and their causes:

Acute pain: recent treatment or procedures

Chronic pain: usually caused by the condition; possible impaired memory, attention

Somatic pain: tissue, tendon, or bone injury from surgery, trauma, inflammation, tumor

Visceral pain: organ damage or tumor infiltration

Neuropathic pain: tumor infiltration of peripheral nerves, roots, spinal cord; treatment side effects

NEUROPATHIC

Signs and symptoms:

Motor: weakness, fatigue, wasting, cramps, twitching, decreased reflexes, myokymia

Sensory: numbness, tingling; burning or stabbing pain; gait and balance difficulty; temperature intolerance; hyperalgesia

Other: skin, hair, or nail changes; foot and leg ulcers, infections

Investigations: nerve conduction studies; EMG

COMPLEX REGIONAL PAIN SYNDROME

Signs and symptoms: chronic unilateral pain in an arm or leg; history of trauma to the limb (most cases involve trauma; others may involve surgery, stroke, heart attack, or diabetes); pain out of proportion to the initial injury

Early symptoms in the affected limb: pain; swelling; redness; changes in skin temperature (from sweaty and hot to cold); cold, touch sensitivity

Later symptoms in the affected limb: changes in skin color (pallor), texture (thin, shiny, tender), hair growth, and nail growth; muscle spasms

Investigations: sympathetic nervous system tests to detect disturbances; bone scan to detect possible bone changes; x-rays for later stage bone-mineral assessment

Keys to patient encounter

This clinical presentation has a wide differential diagnosis. To narrow the possible diagnosis, determine whether the pain is localized or diffuse, and acute or chronic, and note specific findings on physical exam.

Key concerns

Differentiate symptoms from the following sources: bone, muscle, nerve, blood vessels.

Identify patients who require urgent action.

History

HISTORY OF PRESENT ILLNESS

Ask where the pain is, when it started, how constant it is, and what triggers it. Ask about other symptoms the patient has (e.g., weakness, malaise). Ask about trauma. Ask how the pain affects function, including work and recreation.

SOCIAL HISTORY

Ask about the patient's occupation and recreation routines, listening for evidence of repetitive stress or pressure (relevant to tendinopathy and bursitis).

Physical exam

Examine the area of the pain, looking for tenderness, masses, erythema, and swelling.

Investigations

X-ray of the affected area

Other specific tests as indicated (see the differential diagnosis)

Management

Urgent intervention is required for patients with obvious fractures or dislocations, and with signs and symptoms consistent with necrotizing fasciitis or compartment syndrome.

MUSCULOSKELETAL PRESENTATIONS

Oligoarthralgia (pain in 1 to 4 joints)

Differential diagnosis

ACUTE JOINT PAIN

Injury (e.g., meniscal tear)

JOINT INJURY IN GENERAL

Signs and symptoms: history of trauma (e.g., sports injury, bicycle accident); joint pain made worse by activity and relieved by rest (as opposed to resting joint pain in inflammatory conditions); joint swelling, redness, warmth, bruising; movement difficulty around the joint

Investigations: x-ray, MRI, CT scan

MENISCAL TEAR

Signs and symptoms: knee pain, effusion; history of changing speed and direction at the same time; mechanical symptoms (locking, popping, catching, buckling); persistent focal joint line tenderness

Infection

Common pathogens in joint infections include *S. aureus* and *Streptococcus*.

Infants and younger children may be asymptomatic.

Signs and symptoms: symptoms in 1 joint (usual); acute joint pain, tenderness, warmth, redness; restricted joint motion; loss of joint function; fever; sweating; rigor; abscesses; hemorrhagic pustules; symptoms of endocarditis (e.g., fatigue, new heart murmur, night sweats, shortness of breath, petechiae)

Locations: knee (most common: about 50 % of cases), hip, shoulder, elbow

Risk factors: advanced age; IV drug use; underlying joint injury; prosthetic joint; skin conditions (e.g., psoriasis, eczema); immunocompromise (e.g., diabetes, kidney disease, liver disease, use of immunosuppressants)

Investigations: synovial fluid analysis (cell counts, Gram stain, culture, WBCs); blood cultures

Crystal

PSEUDOGOUT (CALCIUM PYROPHOSPHATE DIHYDRATE DEPOSITION DISEASE)

Signs and symptoms: older than 65 (usual); severe joint pain with stiffness, tenderness, swelling, erythema that peaks in 6 to 24 hours

Location: knee, wrist, hand, pelvis, hip (common)

History of illness, surgery, medication (bisphosphonates, intraarticular hyaluronic injections, granulocyte colony-stimulating factor)

Investigations: analysis of synovial fluid or biopsy specimen to detect calcium pyrophosphate dihydrate crystals; x-ray, US to detect chondrocalcinosis

GOUT

Chronic gout is characterized by recurrent severe acute attacks from monosodium urate crystals in joints.

Signs and symptoms: severe joint pain, erythema, warmth, swelling that peaks in 24 to 48 hours

Locations: first metatarsophalangeal joint (most common), midfoot, ankles, knees (gout is uncommon in axial joints)

Progressing chronic gout: possible persistent arthritis and white-yellow intradermal deposits

Risk factors: obesity, hypertension, alcohol use, high purine diet (e.g., high in meat and seafood), use of antihypertensives (e.g., diuretics, beta-blockers)

Investigations: urate crystal detection (e.g., synovial fluid analysis; US of joint or tophus); blood tests (CBC, BUN, creatinine)

Hemarthrosis (e.g., clotting disorder)

Hemarthrosis occurs in patients with hemophilia and other clotting disorders.

Signs and symptoms: personal or family history of hemophilia; joint tingling, tightness followed by joint swelling, warmth, pain

Locations: ankles, knees, elbows (most common); shoulders, wrists, hips (less common)

Late symptoms: pain at rest; extreme loss of motion

Investigations: coagulation profile (PT/INR, aPTT, platelet count, von Willebrand factor assay)

Diagnosis of clotting disorder: factor IX inhibitor (hemophilia B), factor VIII activity (hemophilia A), gene mutation testing

Acute reactive arthritis

Symptoms: acute, asymmetric pain in 1 to 4 joints; inflammation of ligaments or tendons; tendonitis; swollen toes, fingers; recent or current mild, bilateral conjunctivitis; recent GI, GU, or respiratory infection; fever; malaise; weight loss; morning stiffness lasting > 1 hour

Locations: knee, ankle, and/or heel (usual) (it is uncommon in the upper limbs)

Investigations: positive HLA-B27; elevated acute phase reactants; serology, urinalysis, stool cultures to detect recent infection

CHRONIC JOINT PAIN

Osteoarthritis

This is breakdown of joint cartilage and underlying bone.

Signs and symptoms: joint pain and stiffness following exercise initially and progressing to permanence (over years)

Joint symptoms: often asymmetrical; swelling; impaired function; instability; buckling; bone tenderness and/or enlargement; crepitus

Locations: ends of the fingers; bases of the thumbs; the neck, lower back, knees, hips

Risk factors: older age; female; obesity; joint injuries; abnormal joint or limb development; family history of osteoarthritis

Investigations: x-ray

Periarticular disease (e.g., bursitis, tendinosis)

BURSITIS

This is inflammation of the bursae, which are sacs that cushion bones and the structures surrounding joints.

The most common cause is repetitive pressure on bursae (e.g., kneeling, leaning on the elbows, sitting for long periods on hard surfaces).

Investigations: x-ray, US, or MRI to rule out other causes; blood tests or analysis of fluid from inflamed bursae to identify the cause

TENDINOSIS

This is cellular-level damage to tendons that results from chronic overuse, and involves the generation of new blood vessels to the injury. It can develop from untreated tendonitis.

Signs and symptoms: tendon pain that persists for weeks or months; history of chronic repetitive low-grade trauma or overuse (common); history of sports injury (common); pain on palpation of the affected tendon; pain with tendon loading

> Achilles tendon: heel pain (this is common in runners)
>
> Biceps: anterior shoulder pain in the bicipital groove that is worse on flexing the shoulder or supination of the forearm
>
> Lateral epicondylitis ("tennis elbow"): pain of the lateral elbow that is worse on grasping and twisting
>
> Medial epicondylitis ("golfer's elbow"): pain of the medial elbow
>
> Patellar ("jumper's knee"): male (more common); history of sports involving jumping and running (common); pain on standing up from sitting, and climbing stairs or hills
>
> Rotator cuff, shoulder: dull, aching shoulder pain that is difficult to localize and radiates into the upper arm; painful range of motion; pain that is worse at night

Pediatric disorder (e.g., slipped epiphysis, Osgood-Schlatter disease)

SLIPPED CAPITAL FEMORAL EPIPHYSIS

This is the most common hip disorder in adolescents.

It requires accurate diagnosis and immediate treatment.

Symptoms: hip pain (sometimes groin, thigh, or knee pain) that becomes worse with physical activity; altered gait (limping; walking with a leg turned outward; waddling walk)

Risk factors: obesity, hypothyroidism, growth hormone deficiency, Down syndrome, prior radiation therapy

Investigations: x-ray (anteroposterior and lateral views of the bilateral hips)

> Anteroposterior view shows a blurry junction between the metaphysis and the growth plate.
>
> Both views show the line of Klein passing outside the epiphysis (instead of intersecting it) or passing just at its superior edge.

OSGOOD-SCHLATTER DISEASE

This is a common cause of anterior knee pain in adolescents.

Signs and symptoms: gradual-onset knee pain with swelling in nearby tibial tuberosity, which is tender on palpation; unilateral (usual); stiffness in the hamstring, rectus femoris; symptoms exacerbated by running, jumping, and direct pressure (e.g., kneeling); fluctuating symptoms for 12 to 24 months

Investigations: x-ray to exclude other causes

POINTER

Common causes of joint pain

The 3 main underlying causes of joint pain are:

Trauma

Inflammation

Mechanical disorders

Keys to patient encounter

Key concerns

Differentiate joint disease from other anatomic causes (i.e., determine the source of pain: joint or other tissues).

Identify patients who need immediate, definitive management or referral.

History

HISTORY OF PRESENT ILLNESS

Ask which joints are painful, when the pain started, and how constant it is. Ask about other symptoms the patient has.

Listen for evidence consistent with entities that require immediate management (e.g., recent-onset knee pain with fever in infection); and evidence consistent with particular entities (e.g., recurrent episodes of severe pain at the base of a toe in gout; recent trauma).

Ask how the pain affects function, including work and recreation.

PAST MEDICAL HISTORY

Ask about skin disease, diabetes, kidney disease, and liver disease (relevant to infection); and clotting disorders (relevant to hemarthrosis).

MEDICATIONS

Ask about immunosuppressant drugs.

SOCIAL HISTORY

Ask about the patient's occupation and recreation routines, listening for evidence of repetitive stress or pressure (relevant to tendinopathy and bursitis).

POINTER

Red flags in joint pain

Immediate management is required in acute joint pain with any of the following features:

Fever

Tachycardia

Signs of endocarditis

Physical exam

Vital signs: Look for fever.

Affected joints:

- Look for swelling, redness, warmth, and bruising.
- Palpate the surrounding soft tissues.
- Test the joint's active and passive range of motion.

Cardiovascular: Auscultate the heart looking for murmurs (relevant to endocarditis).

Investigations

CBC in suspected infection

CRP in suspected inflammation

Serum uric acid in suspected gout

Joint aspiration in suspected gout or infection for culture, cell count, and crystals

X-ray or MRI (consider this)

Management

Management depends on the probable entity.

MUSCULOSKELETAL PRESENTATIONS

Polyarthralgia (pain in more than 4 joints)

Differential diagnosis

INFLAMMATORY JOINT PAIN (E.G., RHEUMATOID ARTHRITIS, JUVENILE POLYARTHRITIS)

Rheumatoid arthritis

This is a chronic, systemic, inflammatory disease that involves synovial joints.

Signs and symptoms: symmetrical symptoms; pain, stiffness (morning stiffness); swelling in multiple joints that improves with movement; symptoms that progress from the periphery to proximal joints; decreased grip strength; fatigue; fever; weight loss; impaired ADLs; joint deformities and locomotor disability (later disease); rheumatoid nodules in the fingers, knuckles, elbows, forearms, knees, backs of heels (in about 25% of patients)

> Commonly affected joints: metacarpophalangeal and proximal interphalangeal joints of the fingers; interphalangeal joints of the thumbs and wrists; metatarsophalangeal joints of the toes
>
> Other joints: synovial joints of the upper and lower limbs (elbows, shoulders, ankles, knees)

Investigations: blood tests (to detect autoantibodies of rheumatoid factors and/or anticitrullinated peptide/protein antibodies; anemia; thrombocytosis; elevated ESR; elevated CRP); tests of synovial joint fluid (leukocyte count of 1500–25,000/mm^3 with predominance of polymorphonuclear cells); x-rays of the hands and feet to detect narrowing joint spaces, and erosions of bone and cartilage

Juvenile polyarthritis

Signs and symptoms: symptoms for > 6 weeks; symptoms in ≥ 5 joints within 6 months; joint pain, tenderness; reduced range of motion; refusal to walk or use affected joints; guarding of affected joints; limping; irritability; malaise; fatigue; diffuse pain; low-grade fever

> Rheumatoid factor–positive subtype: similar symptoms to adult rheumatoid arthritis; involvement of small joints; symmetrical symptoms; rheumatoid nodules

Rheumatoid factor–negative subtype: asymmetrical symptoms; involvement of fewer joints (knees, wrists, ankles); fewer rheumatoid nodules

Diagnosis: blood tests (IgM rheumatoid factor; CBC, to rule out septic arthritis or acute lymphoblastic leukemia; ESR; ANA; CRP); imaging (US, MRI, x-ray)

MECHANICAL JOINT PAIN (E.G., OSTEOARTHRITIS)

Osteoarthritis

This is breakdown of joint cartilage and underlying bone.

Signs and symptoms: joint pain and stiffness following exercise initially and progressing to permanence (over years)

Joint symptoms: often asymmetrical; swelling; impaired function; instability; buckling; bone tenderness and/or enlargement; crepitus

Locations: ends of the fingers; bases of the thumbs; the neck, lower back, knees, hips

Risk factors: older age; female; obesity; joint injuries; abnormal joint or limb development; family history of osteoarthritis

Investigations: x-ray

NONARTICULAR DISEASE (E.G., FIBROMYALGIA, POLYMYALGIA RHEUMATICA)

Fibromyalgia

This is a diagnosis of exclusion.

Signs and symptoms: female (more common); chronic, widespread pain for ≥ 3 months; pain that is bilateral, and above and below the waist; aching pain; fatigue; long sleep; restless leg syndrome; sleep apnea; impaired concentration, memory; dizziness; cramping (e.g., menstrual, abdominal); morning stiffness; numbness, tingling in the extremities; tender points; urinary symptoms (difficult or painful urination; irregular urination); sensitivity to noise, light, temperature

Coexisting conditions (often): headaches, irritable bowel syndrome, interstitial cystitis

Polymyalgia rheumatica

Signs and symptoms: older than 50 (always); female (more common); northern European descent (higher incidence); history of giant cell temporal arteritis (many patients have this, but it may not be active at the same time as polymyalgia rheumatica); symmetrical symptoms (usual); shoulder pain (more common), hip pain, neck pain; stiffness (morning stiffness usually lasts ≥ 30 minutes, with inability to abduct shoulders past 90 degrees); pain that is worse with movement; synovitis and bursitis (many patients have distal musculoskeletal manifestations)

Investigations: elevated ESR (≥ 50 mm/h); elevated serum CRP

Keys to patient encounter

Key concerns

Differentiate joint disease from other causes of pain.

Differentiate inflammatory from mechanical causes.

History

Ask when the pain started and where it is. Listen for joint pain versus nonarticular pain.

In joint pain, determine what joints are involved (the symmetrical involvement of many joints suggests RA) and whether the pain is always in the same joints (polyarthralgia that migrates suggests an inflammatory arthritis, such as RA). Ask about factors that make the pain better and worse (pain that is better with movement suggests an inflammatory cause; pain that is worse with movement or use suggests a mechanical cause). Ask about a daily pattern of pain or stiffness (morning pain and stiffness suggests an inflammatory cause). Ask about associated symptoms and listen for evidence consistent with specific entities (e.g., fatigue, fever, and weight loss in rheumatoid arthritis; joint swelling in osteoarthritis). Ask how the pain affects function, including work and recreation.

Physical exam

Affected joints:

- Look for warmth, erythema, and swelling.
- Assess range of motion.

Rheumatoid nodules: Common locations are hands, feet, fingers, knuckles, elbows, forearms, knees, and backs of heels.

Investigations

CRP
X-rays of affected joints
Other specific tests as indicated (see the differential diagnosis)

Management

Refer patients with inflammatory arthritis to a rheumatologist. Treat patients with osteoarthritis with analgesics (acetaminophen or NSAIDs), and counsel exercise and weight control.

NAIL PRESENTATIONS

Nail presentations

Differential diagnosis

LOCAL NAIL PROBLEMS

Paronychia

Signs and symptoms: tenderness or redness of the nail or surrounding skin; blisters or pustules; detachment of the nail; changes in nail color, texture, or shape

History of nail biting; cuticle injury (e.g., aggressive pushing down of cuticles during manicures); hands in water for long periods

Investigations: biopsy to detect nail fungi

Herpetic whitlow

Signs and symptoms: pain and swelling of the terminal phalange of a finger (typical; it may affect > 1 finger; it may affect toes)

Investigations: tests to detect HSV-1 or HSV-2 (Tzanck; viral cultures of vesicle fluid; serum antibody titers; fluorescent antibody testing; DNA PCR hybridization)

Ingrown toenail

Signs and symptoms: redness and swelling of the surrounding skin; overgrowth of skin around the nail; pain; bleeding; oozing pus

History of chronic infections, diabetes, injury to foot, or new footwear

ASSOCIATED WITH AN UNDERLYING CONDITION

Clubbing

Signs and symptoms: gradual swelling of the terminal phalanges of the fingers or toes; concave nails (Schamroth sign); **no** associated pain

History of associated underlying disease: pulmonary disease, cardiovascular disease, neoplastic disease, infection, hepatobiliary disease, endocrine disease, GI disease

Investigations: CBC to detect elevated WBCs; imaging to detect abnormalities associated with hypoxia (chest x-ray, cardiovascular imaging)

Psoriasis

Signs and symptoms: nail pitting; current or prior erythematous scaly rashes; family history of psoriasis or similar skin conditions; history of other autoimmune diseases

Investigations (usually diagnosed clinically): biopsy

Subungual melanoma

Signs and symptoms: changes to the nail of the thumb or big toe (more common); symptoms that develop over weeks to months; widening of the nail (especially at the cuticle); changes in nail color (e.g., brown or black streaks) that eventually spread to the nail fold (Hutchison sign)

Risk factors: darker skin

Investigations: biopsy

Keys to patient encounter

Key concern

Determine whether a condition is benign, malignant, or associated with an underlying condition.

History

HISTORY OF PRESENT ILLNESS

Ask when the patient first noticed the nail changes and what characterizes the changes. Listen for recent-onset versus long-standing changes (long-standing changes suggest an underlying condition); and for associated pain (this suggests a local nail problem as opposed to an underlying condition). Ask about a history of trauma to the affected nails.

PAST MEDICAL HISTORY
Ask about hypoxia (clubbing) and psoriasis.

Physical exam

Nails

Full physical

Investigations

IN SUSPECTED MELANOMA
Biopsy

IN SUSPECTED FUNGAL INFECTION
KOH analysis of fungal scrapings or nail clippings

IN SUSPECTED HYPOXIA
Chest x-ray

ABG

Pulmonary function tests

Management

Treat paronychia with antibiotics, and incision and drainage of any abscess. Onychomycosis is most commonly due to tinea infection, and can be treated with amorolfine nail lacquer, or with oral terbinafine, itraconazole, or fluconazole. Treat ingrown nails with partial or complete nail resection: counsel the patient to avoid tight fitting footwear to prevent recurrence. Psoriatic nail changes do not have a specific treatment other than general psoriasis management. Painful or large subungual hematomas are treated by drilling a hole with a 19-gauge needle, or creating a hole in the nail with a heated paperclip. Suspected subungual melanomas require biopsy, and referral to a dermatologist or plastic surgeon.

Numbness, tingling, altered sensation

Differential diagnosis

PERIPHERAL NEUROPATHY (E.G., DIABETIC NEUROPATHY, CARPAL TUNNEL SYNDROME, RADICULOPATHY)

PERIPHERAL NEUROPATHIES IN GENERAL

Signs and symptoms:

Motor: weakness, fatigue, wasting, cramps, twitching, myokymia, decreased reflexes

Sensory: numbness, tingling; burning or stabbing pain; gait and balance difficulty; temperature intolerance; hyperalgesia

Diabetic neuropathy

Signs and symptoms: polydipsia, polyuria, and/or weight loss; autonomic neuropathy effects (in addition to general motor and sensory symptoms, listed above) including indigestion, nausea, diarrhea, constipation, dizziness, difficulty urinating, erectile dysfunction, vaginal dryness

Carpal tunnel syndrome

This is caused by compression or irritation of the median nerve within the carpal tunnel.

Signs and symptoms: numbness, tingling, weakness in the arm and hand

Risk factors: previous wrist injury or surgery; female; history of inflammatory conditions (e.g., RA); fluid retention from pregnancy (this resolves after delivery) or menopause; workplace factors such as working with vibrating tools, work that requires prolonged or repetitive flexing (e.g., assembly-line work), and working in cold temperatures

Investigations: x-ray (wrist, arm, or hand); EMG; nerve conduction study of the median nerve

Radiculopathy

ACUTE LUMBOSACRAL (LOWER BACK) RADICULOPATHY

Signs and symptoms:

L5 radiculopathy: back pain that radiates down the lateral side of the leg into the foot; reduced strength on flexing the foot in any direction (up, down, in, out); reduced sensation on the lateral side of the lower leg and upper foot (when testing sharp sensation in the web space between the first and second digits)

S1 radiculopathy: pain that radiates from the back down the posterior side of the leg into the foot; weakness on flexing the foot down, extending the leg, flexing the knee; reduced sensation on the posterior side of the leg and lateral edge of the foot; loss of ankle reflex

CERVICAL (NECK) RADICULOPATHY

Signs and symptoms: pain in the neck (acute or chronic), upper limbs, shoulders, interscapular region, chest, breast, face; possible mild sensory loss

CENTRAL NERVOUS SYSTEM (E.G., MULTIPLE SCLEROSIS)

Multiple sclerosis

Signs and symptoms: variable depending on lesion location

Spinal cord: sensory or motor dysfunction; Lhermitte sign (paresthesias radiating down the extremities or trunk with neck flexion); bowel, bladder or erectile dysfunction

Brainstem: double vision; swallowing, speech difficulties; vertigo; pseudobulbar palsy

Cerebrum: cognitive impairment; depression; upper motor neuron signs; unilateral motor or sensory deficits

Cerebellum: problems with balance and coordination; vertigo

Other symptoms: tonic spasms; fatigue; pain; exercise intolerance; temperature sensitivity; painful unilateral loss of visual acuity

Risk factors: younger than 50, female

Investigations: brain and spinal cord MRI, including advanced MRI techniques, with established occurrence of multiple episodes; CSF analysis

DERMATOLOGICAL CONDITION (E.G., HERPES ZOSTER, ANGIOEDEMA)

Herpes zoster (cutaneous)

Signs and symptoms: unilateral dermatomal rash that does not cross the midline (i.e., reaction from a single nerve root or ganglion); involvement of thoracic, trigeminal, lumbar, and cervical dermatomes (common); rash that is often preceded by prodromal pain, itching, tingling, intense pain to light touch; continuous or episodic symptoms

Rash progression: red macules to papules to clear vesicles (1 to 5 days) to pustules (1 week) to lesion ulceration and crusting (second week) to lesion healing (2 to 4 weeks)

Angioedema

Common triggers include allergies and environmental factors (heat, cold, sunlight, water, pressure on the skin, emotional stress, and exercise).

Signs and symptoms: symptoms that can be chronic (frequent, unpredictable recurrence); involvement of the dermis, subcutaneous tissue, mucosa, submucosa; swelling with pain or burning that can affect the eyes, cheeks, lips, hands, feet, genitals, inside the throat

Investigations: CBC with differential, liver function tests, CRP, ESR, complement protein C4

MENTAL DISORDER (E.G., PANIC ATTACKS)

Panic attacks[1(pp189–234)]

Panic attacks can arise from anxiety disorders, such as generalized anxiety disorder, panic disorder, separation anxiety disorder, social anxiety disorder, and specific phobia. In panic disorder, panic attacks occur spontaneously. In other anxiety disorders, panic attacks can have specific triggers (e.g., phobic objects in specific phobia).

Signs and symptoms: history of anxiety disorder and/or symptoms consistent with a panic attack; history of social or emotional triggers for symptoms (possible); lack of evidence for other causes, including hyperthyroidism (anxiety can mimic other conditions and is therefore a diagnosis of exclusion)

Panic attack: symptoms that peak within minutes; symptoms that can include palpitations, accelerated heart rate, shortness of breath, chest pain, dizziness, numbness or tingling, fear of losing control, fear of dying

Keys to patient encounter

History

HISTORY OF PRESENT ILLNESS

Ask about the distribution of the symptoms (this should point to a likely diagnosis). Ask about symptoms of panic attacks (recurrent surges of intense fear or discomfort that peak within minutes).

PAST MEDICAL HISTORY

Ask about diabetes (personal or family history) and anxiety disorders.

SOCIAL HISTORY

Ask about the patient's occupation, looking for possible workplace injury (e.g., repetitive tasks).

Physical exam

Neurological: Perform a regional exam of the affected area.
Dermatological: Look for rash (relevant to herpes zoster).

Investigations

HbA_{1c}
Nerve conduction studies in suspected carpal tunnel syndrome (consider this)

Management

Manage any underlying conditions. Consider referral to a plastic surgeon for patients with carpal tunnel syndrome.

REFERENCE

1. American Psychiatric Association. Diagnostic and statistical manual of mental disorders. 5th ed. Arlington, VA: American Psychiatric Association; 2013. 991 p.

ORAL CONDITIONS

Oral conditions

Differential diagnosis

MOUTH PROBLEMS IN GENERAL

Dental caries and periodontal infections are common.

CONGENITAL CONDITION (E.G., CLEFT PALATE)

Cleft palate

Signs and symptoms: drooling; difficulty swallowing; hypernasal voice resonance; difficulty hearing; frequent ear infections; visible congenital facial or oral malformation

ACQUIRED CONDITION

Infection (e.g., candidiasis)

CANDIDIASIS

This is a fungal infection (*Candida*) that is usually diagnosed clinically.

Signs and symptoms: white plaques in the mouth and throat; feeling of "cotton in the mouth"

Risk factors: dentures; use of inhaled corticosteroids; immunosuppression

Malignancy (e.g., adenocarcinoma, leukoplakia)

ADENOCARCINOMA

Signs and symptoms: mass on the side of the face, below the jaw, or in the mouth; pain; swallowing difficulty; fluid draining from an ear

Risk factors: male (more common); older age; exposure to radiation (e.g., radiation treatment to the head and neck)

LEUKOPLAKIA

This is usually benign (but see risk factors for progression to malignancy, below).

Signs and symptoms: white lesions of the oral mucosa (surface texture and color may be homogeneous); tobacco use, including smoking, but especially chewing tobacco (common); asymptomatic (usual); discomfort, pain

Risk factors for lesions to become malignant: verrucous type; association with erosion or ulceration; presence of a nodule in the lesion; texture that is hard, or lesion with a hard periphery; located in the anterior floor of the mouth, on the undersurface of the tongue

Poor oral hygiene (e.g., caries, periodontal disease)

Signs and symptoms: obvious dental caries

> Gingivitis: gingival redness, swelling; gingival bleeding on brushing, flossing, or examination with periodontal probe
>
> Periodontitis: attachment loss; loose teeth; alveolar bone loss

Trauma (e.g., abuse)

The oral cavity may be a central focus for physical abuse due to its significance in communication and nutrition.

Signs and symptoms: contusions, burns, lacerations in the mouth (lips most common); fractured, displaced, avulsed teeth; facial bone and jaw fractures; injury from gags at the corners of the mouth (bruises, lichenification, scarring)

Toxic ingestion

Common toxins causing oral ulcers include methotrexate and other cytotoxic chemotherapy agents; bisphosphonates; nicorandil; propylthiouracil; NSAIDs; and recreational drugs such as cocaine.

Xerostomia (e.g., age, medications)

Signs and symptoms: oral mucosal dryness; use of drugs that cause xerostomia (e.g., TCAs, antipsychotics, antihistamines)

Systemic disease (e.g., lichen planus, Behçet disease)

LICHEN PLANUS

This is a common, chronic inflammatory condition of the skin (common locations: inner wrists, forearms, lower legs, lower back) and mucous membranes (locations: mouth, vagina).

Signs and symptoms (mouth): lacy white lines (Wickham striae) on the inner cheeks; tender red patches in the mouth, which can cause burning sensations, food sensitivity (hot, acidic, spicy), and chewing or swallowing difficulty; recurrent ulcers (rare)

Investigations: biopsy

BEHÇET DISEASE

This is a rare entity that causes inflammation of the body's blood vessels. It is diagnosed clinically.

Signs and symptoms: mouth sores that recur at least 3 times over 12 months (most common symptom); recurring genital sores; uveitis; skin rash

Risk factors: age 20 to 30 (more common); male (more severe); Middle Eastern or Asian descent

Keys to patient encounter

Key concern

Identify patients who require specialized care.

History

HISTORY OF PRESENT ILLNESS

Ask when the mouth symptoms started and how often they occur. Examples of characteristic symptoms include:

Candidiasis: "cotton in the mouth"

Gingivitis: gum bleeding

Periodontitis: loose teeth

Toxic ingestion: oral ulcers

Behçet disease: intermittent symptoms (most causes manifest with constant symptoms)

PAST MEDICAL HISTORY

Ask about cancers of the head and neck (these are relevant for radiation exposure), cleft palate, lichen planus, and Behçet disease.

MEDICATIONS AND DRUGS

Ask what medications and recreational drugs the patient uses. Listen for evidence relevant to particular entities, such as corticosteroids in candidiasis, chemotherapy and cocaine in toxic ingestion, and TCAs in xerostomia (see the differential diagnosis).

Physical exam

Mouth:

- Look for masses and mucosal abnormalities.
- Examine the teeth for decay or signs of trauma.

Neck: Look for masses and enlarged lymph nodes.

Investigations

Consider the need to investigate for potential systemic diseases. Take a tissue sample of any visible lesions.

Management

Management depends on the specific entity diagnosed. Consider the need for referral to a dentist or oral surgeon.

PAIN, GENERALIZED AND NEUROPATHIC

Central or peripheral neuropathic pain

Differential diagnosis

METABOLIC CONDITION (E.G., DIABETIC NEUROPATHY)

Diabetic neuropathy

Signs and symptoms: symptoms in the legs and feet (most common); symptoms worse at night; numbness; tingling, burning sensations; sharp pains, cramps; hypersensitivity to touch; muscle weakness; loss of reflexes, especially in the ankles; loss of balance, coordination; foot ulcers, infections, deformities

Diabetes: personal or family history of diabetes; history of diabetic complications and/or inadequate monitoring; polydipsia, polyuria, and/or weight loss

Investigations: neuromuscular signal conduction tests

NERVE ENTRAPMENT (E.G., CARPAL TUNNEL SYNDROME, LYMPHOMA, TRIGEMINAL NEURALGIA)

NERVE ENTRAPMENT OR COMPRESSION IN GENERAL

Signs and symptoms:

Initial: numbness, pain, tingling; positive Tinel sign

Subsequent: impaired function and muscle weakness; possible muscle atrophy

Investigations: nerve conduction studies

Carpal tunnel syndrome

This is caused by compression or irritation of the median nerve within the carpal tunnel.

Signs and symptoms: numbness, tingling, weakness in the arm and hand

Risk factors: previous wrist injury or surgery; female; history of inflammatory conditions (e.g., RA); fluid retention from pregnancy (this resolves after delivery) or menopause; workplace factors such as working with vibrating tools, work that requires prolonged or repetitive flexing (e.g., assembly-line work), and working in cold temperatures

Investigations: x-ray (wrist, arm, or hand); EMG; nerve conduction study of the median nerve

Lymphoma

Enlarged lymph nodes may press on nerves, causing limb pain.

Signs and symptoms (non-Hodgkin lymphoma): constitutional symptoms (fatigue, fever, night sweats, weight loss), enlarged lymph nodes, chest pain, coughing, shortness of breath

> Hodgkin lymphoma (less common): constitutional symptoms (fatigue, fever, night sweats, weight loss); enlarged lymph nodes; itching or pain on drinking alcohol, or increased sensitivity to alcohol

Investigations: blasts or cancer cells on peripheral blood smear; excess blasts or cancer cells on bone marrow examination

Trigeminal neuralgia

Compression of the trigeminal nerve near the brain stem may occur due to the effects on a nearby blood vessel because of trauma, stroke, or MS.

Signs and symptoms: severe, sudden, shock-like unilateral facial pain that last seconds to minutes with possible multiple episodes over hours; spontaneous pain or pain triggered by touch, air currents, eating, talking

INFECTION (E.G., POSTHERPETIC NEURALGIA)

Postherpetic neuralgia

This involves pain > 4 months after the initial onset of rash from herpes zoster.

Signs and symptoms: advanced age (more common); involvement of thoracic (T4 to T6), cervical, trigeminal nerves; burning, sharp, stabbing pain that is constant or intermittent in areas of lost or impaired sensation; pain triggered by nonpainful stimuli (e.g., light touch); areas lacking sensation; deficits of thermal, tactile, pinprick, and vibration sensations with affected dermatomes

> Severe: impaired sleep; decreased appetite; diminished libido

CENTRAL PAIN (E.G., PHANTOM LIMB PAIN, SPINAL CORD INJURY)

This is a delayed reaction that may come from amputation (phantom limb pain), spinal cord injury, trauma, tumors, stroke, and diseases such as MS and Parkinson disease.

Signs and symptoms: pain that is unrelenting, moderate to excruciating, localized or diffuse (localized in the case of phantom limb pain); burning sensations (common); pain with peculiar qualities (e.g., "skin coming off," "boring into bone marrow"); pain that is made worse by touch, movement, emotions, changes in temperature

Other: nausea, vomiting, hyperventilation, hypertonia

SYMPATHETIC PAIN (E.G., REFLEX SYMPATHETIC DYSTROPHY)

Reflex sympathetic dystrophy (complex regional pain syndrome)

Signs and symptoms: chronic unilateral pain in an arm or leg; history of trauma to the limb (many cases involve trauma; others may involve surgery, stroke, heart attack); pain out of proportion to the initial injury

Early symptoms in the affected limb: pain; swelling; redness; changes in skin temperature (from sweaty and hot to cold); cold, touch sensitivity

Later symptoms in the affected limb: changes in skin color (pallor), texture (thin, shiny, tender), hair growth, and nail growth; muscle spasms

Investigations: sympathetic nervous system tests to detect disturbances; bone scan to detect possible bone changes; x-ray for later stage bone-mineral assessment

Keys to patient encounter

History

Ask about the location of the pain, its quality (e.g., sharp, dull, throbbing), its severity (on a scale of 1 to 10), where it radiates, and what makes it better or worse. Ask about other symptoms the patient has. The evidence should considerably narrow the differential diagnosis. Ask about psychosocial and functional impairment as a result of the pain.

Physical exam

Examine the affected area, paying particular attention to neurovascular examination.

Investigations

HbA_{1c} to rule out diabetic neuropathy (consider this in most patients)

Nerve conduction studies to confirm suspected peripheral neuropathy (e.g., carpal tunnel syndrome) and evaluate the urgency for surgery
Chest x-ray to rule out lymphoma (consider this)
Vascular studies in patients with signs of vascular insufficiency

Management

Treat any underlying conditions (e.g., diabetes, carpal tunnel syndrome). Discuss pharmacotherapy options. Counsel the patient regarding exercise and activity modification.

PAIN, GENERALIZED AND NEUROPATHIC

Generalized pain disorders

Differential diagnosis

FIBROMYALGIA OR CHRONIC FATIGUE SYNDROME

Fibromyalgia

This is a diagnosis of exclusion.

Signs and symptoms: female (more common); chronic, widespread pain for ≥ 3 months; pain that is bilateral, and above and below the waist; aching pain; fatigue; long sleep; restless leg syndrome; sleep apnea; impaired concentration, memory; dizziness; cramping (e.g., menstrual, abdominal); morning stiffness; numbness, tingling in the extremities; tender points; urinary symptoms (difficult or painful urination; irregular urination); sensitivity to noise, light, temperature

Coexisting conditions (often): headaches, irritable bowel syndrome, interstitial cystitis

Chronic fatigue syndrome

Signs and symptoms: extreme fatigue unexplained by any underlying medical condition; symptoms that do not improve with rest; symptoms for ≥ 6 months

PQ

Other symptoms: loss of memory or concentration; sore throat; enlarged lymph nodes (neck, armpits); muscle pain; pain that moves among joints without swelling or redness; headache of a new type, pattern, or severity; unrefreshing sleep; extreme exhaustion lasting > 24 hours after mental or physical exertion

POLYMYALGIA RHEUMATICA

Signs and symptoms: older than 50 (always); female (more common); northern European descent (higher incidence); history of giant cell temporal arteritis (many patients have this, but it may not be active at the same time as polymyalgia rheumatica); symmetrical symptoms (usual); shoulder pain (more common), hip pain, neck pain; stiffness (morning stiffness usually lasts ≥ 30 minutes, with inability to abduct shoulders past 90 degrees); pain that is worse with movement; synovitis and bursitis (many patients have distal musculoskeletal manifestations)

Investigations: elevated ESR (≥ 50 mm/h); elevated serum CRP

MENTAL HEALTH DISORDER (E.G., DEPRESSION, SOMATIC SYMPTOM DISORDER)

Major depressive disorder[1(pp160–161)]

Signs and symptoms: symptoms that are present most of the time for ≥ 2 weeks; symptoms with significant impact on day-to-day life

Key symptoms: depressed mood and/or loss of interest in usual activities

Other symptoms: significant weight change; sleep disturbance; slowed or agitated mental processes; loss of concentration; recurrent thoughts of death or suicide

Risk factors: family history of mental health disorders (depression, anxiety, suicide); personal history of other mental health disorders; substance abuse; chronic illness (e.g., cancer, stroke, chronic pain)

Somatic symptom disorder[1(p311)]

Signs and symptoms: disproportionate and persistent thoughts about the seriousness of a health concern, and/or excessive and persistent anxiety about a health concern, and/or excessive time or energy devoted to a health concern; presence of symptoms for ≥ 6 months (the health concern involved may change); symptoms with significant impact on day-to-day life

Keys to patient encounter

Key concern

Differentiate articular from nonarticular pain.

History

HISTORY OF PRESENT ILLNESS

Causes of generalized pain can be difficult to separate.

Start by asking about the patient's symptoms. Examples of characteristic symptoms include:

Fibromyalgia and polymyalgia rheumatica: morning stiffness (ask specifically about this symptom)

Polymyalgia rheumatica: shoulder pain and pain that is worse with movement

Chronic fatigue syndrome: enlarged lymph nodes

Major depressive disorder: depressed mood combined with possible weight loss and/or suicidal thoughts (ask specifically about these symptoms)

PAST MEDICAL HISTORY

Ask about giant cell temporal arteritis (relevant for polymyalgia rheumatica) and mental health disorders.

FAMILY HISTORY

Ask about mental health disorders.

Physical exam

Musculoskeletal: Look for areas of tenderness.

Temporal arteries: Palpate for tenderness.

Investigations

ESR or CRP

Temporal artery biopsy in suspected temporal arteritis

POINTER

Treating fibromyalgia

The best way to treat fibromyalgia is through a multidisciplinary approach. A number of medications have been used with varying results, including antidepressants, NSAIDs, muscle relaxants, and antiepileptics. If medications are used at all, they should be combined with physical exercise and cognitive behavioral therapy.

Management

Polymyalgia rheumatica and temporal arteritis require immediate treatment with steroids. Patients with suicidal ideation (in major depressive disorder) may require hospitalization.

REFERENCE

1. American Psychiatric Association. Diagnostic and statistical manual of mental disorders. 5th ed. Arlington, VA: American Psychiatric Association; 2013. 991 p.

PEDIATRICS

Attention, learning, and school problems

Differential diagnosis

DEVELOPMENTAL DISORDERS (E.G., ATTENTION DEFICIT HYPERACTIVITY DISORDER, SPECIFIC LEARNING DISORDER, AUTISM SPECTRUM DISORDER)

DEVELOPMENTAL DISORDERS IN GENERAL

Signs and symptoms: family history of developmental delay, disorders, or impairments; history of complications during gestation (e.g., toxin exposure such as alcohol or smoking) and/or delivery, including premature birth; growth abnormalities; neurological abnormalities; dysmorphic features; hypothyroidism; lead poisoning

Attention deficit hyperactivity disorder[1(pp59–60)]

Signs and symptoms (children younger than 17 years): hyperactive-impulsive symptoms and/or inattention symptoms; symptoms that are present before age 12; symptoms with significant impact on the child's day-to-day life in a variety of contexts (e.g., home, school)

> Hyperactive-impulsive symptoms (examples): excessive fidgeting, talking, restlessness; inability to play quietly or wait turns

Inattention symptoms (examples): marked frequency of careless mistakes, not listening, forgetfulness, distractibility; marked difficulty with activities that require organization, sustained attention

Specific learning disorder[1(pp66–67)]

Specific learning disorder is often identified during school years, but may only become a problem in later academic life, with heavier workloads and timed tests.

Signs and symptoms: significantly impaired key academic skills (e.g., reading, spelling, grammar, punctuation, numbers, and math); persistent impairments (e.g., impairments endure for months and despite steps to remediate)

Autism spectrum disorder[1(pp50–51)]

Signs and symptoms: deficits in social interaction and communication; repetitive, stereotyped behaviors (motor and/or vocal); restricted interests; sensory problems; presence of symptoms in all contexts (e.g., home, school); presence of symptoms from early childhood

SENSORY IMPAIRMENT (E.G., HEARING OR VISION IMPAIRMENT)

SENSORY IMPAIRMENT IN GENERAL

Signs and symptoms: differences in development compared to other children; problems with social interactions with other children

Hearing impairment

Signs and symptoms: problems identifying the source of a sound; language or speech delays; blocked (from impacted wax or mass) or nonmobile (from chronic effusion) tympanic membranes

Vision impairment

Signs and symptoms: frequent injuries; problems with self-feeding; abnormal pupil reflexes or optic fundi (possible)

NEUROLOGICAL DISORDERS (E.G., SEIZURE DISORDER, FETAL ALCOHOL SPECTRUM DISORDER)

NEUROLOGICAL DISORDERS IN GENERAL

Signs and symptoms: family history of neurological disorders; history of complications during gestation (e.g., toxin exposure such as alcohol or smoking) and/or delivery; growth abnormalities; dysmorphic features; hypothyroidism; lead poisoning

Seizure disorder

Signs and symptoms: personal or family history of seizures; behavioral and other abnormalities

Fetal alcohol spectrum disorder

Signs and symptoms: history of exposure to alcohol in utero

Pathognomonic dysmorphic features: small eye openings; thin upper lip; smooth philtrum; maxillary hypoplasia; small lower jaw; short upturned nose; flat nasal bridge; abnormal ear position or formation

Other features: growth deficits before and after birth (at birth: low weight; short length; head circumference ≤ tenth percentile); defects in the heart, kidneys, bones; deformities in joints, limbs, extremities; neurobehavioral impairments

MENTAL HEALTH DISORDERS

Signs and symptoms: personal or family history of psychiatric conditions (e.g., anxiety, major depressive disorder); excessive worry; loss of interest in friends and usual activities; changes in sleep habits; hallucinations or delusions; suicidal thoughts; history of adverse experience (emotional, physical, or sexual abuse; recent stress such as death of a friend or family member), or substance abuse

PSYCHOSOCIAL STRESSORS (E.G., HUNGER, ADVERSE CHILDHOOD EXPERIENCE)

Hunger can be a sign of neglect. Other signs and symptoms of neglect include not attending school regularly; poor hygiene, dental care; reports by the child suggesting lack of physical and/or emotional care at home.

Examples of adverse experiences include abuse, and death of a friend or family member.

CHRONIC MEDICAL DISEASE (E.G., OBSTRUCTIVE SLEEP APNEA)

Obstructive sleep apnea

Signs and symptoms: excessive or loud snoring; disturbed sleep (e.g., not feeling rested in the morning); obesity (common); allergic rhinitis (sneezing, runny nose, eye irritation); morning headache; palpable masses in the oral cavity or neck

Investigations: sleep study (polysomnography); hypertrophic adenoid tissue on lateral neck x-ray

DISORDERS RELATED TO SUBSTANCE ABUSE AND ADDICTION

Signs and symptoms: personal or family history of substance abuse; excessive worry; loss of interest in friends and usual activities; adverse experience (e.g., abuse, death of a friend or family member); physical evidence (track marks on the arms, nasal septum perforation); tachycardia; tremor and/or sweating

Keys to patient encounter

Key concern

Provide interdisciplinary management and ongoing supportive care.

History

HISTORY OF PRESENT ILLNESS

Establish what problems the child is experiencing. Ask at what age the problems began, in what contexts they occur, and how they affect the child's school performance and relationships with family and friends. Ask about sleep schedule, screen time at night, and sleep disturbances (snoring and obstructive sleep apnea). Examples of specific characteristic features include:

ADHD: symptoms of hyperactivity or inattention at school and at home that began before age 12, and that significantly impair the child's academic performance

Hearing impairment: delayed speech development compared to other children and problems interacting with other children

Mental health disorder: excessive worry, sleep disturbance, and loss of interest in friends and activities

PAST MEDICAL HISTORY

Determine the child's gestation, birth, and developmental history. Ask about prenatal exposures (e.g., tobacco, drugs, alcohol), and complications during the pregnancy or delivery (e.g., perinatal infections). Ask whether the child was premature. Ask how the child's development compares with children of the same age.

Ask whether the child has been diagnosed with any developmental, neurological, sensory, or psychiatric disorders, or with hypothyroidism.

FAMILY HISTORY

Ask about developmental, neurological, and mental health disorders. Ask about substance abuse.

SOCIAL HISTORY

Ask about a history of child abuse and recent psychosocial stressors such as a death in the family. Ask about potential substance abuse by the child.

Physical exam

Height, weight, head circumference: Plot these on a growth chart.

Vital signs

General inspection:

- Look for dysmorphic features.
- Assess for signs of neglect and abuse.

Neurological

Vision

Hearing

Investigations

Serum lead level

Thyrotropin (TSH)

Hearing assessment by an audiologist

Vision assessment by an optometrist

Genetic testing and/or consultation in children with dysmorphic features (consider this)

Overnight polysomnography in suspected obstructive sleep apnea

BEHAVIOR ASSESSMENT

Assess the child for developmental disorders and coexisting conditions with behavior-rating scales, filled out by parents, family members, teachers, or caregivers, as appropriate. Ask to examine school report cards and examples of schoolwork.

Management

Identify any modifiable conditions (toxic exposure, neglect), and treat any coexisting medical conditions (e.g., hypothyroidism, obstructive sleep apnea).

All cases of attention and learning disorders require a multidisciplinary approach involving family, educators, and ongoing supportive care.

In patients with ADHD, prescribe psychostimulant medication (monitor appetite, weight, and BP), refer for behavioral therapy, and consider referral to a multidisciplinary clinic for ADHD.

There is no specific treatment for autism. Management includes behavioral therapy and treating any associated conditions (e.g., depression, ADHD).

Management of fetal alcohol spectrum disorder includes supports for learning and behavior, and addressing any ongoing maternal addiction issues.

REFERENCE

1. American Psychiatric Association. Diagnostic and statistical manual of mental disorders. 5th ed. Arlington, VA: American Psychiatric Association; 2013. 991 p.

PEDIATRICS

Brief resolved unexplained event (BRUE)

Key concerns

Evaluate risk factors and possible causes.

In idiopathic BRUE, use risk categorization to determine the need for further investigations.

Differential diagnosis

BRUE IN GENERAL

The American Pediatric Society defines BRUEs as nonspecific, resolved events in infants aged 1 year or younger that last < 1 minute, and typically last 20 to 30 seconds. BRUEs are idiopathic in most infants, and may involve cyanosis, breathing abnormalities (decreased, absent, irregular breathing), and hyper- or hypotonia.

MISINTERPRETATION OF NORMAL INFANT PHYSIOLOGY

Examples include transient choking because of rapid feeding, or because of coughing during feeding, and periodic pauses in breathing of 5 to 15 seconds.

INFECTIOUS DISEASE (E.G., RESPIRATORY INFECTION, SEPSIS, MENINGITIS, ENCEPHALITIS)

Respiratory syncytial virus

This is the most common cause of respiratory infection in infants.

Signs and symptoms:

> Initial: apnea (common in infants younger than 6 months); upper respiratory symptoms (e.g., cough, nasal congestion), fever (common in infants older than 6 months and in children)
>
> Subsequent (these develop over a few days): shortness of breath; cough; wheezing and/or crackles on chest auscultation

Investigations (it is generally diagnosed clinically): rapid antigen test of nasal washing or swab; RT-PCR; viral culture

Sepsis

Definition: infection with systemic inflammatory response, dysfunction of ≥ 1 organ system

In neonates, infection usually occurs by vertical transmission. Examples include group B streptococci, *E. coli*, *S. aureus*, *L. monocytogenes*, *S. viridans*, *H. influenzae*, CMV, RSV, human metapneumovirus, parainfluenza virus, human coronavirus, HSV, HIV, *C. albicans*, *C. parapsilosis*, and *Aspergillus*.

Signs and symptoms: fever, tachycardia, tachypnea, poor muscle tone, poor feeding, vomiting, jaundice, abdominal distention, poor perfusion

> Severe: oliguria; mental status changes; shortness of breath; extreme hypotension unresponsive to fluid replacement (this indicates septic shock)

Risk factors: compromised immune system; wounds, burns; catheterization, intubation

> Maternal factors: chorioamnionitis (intrauterine onset of infection); intrapartum maternal temperature ≥ 38° C; < 37 weeks gestation; membrane rupture > 18 hours before delivery

Investigations: CBC with differential (elevated neutrophils is a common finding); CRP; blood culture; cultures of other fluids (CSF, urine)

Encephalitis

Viral infection is the most common cause: HSV-1, HSV-2; EBV; VZV; Enterovirus (e.g., Coxsackievirus); and insect-borne viruses (e.g., West Nile disease, Lyme disease).

Signs and symptoms: seizures, altered mental status (e.g., decreased level of consciousness, lethargy, personality change, behavior change), fever, headache, nausea, vomiting

Infants and neonates: poor feeding, irritability, lethargy

Investigations: blood tests (CBC, differential, platelets, electrolytes, glucose, BUN, creatinine, aminotransferases, coagulation); MRI (to detect brain edema; inflammation of the cerebral cortex, gray-white matter junction, thalamus, basal ganglia); CSF tests (perform LP after results of MRI; order CSF protein, glucose, cell count, differential, Gram stain, bacterial culture); EEG (usually abnormal) to differentiate from nonconvulsive seizure activity

CARDIOPULMONARY ABNORMALITIES (CENTRAL OR OBSTRUCTIVE SLEEP APNEA, ARRHYTHMIA)

Central or obstructive sleep apnea

Obstructive sleep apnea involves a mechanical blockage from soft tissues in the throat. It is a common cause of airway obstruction in infants and children, and is underdiagnosed. Central sleep apnea involves episodes of absent respiration without mechanical obstruction.

Signs and symptoms: recurring pauses in breathing of ≥ 20 seconds; possible cyanosis, hypotonia, bradycardia, and/or pallor

Central sleep apnea: absence of chest wall motion; premature birth (more common)

Obstructive sleep apnea: enlarged tonsils, adenoids; obesity; craniofacial abnormalities (e.g., micrognathia); mucopolysaccharidoses; conditions that affect muscle tone (e.g., Down syndrome, cerebral palsy, muscular dystrophy)

Arrhythmia

Signs and symptoms: family history of sudden, unexplained death (parent, sibling); irritability; pallor; disinterest in feeding; bradycardia, tachycardia, or arrhythmia

Investigations: ECG

NEUROLOGIC DISEASE (E.G., EPILEPSY)

Epilepsy

Epilepsy is difficult to diagnose in infants.

Signs and symptoms: episodes of jerking movements with possible changes in expression, breathing, and/or heart rate; recurring episodes with the same symptoms and duration; episodes that occur during awake hours and during sleep; episodes that do not resolve with caregivers' attempts to resolve; episodes that interrupt other activities (e.g., feeding)

CHILD ABUSE (E.G., INTENTIONAL SUFFOCATION, NONACCIDENTAL HEAD INJURY)

CHILD ABUSE (INFANTS) IN GENERAL

The suspicion of child abuse rises with repeated BRUEs with no medical cause and with evidence of other injuries (e.g., burns, bruises, fractures).

Signs and symptoms (in caregivers): inconsistency in descriptions of the circumstances surrounding the BRUE; inappropriate expectations about infant behavior

Risk factors: history of substance abuse by the parents or caregiver; unstable living situation of the parents or caregiver

Abusive head trauma

Signs and symptoms: extreme irritability or sleepiness; disrupted breathing; disinterest in feeding; vomiting, seizures; loss of consciousness

METABOLIC DISEASE (E.G., INBORN ERROR OF METABOLISM)

Inborn error of metabolism

Signs and symptoms: failure to thrive; family history of metabolic disease (e.g., glycogen storage disease, Gaucher disease, Niemann-Pick disease)

OTHER (E.G., TOXIC INGESTION, POISONING)

Poisoning

The common cause is OTC cold medication.

Other causes recorded in cases of BRUE include acetaminophen, amphetamine, benzodiazepines, cocaine, codeine, meperidine, methadone, phenobarbital, and phenothiazine.
Investigations: urine toxicology screen

Keys to patient encounter

Key concerns

Evaluate risk factors and possible causes.

In idiopathic BRUE, use risk categorization to determine the need for further investigations.

History

HISTORY OF PRESENT ILLNESS

Ask about the child's symptoms during the episode, how long the episode lasted, and how often similar episodes have happened. Listen for symptoms consistent with particular entities (e.g., breathing pauses in apnea; jerky movements in epilepsy); episodes lasting longer than 1 minute; and recurrent episodes. Ask whether the infant required CPR.

Ask how child's health was before and after the episode. Listen for symptoms of infection (e.g., fever, cough); persistent symptoms that suggest enduring disorders (e.g., persistent irritability, persistent disinterest in feeding); and use of cold medications and acetaminophen.

PAST MEDICAL HISTORY

Ask about Down syndrome and cerebral palsy (these can contribute to sleep apnea).

In neonates, ask whether the child was premature and about risk factors for vertical transmission of infection (e.g., intrapartum maternal fever, early membrane rupture in labor and delivery). In premature delivery, ask about risk factors for BRUE: birth at less than 32 weeks gestation and/or current postconception age less than 45 weeks.

FAMILY HISTORY

Ask about heart abnormalities (e.g., long QT syndromes) and MD. Ask about sudden death in first-degree relatives.

SOCIAL HISTORY

Ask the parents or caregivers about their living arrangements and relationship situation. Ask whether they have diagnosed psychiatric disorders. Ask about their alcohol use and recreational-drug use.

Physical exam

Vital signs: Look for fever.

General inspection: Examine the skin for unexplained bruising and look for a torn labial or lingual frenulum (these are signs of possible child abuse).

Cardiovascular: Auscultate the heart for abnormal sounds, rate, and rhythm.

Respiratory: Auscultate the lungs for wheezing and respiratory symptoms.

Investigations

Respiratory virus and pertussis

IN PATIENTS AT HIGHER RISK OF BRUE

See the pointer for BRUE risk factors.

Overnight polysomnograph

CBC

Urinalysis

Urine culture

Chest X-ray

CSF analysis and culture

Workup for inborn errors of metabolism: serum lactic acid, serum HCO_3^-,

---

POINTER

Risk factors for BRUE

FROM THE AMERICAN PEDIATRIC SOCIETY

Lower risk: first BRUE; older than 60 days; full term (if premature, gestational age at birth 32 or more weeks and current postconceptional age 45 or more weeks); event duration less than 1 minute; **no** cardiopulmonary resuscitation necessary; **no** abnormal findings from the history or physical exam

Higher risk: younger than 2 months; premature (gestational age at birth less than 32 weeks and current postconceptional age less than 45 weeks); more than 1 BRUE

---

electrolytes, calcium, ammonia, venous or arterial blood gases, blood glucose, urine organic acids, plasma amino acids, plasma acylcarnitines

Management

Consider a period of brief observation with continuous pulse oximetry for infants with lower-risk BRUE. Admit higher-risk patients for cardiorespiratory monitoring. Refer the parents for CPR training.

PEDIATRICS

Crying or fussing child

Differential diagnosis

CRYING OR FUSSING IN GENERAL

Most crying or fussing expresses a need, and usually stops when the need is met, with fewer and shorter episodes after age 3 months. Serious causes of crying (about 5% of cases) include cardiac, GI, infectious, and traumatic conditions that are potentially life-threatening (HF, intussusception, volvulus, meningitis, and intracranial bleeding due to head trauma).

FUNCTIONAL CAUSES (E.G., HUNGER, IRRITABILITY)

COLIC

Signs and symptoms: excessive crying without any identifiably organic cause that occurs for ≥ 3 hours per day for ≥ 3 days per week for ≥ 3 weeks

TRAUMA

This may include obvious injury or occult injury secondary to abuse.

ILLNESS

Examples include common cold, otitis media, and other infections.

POINTER

Red flags in pediatric crying

Respiratory distress
Bruising or abrasions
Extreme irritability
Fever
Inconsolability

Keys to patient encounter

Key concern

Identify pediatric emergencies.

History

HISTORY OF PRESENT ILLNESS

Ask how long the child has been fussing, how often the child fusses, and how well the parents or caregivers are able to console the child. Ask about associated symptoms. Listen for recurrent versus new-onset fussing (recurrent fussing suggests colic); and inconsolable fussing and fever (these are red flags).

Ask whether the child's usual sleep pattern and feeding pattern has changed recently.

Acute, marked changes in usual behaviors suggest acute illness.

PAST MEDICAL HISTORY

Ask about recent infections and check for missed immunizations.

Physical exam

Examine the child for obvious immediate signs of an emergent condition. Because of the broad differential diagnosis for this clinical presentation, use a systems-check approach to avoid physical omissions.

Head and neck: skull fracture; ocular or nasal foreign body; corneal abrasion; otitis media; oral thrush; tooth decay; stomatitis

CNS: meningitis, encephalitis

Cardiovascular: supraventricular tachycardia, myocarditis

Pulmonary: bronchiolitis, pneumonia, asthma

GI: appendicitis, gastroenteritis, pyloric stenosis, intussusception, volvulus, gastroesophageal reflux

GU: UTI, testicular torsion, incarcerated inguinal hernia

Musculoskeletal: fracture or dislocation, osteomyelitis, arthritis

Dermatological: skin infection or abscess, insect bite, anal fissure

Sepsis

Investigations

Investigations depend on the probable diagnosis determined through the history and physical exam. Imaging of the chest, heart, GI tract, and head may be required.

Management

Management depends on the specific entity diagnosed. If no organic disease is detected, counsel the parents to continue to observe the child at home, and to return for medical care if new symptoms emerge or the child's condition changes.

Failure to thrive

Differential diagnosis

PRENATAL

See the clinical presentation on IUGR.

POSTNATAL

FAILURE TO THRIVE IN GENERAL

This is the inability of an infant or child to grow adequately or to maintain growth, usually based on at least 1 of the following growth-chart measurements:

- weight: < third percentile for age and sex; < 80% of expected weight for height and age
- height: < fifth percentile for age and sex
- major percentile curves: crosses ≥ 2 over time
- BMI: < fifth percentile for age (see *Notes on labs and assessments*)

Failure to thrive does **not** apply if a child:

- has normal growth velocity, although apparently underweight (e.g., even < second percentile for weight)
- is genetically small
- is small for other reasons (e.g., constitutional growth delay, prematurity, or IUGR), but has normal weight for length and normal growth velocity

Inadequate calorie intake

CAREGIVER

INADEQUATE FEEDING SKILLS

Examples include giving too much juice or pop; preparing formula improperly (e.g., dilution); not providing enough food; providing an inappropriate diet (e.g., a vegetarian diet that is low in protein and essential vitamins); restricting foods (e.g., because of suspected allergies or cultural views); not establishing proper eating protocols (e.g., propping a bottle instead of holding it; allowing distractions such as TV during meals); not responding to the child's hunger cues (e.g., because disengaged or irritable); and not allowing enough time for feeding.

INAPPROPRIATE FOOD FOR AGE

Examples include delayed introduction of solid foods (e.g., the child is exclusively breastfeeding or exclusively drinking milk or formula after age 6 months); too-early introduction of solid food (at younger than 4 months); and lack of knowledge about the dietary needs of infants (e.g., knowing that it is appropriate to introduce soft foods such as rice cereal at 4 to 6 months).

Delayed introduction of solid foods can lead to iron deficiency anemia, food aversion, delayed oral motor function, and atopy.

Too-early introduction of solid foods can lead to new-food intolerance, allergies, and food aspiration.

INSUFFICIENT LACTATION

Causes include maternal stress or fatigue, which decreases milk supply (symptom: poor letdown sensation); history of breast surgery or breast radiation; high androgen or prolactin levels; too-small breasts; medications; decreased frequency of feeds (e.g., due to separation of child and mother); and poor latch.

INFANT

SUCKING OR SWALLOWING DYSFUNCTION

Causes include pain (e.g., dental caries); craniofacial or oral abnormalities (e.g., cleft lip and/or palate; ankyloglossia); and neuromuscular disorder (e.g., dystrophies, hypotonia, cerebral palsy, hydrocephalus).

CHRONIC DISEASE (E.G., INFECTION, METABOLIC DISORDER)

INFECTION

Signs and symptoms: fever (> 38.0°C) or low rectal temperature (< 36.6°C); difficulty feeding; sleepiness; lethargy; irritability; rapid breathing; pallor; jaundice; blue lips or mouth

History of chronic infection (e.g., UTI, TB, HIV), immunodeficiency

METABOLIC DISORDER

Signs and symptoms (these begin a few weeks after birth): lethargy; poor appetite; abdominal pain; vomiting; weight loss; jaundice; developmental delay; seizures; coma; abnormal odor in the urine, breath, sweat, or saliva; chronic renal failure; family history of metabolic disorders (e.g., hypercalcemia, inborn errors of metabolism, storage diseases, diabetes, adrenal insufficiency)

INADEQUATE CALORIC ABSORPTION (E.G., GASTROINTESTINAL REFLUX)

GASTROESOPHAGEAL REFLUX DISEASE

Acid reflux is common in healthy infants aged up to 1 year.

GERD differs from this and is a serious condition.

Signs and symptoms: nonforceful regurgitation into the oral cavity, especially if it is worsening in infants older than 6 months; excessive vomiting; refusal to feed, or irritability during and after feeding; persistent cough, heartburn, gas, belly pain

Investigations: upper GI series (x-ray); pH probe; upper GI endoscopy; gastric emptying study

Increased caloric requirements (e.g., hyperthyroidism, congenital heart disease)

HYPERTHYROIDISM

Signs and symptoms: enlarged thyroid, tachycardia, palpitations, diarrhea, muscle weakness, tremor, hyperactive reflexes, weight loss, sweating, thinning hair

Investigations: decreased thyrotropin (TSH)

CONGENITAL HEART DISEASE

Symptoms: sweating with feeds; feeding intolerance; rapid breathing; fatigue; HF (increased work of breathing; decreased urine output)

Maternal history of diabetes; preeclampsia; older age; multiple gestation; thyroid disorders; CHD; connective tissue disorder; epilepsy; depression; bipolar disorder; use of drugs, alcohol during pregnancy; rubella exposure during pregnancy

Genetic anomaly (infant): trisomy 21, 18, 13; Turner syndrome; Klinefelter syndrome; DiGeorge syndrome; other single gene mutations (e.g., Noonan syndrome, Marfan syndrome, Ehler-Danlos syndrome)

Investigations: echocardiogram to detect cardiac abnormality

Social determinants (e.g., poverty, societal disorder)

Poverty involves restricted family income and, often, social isolation.

Examples of societal disorder include war zones, refugee camps, and disaster areas.

Signs and symptoms of adverse social determinants in children: depression; symptoms of PTSD (e.g., flashbacks); anxiety; poor academic performance; abdominal pain, headache, or other physical symptoms

Risk factors for adverse social determinants: parental psychiatric condition; family discord including domestic abuse; young single mother; parental substance use; medically or developmentally challenging child

Keys to patient encounter

Failure to thrive is most commonly caused by inadequate caloric intake associated with behavioral or psychosocial issues.

Key concern

Identify psychosocial and environmental factors, and disease entities, that give rise to poor infant and child maturation.

History

HISTORY OF PRESENT ILLNESS

Ask about the child's diet, including foods offered to the child, frequency they are offered, and what the child eats in a typical day. Listen for the presence or absence of appropriate food choices for the child's age, adequately frequent meals, and adequate caloric intake.

PAST MEDICAL HISTORY AND FAMILY HISTORY

Ask about chronic conditions and infections (e.g., neuromuscular disorders, HIV, TB, CHD, CF, metabolic disorders).

SOCIAL HISTORY

Ask the parents or caregivers about their income, living situation, and experience of traumatic events. Ask whether they have concerns about violence, addictions, or child abuse in their home, and whether they have a history of psychiatric disorders. Listen for evidence of social risk factors (poverty; unstable living situation; exposure to disasters or other trauma; child abuse; caregivers with a history of substance abuse and/or psychiatric disorders).

Physical exam

Height, weight, and head circumference: Plot these on a growth curve.

Full physical: Stay alert to signs of abuse (e.g., burn marks, ligature marks, bruising) and neglect (e.g., poor hygiene, poor dental care).

Investigations

In the absence of localizing features, investigations usually have little useful information to contribute in the diagnosis or management of failure to thrive. However, a major role of testing is to rule out underlying organic illness. Consider:

CBC for infection, anemia, immune deficiency

Urinalysis for infection

Serum electrolytes and creatinine for renal dysfunction

Liver function for protein wasting (see *Notes on labs and assessments*)

OTHER SPECIFIC TESTS

Consider tests for specific disorders if the history or physical exam reveal relevant signs or risk factors. For example:

Sweat chloride for CF

HIV

Stool for fecal fat

Management

Report cases of abuse or neglect to child protection services or police. Apply a multidisciplinary approach including dietary counseling, social services support, and home nursing visits. Consider referral to a pediatrician and hospitalization for severe cases.

POINTER

Incidence of failure to thrive

Failure to thrive is seen in 5% to 10% of children in primary care settings in the United States.

PEDIATRICS

Hypotonic infant

Differential diagnosis

HYPOTONIC INFANT IN GENERAL

Signs and symptoms: reduced muscle tone and tension; "floppy infant" (infant seems like a rag doll when held); loosely extended elbows and knees while resting (normal position is flexed); poor head control; decreased spontaneous activity; decreased muscle resistance to stretch

NEUROLOGIC CONDITION (E.G., PERINATAL ASPHYXIA, SPINAL MUSCULAR ATROPHY, MYASTHENIA GRAVIS)

Perinatal asphyxia

This condition can result in hypoxic damage to most organs. Brain damage is of most concern.

Signs and symptoms: neurologic symptoms (low level of consciousness; seizures; stupor); symptoms of respiratory distress (cyanosis; low perfusion, responsiveness, muscle tone, reflexes, respiratory effort); generalized hypotonia; bradycardia; acidosis

Investigations: US of the head, MRI to detect brain injury, EEG to assess seizures

Spinal muscular atrophy

Signs and symptoms: severe weakness that is symmetrical, progressive, more proximal than distal, in the arms more than the legs; poor head control; bilateral facial weakness; impaired tendon reflexes

Other: hypotonia; severe joint contractures; respiratory failure; atrial septal defects; weak cry and cough; poor feeding

Investigations: genetic testing

Myasthenia gravis

Signs and symptoms: ocular weakness (most common presentations: asymmetric drooping eyes; weakness in eye closure; double vision); painless, fluctuating, asymmetric muscle weakness (this may lead to respiratory failure); poor suck, head control; weak limbs

Investigations: serum anti-acetylcholine receptor antibody, single fiber electromyography

DISORDERS OF SKELETAL MUSCLE (E.G., MUSCULAR DYSTROPHY)

Muscular dystrophy

Signs and symptoms (myotonic dystrophy type 1): family history of MD; severe hypotonia and weakness; poor feeding; respiratory difficulties; positional malformations (e.g., club foot); delayed motor and intellectual development

Prenatal signs: reduced fetal movements or excess amniotic fluid

Investigations: genetic testing

GENETIC OR METABOLIC CONDITION (E.G., PRADER-WILLI SYNDROME, HYPOTHYROIDISM)

Prader-Willi syndrome

Signs and symptoms (adults and children in general): excess fat in the central body; small hands and feet; prominent nasal bridge; thin upper lip; downturned mouth; almond-shaped eyes; high narrow forehead; tapered fingers; soft, easily bruised skin; light skin and hair compared to family members; incomplete sexual development; frequent skin picking; delayed motor development

Prenatal and neonate: reduced fetal movement; abnormal fetal position; excessive amniotic fluid; breech or cesarean birth; lethargy; hypotonia; poor sucking; hypogonadism

Children: delayed intellectual development; excessive sleeping; strabismus; scoliosis; cryptorchidism; speech delay; poor physical coordination; hyperphagia; excessive weight gain; sleep disorders; delayed puberty; short stature; obesity; extreme flexibility

Adults: infertility; hypogonadism; sparse pubic hair; obesity; hypotonia; learning and cognitive disabilities; diabetes (often)

Investigations: DNA-based methylation testing for Prader-Willi syndrome and Angelman syndrome

Hypothyroidism

Signs and symptoms in infants:

Early signs: jaundice; frequent choking; large, protruding tongue; puffy face

Later signs: constipation; poor muscle tone; sleepiness

Risk factors: family history of thyroid disease or autoimmune disease

SYSTEMIC ILLNESS (E.G., SEPSIS, DEHYDRATION)

Sepsis

Definition: infection with systemic inflammatory response, dysfunction of ≥ 1 organ system

Infection usually occurs by vertical transmission. Examples include group B streptococci, *E. coli*, *S. aureus*, *L. monocytogenes*, *S. viridans*, *H. influenzae*, CMV, RSV, human metapneumovirus, parainfluenza virus, human coronavirus, HSV, HIV, *C. albicans*, *C. parapsilosis*, and *Aspergillus*.

Signs and symptoms: fever, tachycardia, tachypnea, poor muscle tone, poor feeding, vomiting, jaundice, abdominal distention, poor perfusion

Severe: oliguria; mental status changes; shortness of breath; extreme hypotension, unresponsive to fluid replacement (this indicates septic shock)

Risk factors: compromised immune system; wounds, burns; catheterization, intubation

Maternal factors: chorioamnionitis (intrauterine onset of infection); intrapartum maternal temperature ≥ 38° C; < 37 weeks gestation; membrane rupture > 18 hours before delivery

Investigations: CBC with differential (elevated neutrophils is a common finding); CRP; blood culture; cultures of other fluids (CSF, urine)

Dehydration

Dehydration presenting with hypotension requires immediate aggressive isotonic fluid treatment.

Signs and symptoms: diminished skin turgor on skin pinch; decreased peripheral perfusion, delay in capillary refill; hypotension; increased pulse and respiratory rate; oliguria; irritability

Investigations: comparison of body weight change before and after rehydration; hypernatremia; elevated serum osmolality

Keys to patient encounter

Key concern

Hypotonic infants always require urgent attention.

History

HISTORY OF PRESENT ILLNESS

Ask what symptoms the baby has and for how long. Ask how often the baby has a wet diaper and what the baby's stools are like. Listen for evidence of respiratory problems, neurologic symptoms, jaundice, constipation, fever, and dehydration.

PAST MEDICAL HISTORY

Ask about the mother's obstetrical history, including total number of pregnancies, number of miscarriages, and complications during the pregnancy and delivery for this child. Listen for a history of repeated spontaneous abortions, and risk factors for infection (e.g., premature birth, intrapartum maternal fever, early membrane rupture in labor and delivery).

Ask about the baby's birth weight and Apgar score. Ask about the baby's health after delivery.

FAMILY HISTORY

Ask about genetic disorders.

Physical exam

Perform a thorough physical exam, including a neurological and musculoskeletal exam, and an assessment for dysmorphic features.

Investigations

CBC and inflammatory markers to rule out sepsis

Serum electrolytes

Serum glucose

CK to look for muscle disorders

ABG

CT scan or MRI of the brain and spine to detect structural abnormalities

LP for CNS analysis to rule out neuroinfection

POINTER

Prognosis in hypotonic infants

Neonates with severe neuromuscular symptoms (e.g., respiratory insufficiency, and lack of swallowing and tendon reflexes) have a very poor prognosis.

OTHER SPECIFIC INVESTIGATIONS

Nerve conduction and electromyogram studies as indicated

Muscle or nerve biopsy as indicated

Genetic studies if the diagnosis is not apparent or there is multisystem involvement

Management

In addition to immediate supportive care, refer the patient to a neonatologist or pediatric neurologist. As these children will usually require long-term support, also ensure multidisciplinary follow-up.

PEDIATRICS

Neonatal distress

Differential diagnosis

CONDITIONS RELATED TO PREMATURITY

Respiratory distress syndrome

This is common in premature neonates due to deficiency of pulmonary surfactant.

Signs and symptoms: tachypnea, grunting, chest retractions, nasal flaring, cyanosis, apnea

Investigations: chest x-ray to detect ground-glass appearance, air bronchograms, low lung volume, absence of thymus

Apnea

This may be preceded by squirming, crying, and eye opening.

Signs and symptoms: possible airway obstruction; bradycardia; cyanosis, BP fluctuation

Persistent pulmonary hypertension

Signs and symptoms (labile hypoxemia): large variations in peripheral capillary oxygen saturation and arterial PaO_2; single loud S2 and systolic murmur on auscultation

Investigations: chest x-ray, ECG

Patent ductus arteriosus

Signs and symptoms: nonspecific signs (pulmonary edema, loss of lung compliance); systolic or systolic-diastolic murmur at the upper left sternal border; "machinery murmur" (continuous heart murmur, louder in the left upper chest or infraclavicular area)

Bronchopulmonary dysplasia

Signs and symptoms: paradoxical breathing pattern (diaphragm dysfunction); rales, coarse rhonchi, wheezing on auscultation

Investigations: chest x-ray or CT scan

Neonatal hypoxic-ischemic encephalopathy

Signs and symptoms: depressed tone, reflexes, respiration; fetal umbilical artery acidemia

PULMONARY CONDITION (E.G., MECONIUM ASPIRATION, PNEUMOTHORAX)

Meconium aspiration syndrome

Signs and symptoms: symptoms that develop within 15 minutes of birth; respiratory distress (tachypnea, grunting, chest retractions, nasal flaring, cyanosis, apnea); neonatal depression (bradycardia; decreased respiratory effort and muscle tone); presence of meconium below the vocal cords, or heavy meconium staining in amniotic fluid

Maternal risk factors for meconium-stained amniotic fluid: diabetes, chronic respiratory or cardiovascular disease, preeclampsia, heavy smoking, postterm delivery, cesarean delivery

Investigations: chest x-ray, pulse oximetry

Pneumothorax

Signs and symptoms: respiratory distress (tachypnea, grunting, chest retractions, nasal flaring, cyanosis, apnea), absence of breath sounds on auscultation

Investigations: chest x-ray; transillumination of the chest to detect pockets of air

DECREASED RESPIRATORY DRIVE (E.G., MATERNAL MEDICATIONS, ASPHYXIA)

Maternal medications

Examples of medications include depressants, narcotics (abused or prescribed), barbiturates, local anesthesia, alcohol, and magnesium.

Neonatal asphyxia

Hypoxic damage can happen to most organs. Brain damage is of most concern.

Signs and symptoms: bradycardia; cyanosis; low perfusion, responsiveness, muscle tone, reflexes; respiratory effort; possible meconium aspiration (see above); acidosis; seizures

CARDIOVASCULAR CONDITION (E.G., ANEMIA, CONGENITAL HEART DISEASE)

Anemia

Causes of anemia in neonates include hemolytic anemia, autoimmune hemolytic anemia, transfusion reaction, and alpha-thalassemia.

Signs and symptoms: jaundice, generalized edema, hepatomegaly, splenomegaly, tachycardia, tachypnea

Investigations: fetal hematocrit or hemoglobin via umbilical cord blood sampling, or direct neonatal blood tests; RBCs; peripheral blood smear; blood antigen typing for incompatibility with maternal IgG

Congenital heart disease

Types of defects include hole in the heart, obstructed flow, blood vessel abnormalities, valve abnormalities, underdeveloped heart, and possibly a combination of defects.

Signs and symptoms: failure to thrive; feeding intolerance; tachypnea; sweating, especially with feeding; cyanosis; slow capillary refill; regional swelling; uneven BP in all 4 limbs

Heart: characteristic gallop rhythm, pathologic murmurs

Investigations: echocardiogram, ECG

INFECTION

Infection usually occurs by vertical transmission. Examples include group B streptococci, *E. coli*, *S. aureus*, *L. monocytogenes*, *S. viridans*, *H. influenzae*, CMV, RSV, human metapneumovirus, parainfluenza virus, human coronavirus, HSV, HIV, *C. albicans*, *C. parapsilosis*, and *Aspergillus*.

Signs and symptoms: chest retractions; tachycardia or bradycardia; nasal flaring; grunting; apnea; rash; lethargy; hypothermia or fever; irritability; poor perfusion; hypotension; acidosis; diarrhea; poor feeding; bulging fontanelle; seizures; DIC; jaundice

Risk factors for sepsis (from mother): chorioamnionitis (intrauterine onset of infection); intrapartum maternal temperature ≥ 38° C; < 37 weeks gestation at delivery; membrane rupture > 18 hours before delivery

Investigations: CBC; CRP; culture or antigen tests (urine, CSF, throat swab, other fluids)

Keys to patient encounter

Key concerns

Assess the need for, and initiate, resuscitation.

Identify causal and ongoing pathologies.

Determine if the infant needs level 2 or 3 neonatal intensive care.

Airway and hemodynamic status

The first task is to determine if the child is in respiratory distress. Assess the patient's ABCs. Note the presence of tachypnea (respiration rate higher than 60 breaths per minute) and/or tachycardia (heart rate higher than 160 beats per minute). Initiate resuscitation as necessary.

History

Perform a history and physical exam at the same time.

HISTORY OF PRESENT ILLNESS

Ask whether the onset of symptoms was sudden or gradual, and whether the baby's respiration is improving or deteriorating. Ask about associated symptoms of cough, feeding difficulties, and/or regurgitation.

PAST MEDICAL HISTORY

Ask about the mother's group B streptococcus status. Ask about problems during labor and delivery (e.g., prolonged rupture of membranes, maternal fever, birth trauma, meconium aspiration, asphyxia). Ask for the baby's Apgar score.

FAMILY HISTORY

Ask about lung disorders and CHD, and a history of early childhood deaths.

Physical exam

Oxygen saturation

General inspection: Observe the baby for cyanosis, pallor, and asymmetric chest wall movement (relevant for tension pneumothorax).

Respiratory:

- Palpate the trachea for displacement, which may indicate tension pneumothorax.
- Auscultate the lungs for abnormal sounds, including absence of sounds.

Cardiovascular: Auscultate the heart for abnormal sounds.

Investigations

ABG (or a cord blood gas test, if the baby is immediately postdelivery)

CBC

Blood cultures

Blood glucose

CRP (this may be elevated in sepsis)

Chest x-ray

Echocardiogram or ECG if indicated.

Management

In addition to resuscitation (if necessary), obtain an emergent referral to a neonatologist and provide ongoing supportive care. Specialized neonatal care for ill newborns is categorized as level 2 (newborns of 32 weeks gestational age or older who are expected to improve rapidly) or level 3 (newborns younger than 32 weeks gestational age who are expected to require subspecialty care). Following stabilization, arrange to transfer the neonate to a facility that provides the appropriate level of care.

PEDIATRICS

Sudden infant death syndrome

Sudden infant death syndrome: risks and protective factors

SIDS IN GENERAL

SIDS appears to arise from the following factors: 1) an underlying genetic or anatomic predisposition, 2) a trigger (e.g., maternal smoking; airflow obstruction), and 3) the coincidence of the first 2 factors with a vulnerable stage of development.

The risk factors and protective factors for SIDS are known.

RISK FACTORS FOR SIDS

Maternal factors

Young maternal age (younger than 20)

Maternal smoking during pregnancy

Maternal alcohol and drug abuse during pregnancy

Late or no prenatal care

Infant factors

Preterm birth or low birth weight

Prone sleeping position

Sleeping on a soft surface, or with bedding accessories (e.g., blankets, pillows)

Sibling of a SIDS victim

Environmental factors

Exposure to secondhand smoke

Bed sharing

Overheating
Swaddling

PROTECTIVE FACTORS

Room sharing
Pacifier use
Breastfeeding
Fan use
Immunizations

Keys to patient encounter

A patient encounter about SIDS is likely to involve parents with a history of a SIDS event in their own family or extended family.

Key concerns

Evaluate fully the possible risk factors and/or causes.
Counsel the family.

History

The goal here is to get a detailed history of the SIDS event.

Ask about the circumstances of the baby's death. In particular, ask about the baby's sleeping position, what the baby's bed was like, and how warm the room was. Ask about secondhand smoke, bed sharing, and swaddling (wrapping baby up).

Take an obstetrical history, looking for maternal risk factors, premature birth, and/or low birth weight.

Ask about a family history of genetic disorders.

Review the autopsy report, if available.

Counseling

Counsel the parents on the risk of recurrence of SIDS. The risk of a SIDS death in the general population is about 1:8500. However, the risk of subsequent SIDS deaths in the same family is considerably higher due to common genetic or environmental factors (as high as 1:100). Note any risk factors present for the previous death from SIDS. Discuss identified protective factors.

Assess the parents' need for short- and long-term bereavement support, and refer them to a psychologist as necessary.

Pelvic pain

Differential diagnosis

PREGNANCY-RELATED CONDITION (E.G., ECTOPIC, MOLAR, ABRUPTION)

Ectopic pregnancy

Signs and symptoms: symptoms of pregnancy and/or positive pregnancy test; pelvic pain; vaginal bleeding; painful intercourse; shoulder pain; palpable tubal mass; pelvic tenderness and pain associated with 1 or both adnexa

Severe symptom: syncope

Risk factors: previous ectopic pregnancy, PID, pregnancy during IUD use

Investigations (pathognomonic): β-HCG above discriminatory zone (> 1500–2000 mIU/mL [1500–2000 IU/L]) **with** transvaginal US findings of a lack of intrauterine gestational sac, complex (mixed solid and cystic) masses in the adnexa, and free fluid in the cul-de-sac

Molar pregnancy (hydatidiform mole)

This is usually benign, but may progress to malignancy.

Signs and symptoms: symptoms similar to early pregnancy (missed menstrual periods; positive pregnancy test; vaginal bleeding; pelvic discomfort, pressure, or pain; hyperemesis gravidarum); uterus that is larger than expected for gestational age on pelvic exam or US

Risk factors: prior molar pregnancy or gestational trophoblastic disease; maternal age younger than 15 or older than 35; prior spontaneous abortion and infertility; vitamin A deficiency

Investigations: β-HCG (this is higher than for intrauterine or ectopic pregnancies of the same gestational age); US

US findings for complete moles may include **no** embryo or fetus; **no** amniotic fluid; central heterogeneous mass with numerous discrete anechoic spaces; and ovarian theca lutein cysts.

US findings for partial moles may include a fetus (this may resemble a missed or incomplete abortion; if viable, it is often growth restricted); amniotic fluid, possibly with reduced volume; placenta with ≥ 1 abnormal findings (enlarged; cystic spaces in a "Swiss cheese" pattern; increased echogenicity of chorionic villi); increased transverse diameter of gestational sac; and **no** theca lutein cysts.

Abruption (placental)

Signs and symptoms: possibly asymptomatic; pregnancy > 20 weeks gestation; abrupt-onset vaginal bleeding; abdominal and/or back pain (mild to moderate); uterine contractions (high frequency, low amplitude); firm uterus that may be rigid and tender; maternal hypotension and nonreassuring fetal heart rate (clinically significant placental separation); disseminated intravascular coagulation

Risk factors: older maternal age, previous abruption, smoking, hypertension, asthma, family history of abruption

Investigations: US

> Classic finding: retroplacental hematoma (this is absent in many patients) with variable appearance (solid, complex; hypo-, hyper-, or isoechoic when compared to placenta)

GYNECOLOGIC CONDITION

Ovary (e.g., ruptured cyst, torsion)

RUPTURED CYST, TORSION

Signs and symptoms: pelvic pain; pain during intercourse; change in bowel habits; nausea, vomiting; fever; worsening or sudden onset of pain (this may indicate ovarian torsion); pelvic tenderness and pain associated with 1 or both adnexa

Investigations: enlarged ovary or ovaries on pelvic US or laparoscopy

Tube (e.g., pelvic inflammatory disease, endometriosis)

PELVIC INFLAMMATORY DISEASE

Signs and symptoms: lower abdominal and pelvic pain; pain during intercourse; fever; urinary symptoms; vaginal discharge; irregular menstruation; pelvic tenderness and pain associated with 1 or both adnexa

> History of gonorrhea, chlamydia, or risk factors for them (multiple partners, unprotected sex); IUD; childbirth; gynecologic procedure

Investigations: cultures for gonorrhea and chlamydia; US (this has normal findings)

ENDOMETRIOSIS

Signs and symptoms: pelvic pain associated with menstruation (very common); excessive bleeding during menstruation; pain during intercourse; pain during urination or bowel movements; tenderness on pelvic exam; normal findings on abdominal exam (common)

Risk factors: family history of endometriosis; nulliparity; personal history of PID

Investigations: US to detect ovarian cysts (common finding); laparoscopy with biopsy

Uterus (e.g., leiomyoma, endometriosis)

LEIOMYOMA

Signs and symptoms: commonly asymptomatic; premenopausal (usual); heavy or prolonged menstrual bleeding; pelvic, abdominal pressure; pain during intercourse; urinary symptoms (incontinence; frequent urination; difficulty emptying the bladder); constipation; pelvic mass or enlarged, irregular uterus on bimanual palpation

Risk factors: family history of leiomyoma; African descent

Investigations: US to detect mass ≥ 1 cm in diameter

ENDOMETRIOSIS—SEE ABOVE

OTHER (DYSMENORRHEA, OVULATION PAIN, DYSPAREUNIA)

Dysmenorrhea (primary)

Primary dysmenorrhea (as opposed to secondary dysmenorrhea) occurs in women without disorders that could account for their symptoms (e.g., endometriosis, adenomyosis, uterine fibroids).

It occurs in 50% to 90% of reproductive-age women, and often improves with age and childbirth.

Signs and symptoms: recurrent pain during menstruation (midline, lower abdominal, suprapubic; mild to severe); **no** demonstrable disease; crampy, intermittently intense, and/or continuous dull ache with possible nausea, diarrhea, fatigue, headache; symptom onset 1 to 2 days before menstruation, diminishing over 12 to 72 hours; normal pelvic exam

Risk factors: younger than 30; smoking; menarche before age 12; longer menstrual cycles, duration of bleeding; irregular or heavy menstrual flow; family history of dysmenorrhea

Ovulation pain

Signs and symptoms: symptom onset 2 weeks before menstrual period; variable symptom duration (minutes to 48 hours); lower abdominal pain, just inside the hip bone, on the left or right side (the location depends on which ovary is active); uncomfortable pressure, twinges, sharp pains, or cramps

Dyspareunia

Signs and symptoms: pain on penetration (sex, tampon insertion); new pain after previously pain-free intercourse

Risk factors: PID, depression, anxiety, history of sexual abuse

SYSTEMIC CONDITION

Urologic (interstitial cystitis, renal colic)

INTERSTITIAL CYSTITIS

Signs and symptoms: increased frequency of urination; painful urination; pelvic pain and/or flank pain; fever; tenderness over the bladder

Investigations: urinalysis (positive for infection)

RENAL COLIC

Signs and symptoms: colicky flank pain; nausea, vomiting; fever; history of kidney stones (common); extreme tenderness at the costovertebral angle on abdominal examination; hematuria

Investigations (to detect stones): KUB x-ray; ureter US, abdominal CT scan

Musculoskeletal (fibromyalgia)

FIBROMYALGIA

This is a diagnosis of exclusion.

Signs and symptoms: female (more common); chronic, widespread pain for ≥ 3 months; pain that is bilateral, and above and below the waist; aching pain; fatigue; long sleep; restless legs syndrome; sleep apnea; impaired concentration, memory; dizziness; cramping (e.g., menstrual, abdominal); morning stiffness; numbness, tingling in the extremities; tender points; urinary symptoms (painful or difficult urination; irregular urination); sensitivity to noise, light, temperature

> Coexisting conditions (often): headaches, irritable bowel syndrome, interstitial cystitis

Gastrointestinal (irritable bowel syndrome, diverticulitis, inflammatory bowel disease, hernia)

IRRITABLE BOWEL SYNDROME[1]

Irritable bowel syndrome is commonly diagnosed by applying the Rome criteria.

Signs and symptoms (Rome criteria): at least 2 symptoms, present for ≥ 1 day/week for ≥ 3 months

> Symptoms: pain associated with 1) defecation, 2) change of stool frequency, and/or 3) change in stool consistency

DIVERTICULITIS

Signs and symptoms: constant left lower quadrant abdominal pain; abdominal tenderness; fever; nausea, vomiting; change in bowel habits (constipation and/or diarrhea)

Risk factors: advanced age; obesity; smoking; poor diet; lack of exercise

Investigations: CT scan

INFLAMMATORY BOWEL DISEASE

Signs and symptoms: younger than 30 (usually); family history of inflammatory bowel disease; fluctuating symptoms with periods of exacerbation and remission; diarrhea (possibly with nocturnal waking); blood in the stool; abdominal pain; weight loss; fever; fatigue; right lower quadrant and periumbilical pain; extraintestinal manifestations (e.g., uveitis, arthritis)

Crohn disease: right lower quadrant mass, uveitis, arthritis

Investigations: elevated CRP (this suggests active inflammation); fecal calprotectin; colonoscopy with biopsy (this is a standard diagnostic procedure); CT scan or MRI (findings: diagnostic structural changes associated with inflammatory bowel disease)

HERNIA (INGUINAL HERNIA)

Signs and symptoms: inguinal swelling that aches and enlarges with straining (usual); nausea, vomiting; constipation (this suggests an incarcerated hernia)

Direct inguinal hernia: palpable bulge above the inguinal canal and **medial** to the internal inguinal ring

Indirect inguinal hernia: palpable bulge above the inguinal canal and **lateral** to the internal inguinal ring

MENTAL HEALTH ISSUES

Major depressive disorder[2(pp160–161)]

Signs and symptoms: symptoms that are present most of the time for ≥ 2 weeks; symptoms with significant impact on day-to-day life

Key symptoms: depressed mood and/or loss of interest in usual activities

Other symptoms: significant weight change; sleep disturbance; slowed or agitated mental processes; loss of concentration; recurrent thoughts of death or suicide

Risk factors: family history of mental health disorders (depression, anxiety, suicide); personal history of other mental health disorders; substance abuse; chronic illness (e.g., cancer, stroke, chronic pain)

Somatic symptom disorder[2(p311)]

Signs and symptoms: disproportionate and persistent thoughts about the seriousness of a health concern, and/or excessive and persistent anxiety about a health concern, and/or excessive time or energy devoted to a health concern; presence of symptoms for ≥ 6 months (the health concern involved may change); symptoms with significant impact on day-to-day life

Sexual, physical, and psychological abuse/domestic violence

People who suffer abuse often don't disclose it.

Pelvic pain in this context is most likely attributable to sexual abuse.

Signs and symptoms of sexual abuse: genital and pelvic bruising and injury; bruising and injury to other parts of the body

Keys to patient encounter

Key concerns

Identify patients with acute pain caused by life-threatening conditions.

Determine if the patient is pregnant.

Stabilize hemodynamically unstable patients.

Airway and hemodynamic status

If the patient is actively bleeding, check their ABCs. Provide emergency management, if indicated.

History

HISTORY OF PRESENT ILLNESS

In women, ask about the patient's usual menstruation pattern and what changes she has noticed. Ask for the date of her last period. Ask about miscarriages and at what stage of pregnancy they occurred, and about complications during previous pregnancies. Determine risk factors for PID (history of sexually transmitted infections, IUD use, multiple sexual partners, gynecological procedures). Ask if the patient could be pregnant.

In all patients, ask what the pain is like and about associated symptoms. Examples of characteristic features include:

Ectopic pregnancy: shoulder pain and vaginal bleeding

Ovarian torsion: abrupt-onset or worsening pain and fever

Endometriosis: pain with menstruation

Renal colic: flank pain

GI condition: changes in bowel habits; constipation or diarrhea

PAST MEDICAL AND PROCEDURAL HISTORY

Ask about gynecological conditions, GI disease, renal disease, fibromyalgia, and mental health disorders. Ask about pelvic surgeries.

Physical exam

Vital signs: Look for fever (this suggests ruptured ovarian cyst, ovarian torsion, PID, urologic infection, or renal colic) and hypotension (this suggests blood loss).

Pelvic: Perform palpation and a speculum exam.

Investigations

β-HCG in patients of childbearing age

Pelvic US (consider this for most patients)

Order specific investigations if the history and physical exam point to a specific etiology

Management

Patients with emergent conditions require immediate referral for surgery. Positive gonorrhea and chlamydia tests require specific antibiotic treatment and reporting to public health authorities. In functional pelvic pain, consider nonopioid analgesics and physiotherapy. Also consider referral to a gynecologist, and to a psychologist for relaxation training, biofeedback, and cognitive behavioral therapy.

REFERENCES

1. Lacey B, Mearin F, Chang L, et al. Rome IV functional gastrointestinal disorders: disorders of gut-brain interaction. 4th ed. Vol. 2. Raleigh, NC: Rome Foundation; 2017. Chapter 11, Functional bowel disorders; 1393–1407.

2. American Psychiatric Association. Diagnostic and statistical manual of mental disorders. 5th ed. Arlington, VA: American Psychiatric Association; 2013. 991 p.

POISONING

Poisoning

Differential diagnosis

COMMON POISONS

Household or work items (e.g., cleaning substances, or other chemical products, cosmetics, plants)

A toxidrome is possible in this context (see the pointer on clinical signs of toxic syndromes).

Anticholinergics (e.g., antihistamines, tricyclics)

Signs and symptoms: possible anticholinergic toxidrome (see the pointer); "red as a beet, dry as a bone, hot as a hare, blind as a bat, mad as a hatter, full as a flask"

Additional symptoms: confusion; blurry vision; dry skin and mucous membranes; constipation (no bowel sounds)

Sympathomimetic (e.g., cold remedies, amphetamines, cocaine)

Signs and symptoms: possible sympathetic toxidrome (see the pointer)

Additional symptoms: hallucinations and/or psychosis; headache; sweating; increased motor activity; seizures; tremor

Depressants (e.g., alcohol, opiates, sedatives, hypnotics)

Signs and symptoms: possible sedative/hypnotic toxidrome (see the pointer)

Additional symptoms: confusion, stupor, or coma; nystagmus; gait disturbance

Cholinergics (e.g., insecticides, nicotine)

Signs and symptoms: possible cholinergic toxidrome (see the pointer); muscarinic symptoms or nicotinic symptoms

Muscarinic symptoms (most common) (mnemonic: **SLUDGE**): **s**alivation, **l**acrimation, **u**rination, **d**iarrhea, **g**astrointestinal pain, **e**mesis

Nicotinic symptoms (less common): tremors; muscle weakness; fasciculations

Serotonergics (e.g., selective serotonin reuptake inhibitors)

Signs and symptoms (serotonin syndrome): agitation, restlessness, confusion, tachycardia, hypertension, dilated pupils, muscle symptoms (loss of control, twitching, rigidity), sweating, diarrhea, headache

Severe: high fever, seizures, arrhythmia, coma

Analgesics (e.g., acetylsalicylic acid, acetaminophen)

SALICYLATE POISONING

Signs and symptoms: history of using skin products that contain salicylates, such as OTC acne remedies; abdominal pain; tinnitus; nausea, vomiting (blood in the vomit); hyperthermia; mental status changes (agitation and seizures; or lethargy, CNS depression, and coma); mixed metabolic acidosis and respiratory acidosis

ACETAMINOPHEN POISONING

Signs and symptoms: nausea, vomiting; lethargy; pallor; liver enlargement and tenderness

Cardiovascular drugs (e.g., digoxin, beta-blockers, calcium channel blockers)

DIGOXIN POISONING

Signs and symptoms: confusion, irregular pulse, fast heartbeat, nausea, vomiting, diarrhea

BETA-BLOCKER POISONING

Signs and symptoms: bradycardia; hypotension or shock; depressed level of consciousness; seizures

POISONING FROM CALCIUM CHANNEL BLOCKERS

Signs and symptoms: bradycardia, hypotension, cardiac arrest

Others (e.g., hallucinogens)

Examples of hallucinogens include amphetamines, cannabinoids, and LSD.

Signs and symptoms: possible hallucinogenic toxidrome (see the pointer)

Additional symptoms: hallucinations, psychosis, sensory distortion

Keys to patient encounter

Key concerns

Determine the nature of the toxicity and exposure.

Provide specific care based on this information.

Airway and hemodynamic status

Check the patient's ABCs. Provide airway and ventilation support if required.

History

If the patient is conscious, ask for a history of ingestion, but consider that the patient may be impaired or not truthful. Always seek collateral information from accompanying caregivers on the ingested substance and dose, if possible.

Physical exam

Vital signs

Full physical: Look for signs of specific toxidromes (see the checklist).

POINTER

Some clinical signs of toxic syndromes (toxidromes)[1]

TOXIDROME	HR	BP	RR	PUP	T
Anticholinergic	up	up	N	D	up
Cholinergic	down	up/down	up/N	C	N
Hallucinogenic	up/N	up/N	N	D/N	N
Sedative/hypnotic	N/down	N/down	N	N/C	down
Sympathetic	up	up	N/down	D	N

Abbreviations: HR, heart rate; BP, blood pressure; RR, respiration rate; PUP, pupils; T, temperature; D, dilated; C, constricted; N, normal.

Investigations

IN ACETAMINOPHEN OR ACETYLSALICYLIC ACID (ASA) POISONING

Serum acetaminophen or ASA

IN UNKNOWN INGESTED SUBSTANCES

ABG

Urine drug screen (consider this, but remember that some substances are commonly missed by this test [e.g., synthetic opioids])

TO CALCULATE SERUM OSMOTIC GAP

Sodium

BUN

Glucose

Ethanol

Blood osmolality

If lab results are reported as mg/dL, the equation for calculating osmolality is:

$$(2 \times Na^+) + (Glucose \div 18) + (BUN \div 2.8) + (Ethanol \div 3.8)$$

If lab tests are reported as mmol/L, the equation is:

$$(2 \times Na^+) + Glucose + BUN + Ethanol$$

TO CALCULATE SERUM ANION GAP

Sodium

Potassium

Chloride

HCO_3^-

The equation for anion gap is:

$$(Na^+ + K^+) - (Cl^- + HCO_3^-)$$

Management

Measure and monitor the patient's vital signs and symptoms, in particular related to cardiac, respiratory, and neurological function. Administer activated charcoal for decontamination or prevention of further absorption. Contact a poison control center. Administer specific antidotes if indicated (e.g., naloxone for opioid overdose, N-acetylcysteine for acetaminophen overdose). In patients with renal failure, or in severe poisoning without a specific antidote, consider referral for dialysis. Consider referral for psychiatric assessment, if indicated.

REFERENCE

1. Baskin LB. Lab literacy for Canadian doctors. Edmonton, Canada: Brush Education Inc.; 2014. Chapter 9, Intoxication and toxidromes; 173–200 (Table 19, 178–179).

PREGNANCY

Early pregnancy loss (spontaneous abortion)

Differential diagnosis

SPONTANEOUS ABORTION IN GENERAL

This is defined as pregnancy loss before 20 weeks gestation, where the fetus or embryo is < 500 g.

Common causes include embryonic chromosomal abnormalities or teratogen exposure.

Signs and symptoms: uterine bleeding (from spotting to heavy bleeding); pelvic pain (severe or dull cramping); small-for-gestational-age uterus (this suggests spontaneous abortion)

Asymptomatic patients: abnormalities incidentally discovered on Doppler or pelvic/transvaginal US (no fetal cardiac activity; abnormal gestational sac and yolk sac)

Risk factors (maternal): age; reproductive factors; medication, drug, substance use; low folate level; high body weight; maternal fever; celiac disease; prior miscarriages

Investigations: decreasing serum β-HCG

GENETIC FACTORS (E.G., CHROMOSOMAL ABNORMALITIES)

Chromosomal abnormalities

Fetal chromosomal abnormalities in number or structure are the most common cause of spontaneous abortions and recurrent pregnancy loss.

Aneuploidy: most common cause; increased risk with each spontaneous abortion

Other causes: mosaicism, translocation, inversion, deletion, fragile sites; single-gene, X-linked, or polygenic disorders

De novo genetic abnormalities: usually not inherited; possible increased risk associated with a first-degree relative with recurrent pregnancy loss of unknown etiology

REPRODUCTIVE TRACT ABNORMALITIES (E.G., UTERINE ANOMALIES)

Uterine abnormalities

These can be congenital or acquired. They interfere with implantation and fetal growth, and are associated with recurrent miscarriages and preterm delivery.

Abnormalities include uterine septum, submucosal leiomyoma, and intrauterine adhesions.

> Women are often asymptomatic.
>
> Removal of the septum increases the live birth rate, even in women who were considered infertile before.

PROTHROMBOTIC FACTORS (E.G., THROMBOPHILIA)

Thrombophilia

This results in recurrent miscarriages and uteroplacental circulation abnormalities.

Signs and symptoms: late or early fetal loss, stillbirths; IUGR; placental disruption; preeclampsia

ENDOCRINOLOGIC FACTORS (E.G., POLYCYSTIC OVARY SYNDROME)

Polycystic ovary syndrome

Signs and symptoms: symptom onset after puberty, with increased rate of hair growth and male-pattern hair growth; irregular menstruation; infertility; obesity; acne

Investigations: LH:FSH ratio (elevated: 2:1 or 3:1) (usual); elevated testosterone; US to detect ovarian cysts; normal prolactin levels; normal thyroid function

IMMUNOLOGIC FACTORS (E.G., ANTIPHOSPHOLIPID SYNDROME)

Antiphospholipid syndrome

This is the only immune condition where spontaneous abortion (sometimes recurrent) is a diagnostic criterion (it also features elevated antiphospholipid antibodies).

Definition: ≥ 1 fetal deaths at ≥ 10 weeks gestation; ≥ 1 preterm deliveries at ≤ 34 weeks gestation due to preeclampsia; ≥ 3 consecutive spontaneous abortions at < 10 weeks gestation

Risk factors: autoimmune condition (e.g., SLE, Sjögren syndrome); syphilis; HIV/AIDS; HCV; Lyme disease; use of hydralazine, quinidine, phenytoin, amoxicillin; family history of antiphospholipid syndrome

Keys to patient encounter

Key concerns

Provide supportive counseling to parents.

Investigate cases of recurrent miscarriage.

History

HISTORY OF PRESENT ILLNESS

Determine the patient's age. Ask how many times the patient has been pregnant, and whether becoming pregnant has been difficult. Ask about miscarriages and at what stage of pregnancy they occurred, and about complications during previous pregnancies. Listen for difficulty in becoming pregnant (this suggests reproductive tract abnormalities or endocrine conditions); IUGR in previous pregnancies (this suggests thrombophilia); preeclampsia in previous pregnancies (this suggests thrombophilia or immunologic factors); and late loss of pregnancy (this suggests immunologic factors).

PAST MEDICAL HISTORY

Ask about celiac disease, polycystic ovary syndrome, SLE, Sjögren syndrome, HIV/AIDS, HCV, Lyme disease, and syphilis.

MEDICATIONS

Ask about hydralazine, quinidine, phenytoin, and amoxicillin.

FAMILY HISTORY

Ask about spontaneous abortions, heritable disorders, and antiphospholipid syndrome.

Physical exam

A key goal of the physical exam is to confirm that early pregnancy loss has occurred.

Vital signs: Look specifically for hypotension (which may indicate bleeding or infection), and fever (which may indicate infection).

Pelvic:

- Look for the amount and site of bleeding, whether the cervix is dilated, and whether fetal tissue has passed.
- Check for cervical motion tenderness and adnexal tenderness.

Abdominal: Look for masses and peritoneal signs.

Investigations

TO CONFIRM ACUTE EARLY PREGNANCY LOSS

Pelvic US

β-HCG

CBC to document baseline hemoglobin and look for anemia secondary to blood loss.

Blood type and antibody screen to identify Rh(D) negative women who have not been previously sensitized

IN RECURRENT MISCARRIAGE

Antiphospholipid antibody screen

Maternal chromosomal analyses

Hysterosalpingogram

Other specific tests if a specific etiology is suspected (e.g., polycystic ovary syndrome)

Management

In acute early pregnancy loss, patients require emergent referral to an obstetrician-gynecologist if there is hemorrhage, hemodynamic instability, or signs of infection. If there is retained tissue, refer patients to an obstetrician-gynecologist for surgical uterine evacuation.

In active pregnancy loss without these warning signs, give misoprostol 800 μg vaginally, with 1 repeat dose as needed within 7 days if there is no response to the first dose. Prescribe pain medications as needed.

Administer Rh(D)-immune globulin in women who are Rh(D) negative and unsensitized (give within 72 hours of the first misoprostol administration).

Perform a follow-up pelvic US within 7 to 14 days to document complete expulsion of uterine contents.

POINTER

Vaginal bleeding and pregnancy loss

About 25% of pregnant women experience vaginal bleeding during the first 2 trimesters and about 50% of these progress to pregnancy loss.

COUNSELING

Provide empathy and support for the parents' grief, and check risk factors for complicated grief (current or previous depression, anxiety, or other mental health disorders; and lack of social supports). Consider referral to a psychologist for parents at risk of complicated grief. Counsel the parents that it is safe to reattempt conception as soon as they are ready physically and psychologically. In spontaneous abortions with unknown etiology, reassure the parents that no evidence supports routine activities as the cause (e.g., stress, heavy lifting, sexual intercourse, bumping the abdomen). As appropriate, consider referral for specialized care (to an obstetrician/gynecologist and/or for medical genetics).

PREGNANCY

Intrauterine growth retardation

Differential diagnosis

IUGR IN GENERAL

This is defined as in-utero growth below the tenth percentile for a baby's gestational age.

MATERNAL CAUSE (E.G., NUTRITIONAL STATUS)

Maternal causes and risk factors include previous IUGR; previous stillbirth; medical conditions (hypertension, diabetes mellitus, renal disease, autoimmune diseases); medications (anticonvulsants, anticoagulants, heparin, antineoplastics, cyclophosphamide); malnutrition; smoking; use of alcohol or illicit drugs; low prepregnancy weight; poverty; younger than 16 or older than 35; use of assisted reproductive technology; and current pregnancy complications (e.g., preeclampsia, threatened miscarriage with heavy bleeding).

FETAL CAUSE (E.G., GENETIC SYNDROME, INTRAUTERINE INFECTION)

Genetic syndrome

Signs and symptoms: family history of a genetic condition or syndrome; karyotype (aneuploidy) abnormalities such as trisomy 21 syndrome, trisomy 13 syndrome, trisomy 18 syndrome, Turner syndrome

Intrauterine infection

TOXOPLASMOSIS

Signs and symptoms: mild, flu-like symptoms lasting weeks to months; history of having cats or changing litter boxes while pregnant, or ingesting undercooked meat or contaminated water

Investigations: low avidity test in acute or recent infection; high avidity test in past infection

CYTOMEGALOVIRUS

Signs and symptoms: history of contact with infected blood and body fluids, including blood transfusions or sexual contact

Investigations: PCR; antigen test

RUBELLA

Signs and symptoms: low-grade fever; rash that begins on the face then spreads to other areas of the body; red or swollen sclera; history of contact with infected persons

Investigations: positive IgM 5 days after rash onset; low IgG rubella antibody on avidity testing for the first few months postinfection

VARICELLA-ZOSTER VIRUS

Signs and symptoms: rash of pruritic blisters ("dew drops on a rose petal") that eventually crust or scab, and that appear first on the face, chest, and back, and then spread over several days; history of fever, fatigue, anorexia, and/or headache 1 to 2 days before the rash (possible); contact with infected persons

> Shingles: unilateral blister rash with crusting and scabbing along a dermatome; history of pain, pruritus, and/or tingling 1 to 5 days before the rash (possible); history of chickenpox or direct contact with shingles blisters

MALARIA

Signs and symptoms: chills followed by fever, headache, and vomiting, then sweating, normal temperature, and fatigue (bouts occur every second or third day depending on the species of *Plasmodium*); weakness; enlarged liver and spleen; mild jaundice; tachypnea; history of living or travelling to an area with endemic malaria and not using insect repellent, antimalarial medications, or bed nets

Investigations: peripheral blood smear to detect parasites in RBCs; PCR to detect organism

SYPHILIS

Signs and symptoms: history of unprotected sex or high-risk sexual behaviors; painless, firm, round ulcers or chancres on the genitals or anus, or in the mouth; nonpruritic red-brown rash on the whole body or on parts of the body (e.g., soles, palms); alopecia; myalgia

> Late stage symptoms: paralysis, numbness, blindness, dementia, loss of coordination, gummatous lesions

Investigations: darkfield microscopy of lesion to detect *T. pallidum* spirochete; VDRL test and treponemal test

HERPES SIMPLEX VIRUS

Signs and symptoms: sexual contact with infected persons who may or may not have visible sores; painful blister(s) on the genitals and rectum, and in the mouth; repeated outbreaks taking several weeks to heal (common)

Investigations: PCR HSV DNA assay (most sensitive); cell culture; Tzanck preparation for cytologic diagnosis

HIV

Signs and symptoms: history of HIV; sexual contact with infected persons

PLACENTAL CAUSE (E.G., MATERNAL SMOKING)

Placental insufficiency

Signs and symptoms: asymmetry sparing the brain, but affecting weight and length (usual); late pregnancy stage (usual); oligohydramnios

Placental malformations

Signs and symptoms: positive US for, or gross identification of, a single umbilical artery; velamentous or marginal cord insertion; circumvallate or bilobed placenta; hemangioma of the placenta

Abruptio placentae

Signs and symptoms: vaginal bleeding; abdominal or back pain with tender uterus; hypotension; tachycardia; fetal distress, including absent heart rate or decelerations with normal fetal presentation

Risk factors: late maternal age; polyhydramnios; history of hypertension or other vascular disease (including coagulopathy); smoking; cocaine use; physical trauma (including abuse); previous abruption; multigestational pregnancy; uterine fibroids

Investigations: low fibrinogen; anemia

Placental ischemia or infarction

Signs and symptoms: preeclampsia; abruptio placentae; history of previous infarction

Keys to patient encounter

Key concerns

Identify modifiable risk factors for IUGR early in pregnancy.

Provide routine monitoring of fetal growth throughout pregnancy.

Provide careful evaluation of neonates who are small for their gestational age to detect a possible IUGR and assess potential causes.

History

Determine risk factors for IUGR. Ask about a family history of genetically inherited disorders; lack of personal immunization for rubella and VZV; and infectious exposures, including toxoplasmosis (exposure to cats, especially cleaning cat litter boxes), CMV (contact with infected blood and body fluids, sexual contact), malaria (travel to endemic areas), syphilis (sexual contact), HSV (sexual contact), and HIV (sexual contact, IV drug use).

Ask about difficulties with this pregnancy and previous pregnancies. Listen specifically for indications of bleeding (in all pregnancies), IUGR (previous pregnancies), and trauma (current pregnancy).

Physical exam

Vital signs

Fundal height

Fetal heart rate with a Doppler monitor

Investigations

Blood tests for infectious causes

Biophysical profile (fetal heart rate, muscle tone, movement, and breathing, and amniotic fluid volume)

Management

Refer the patient to a high-risk obstetrics clinic.

PREGNANCY

Preterm labor

Differential diagnosis

FETAL (E.G., MULTIPLE GESTATION, CONGENITAL ANOMALIES)

Multiple gestation

This is found on US.

Congenital abnormalities

These are often associated with a family history of congenital abnormalities, and are generally found on amniocentesis and/or imaging.

PLACENTAL (E.G., ABRUPTION, PLACENTAL INSUFFICIENCY)

Abruption

This is most likely to occur in the last trimester of pregnancy.

Signs and symptoms: sudden vaginal bleeding (mild to life-threatening), abdominal pain, back pain; uterine tenderness and/or rigidness; rapid uterine contractions (high frequency and low amplitude, or similar to labor); suspicious fetal heart rate pattern

Laboratory findings (during routine prenatal care): increased α-fetoprotein or β-HCG; decreased pregnancy-associated plasma protein A or unconjugated estriol

Risk factors: previous placental abruption; hypertension; smoking; abdominal trauma; substance abuse; premature rupture of the membranes; blood-clotting disorders; multiple gestation; maternal age older than 40

Placental insufficiency

This is usually associated with asymmetry where the brain is spared, but weight and length are affected.

Signs and symptoms: late pregnancy (usual); oligohydramnios; late decelerations on fetal heart rate monitor

UTERINE (E.G., CERVICAL ANOMALIES)

Cervical anomalies

Risk factors:

Acquired (more common): cervical trauma from previous deliveries (e.g., forceps- or vacuum-assisted); previous rapid cervical dilation for gynecological procedures (e.g., uterine evacuation); treatment for cervical intraepithelial neoplasia

Congenital: collagen disorders (e.g., Ehlers-Danlos syndrome); uterine anomalies; maternal diethylstilbestrol (DES) exposure

Investigations: US to measure the length of the cervix; uterine monitoring; swabs of vaginal secretions (not conclusive); maturity amniocentesis

PQ

MATERNAL (E.G., SUBSTANCE ABUSE, CHRONIC ILLNESS, INFECTION)

Signs and symptoms (in general): history of substance abuse, chronic illness (e.g., diabetes), or infection

Infection

BACTERIAL VAGINOSIS

Signs and symptoms: sometimes asymptomatic; vulvovaginal itching; unusual or foul smelling thin gray-white vaginal discharge; burning during urination

Investigations: Gram stain; wet mount microscopy of discharge; vaginal pH > 4.5

CHLAMYDIA TRACHOMATIS

Signs and symptoms: often asymptomatic; vaginal discharge; postcoital or intermenstrual bleeding; difficult or painful urination; pelvic and abdominal pain

Investigations: NAAT; vaginal swab culture; endocervical specimen in speculum exam

URINARY TRACT INFECTION

Signs and symptoms: frequent urination; painful urination; pelvic pain and/or flank pain; fever; tenderness over the bladder

Investigations: urinalysis, urine culture

CHORIOAMNIONITIS

Signs and symptoms: maternal fever; maternal and fetal tachycardia; uterine tenderness; foul-smelling amniotic fluid

Investigations: amniocentesis with confirmation of microbial growth; histology of placenta and umbilical cord

OTHER INFECTIONS

Examples include *U. urealyticum*, *M. genitalium*, vaginal *E. coli*, and chronic HCV.

IATROGENIC (INDICATED INDUCTION OF LABOR—E.G., ECLAMPSIA, INTRAUTERINE GROWTH RETARDATION, PREMATURE RUPTURE OF MEMBRANES)

Eclampsia

Signs and symptoms: BP > 160/110 mmHg; thrombocytopenia; compromised renal function; pulmonary edema; hemolytic anemia; seizures

Intrauterine growth retardation (as indication for induced labor)

This is defined as in-utero growth below the tenth percentile for a baby's gestational age. The timing of delivery of an IUGR fetus is a complex decision taking into account the degree of growth restriction, amniotic fluid volume, biophysical profile, and other factors. In general, delivery (usually by C-section) should occur by 37 to 38 weeks for singleton IUGR fetuses and by 34 to 36 weeks for twin pregnancies.

Factors in decision to deliver: nonreassuring fetal assessment or complete absence of growth over 2 to 4 weeks

Investigations:

US: umbilical artery Doppler; amniotic fluid index; fetal biometry

Blood tests: infection screening; elevated β-HCG in first and second trimester; low pregnancy-associated plasma protein A

Premature rupture of membranes

Signs and symptoms: rupture of the membranes > 1 hour before the onset of labor; gush or slow leak of amniotic fluid

Risk factors: previous preterm birth; infection in the reproductive system; vaginal bleeding during pregnancy; smoking

Investigations: lab tests to confirm amniotic fluid; US to confirm levels of amniotic fluid

Keys to patient encounter

Key concern

Identify patients who need immediate transfer to a facility with neonatal intensive care.

History

Determine the patient's age. Ask how many times the patient has been pregnant. Ask about miscarriages and at what stage of pregnancy they occurred, and about complications during previous pregnancies and this pregnancy.

Listen for evidence of multiple gestation, congenital abnormalities, abdominal trauma, hypertension, diabetes, infection (e.g., fever, vaginal discharge, urinary symptoms), vaginal bleeding during pregnancy, previous placental abruption, previous forceps- or vacuum-assisted deliveries, and previous preterm deliveries. Ask the patient whether they smoke.

Pay particular attention to identifying risk factors for preterm labor: advanced maternal age, smoking, and prior preterm deliveries.

Physical exam

Vital signs: Look for fever and hypertension.

Pelvic:

- Perform a speculum exam to establish the degree of cervical dilation.
- Swab for group B streptococcus.

Abdominal:

- Check for abnormal findings (e.g., uterine tenderness).
- Obtain a fundal height measurement.

Investigations

Urinalysis to look for proteinuria

Urine culture and sensitivity

Fetal fibronectin

Fetal US or monitoring

Management

Refer the patient to an appropriate facility with a NICU. Administer appropriate immediate interventions (antenatal steroids, group B streptococcus prophylaxis, tocolytics). Counsel the parents on the immediate and long-term health problems of premature infants.

PREOPERATIVE MEDICAL EVALUATION

Preoperative medical evaluation

Assessment categories

OPTIMAL MANAGEMENT OF CHRONIC DISEASES (E.G., CORONARY ARTERY DISEASE, DIABETES MELLITUS)

Coronary artery disease

For risks associated with cardiac conditions, see *myocardial risk*, below.

Perioperative management of CAD: see the perioperative management pointer

Investigations: NT-proBNP level in at-risk patients, as identified by the Revised Cardiac Risk Index

Diabetes mellitus

Patients with diabetes mellitus are at higher surgical risk if their diabetes is undetected, uncontrolled, and/or not properly monitored; and if they have comorbid conditions (e.g., CVD, kidney damage, skin conditions, neuropathies).

Signs and symptoms (undiagnosed diabetes mellitus): family history of diabetes; polydipsia, polyuria, and/or weight loss

Perioperative management of diabetes: see the perioperative management pointer

Investigations: HbA_{1c} (in clinically suspected, but undiagnosed, diabetes), glucose, ECG (diabetic patients are at risk of silent myocardial ischemia due to diabetic neuropathy), tests for renal function

IDENTIFICATION OF PERIOPERATIVE RISKS

Cardiopulmonary risk

MYOCARDIAL RISK (E.G., ISCHEMIA, HEART FAILURE, ARRHYTHMIA)

Patients are at higher risk of cardiovascular complications if they have a history of cardiac events (MI, CHF, valvular diseases, angina, arrhythmia, severe pulmonary hypertension); comorbid conditions (e.g., renal insufficiency, diabetes, COPD, hypertension); reduced functional capacity (e.g., tolerance for < 4 METs, such as walking ≤ 2 blocks without stopping); or abnormalities on physical exam (e.g., elevated venous pressure, pulmonary edema, third heart sound).

Other risk factors: dyslipidemia, smoking, current symptoms (e.g., chest pain, shortness of breath, claudication, syncope, presyncope)

Investigations: NT-proBNP

PULMONARY RISK (E.G., CHRONIC OBSTRUCTIVE PULMONARY DISEASE, INFECTION)

CHRONIC OBSTRUCTIVE PULMONARY DISEASE

Signs and symptoms: decreased breath sounds; wheezing; crackles; prolonged expiratory phase

Investigations: chest x-ray; FEV to establish risk in diagnosed COPD

High risk for postoperative complications: $FEV_1 < 40\%$

High risk for mortality in CABG: $FEV_1 < 60\%$

INFECTION

Risk factors for postoperative pulmonary infections include advanced age; planned thoracic or upper abdominal surgery; past or current lung disease; obesity; smoking; poorly controlled asthma; stroke; and chronic steroid use.

Anesthetic

SYSTEMIC RISK (E.G., MALIGNANT HYPERTHERMIA, SLEEP APNEA)

MALIGNANT HYPERTHERMIA (MH)

This is rare and hereditary, and can be fatal. In the context of surgical risk, it is triggered by volatile anesthetics (isoflurane, halothane, sevoflurane, desflurane). People with MH do not react on their first exposure to volatile anesthetics.

Risk factors: first degree relative with MH (50% risk); second degree relative with MH (25% risk); male (higher risk); muscle diseases (central core disease, minicore-multicore myopathy, nemaline myopathy); hypokalemic periodic paralysis; King-Denborough syndrome

Investigations: muscle biopsy for caffeine-halothane contracture test

OBSTRUCTIVE SLEEP APNEA

This can remain undiagnosed until a preoperative evaluation. Patients with this condition are at higher postoperative risk for sleep-disordered breathing, severe hypoxemia, hypercapnia, aspiration pneumonia, ARDS, and PE.

> If also obese, they are additionally at risk of difficulties with endotracheal intubation and postoperative upper airway obstruction.

Signs and symptoms: excessive or loud snoring; disturbed sleep (e.g., not feeling rested in the morning); obesity (common); allergic rhinitis (sneezing, runny nose, eye irritation); morning headache; palpable masses in the oral cavity or neck

Investigations: sleep study (polysomnography); hypertrophic adenoid tissue on lateral neck x-ray

> STOP-BANG questionnaire (patient self-evaluation questionnaire): **STOP-BANG** is a mnemonic for **s**noring, **t**ired, **o**bserved cessation of breathing during sleep by others, **p**ressure (hypertension), **B**MI > 35, **a**ge (older than 50), **n**eck size (large), **g**ender (male).
>
> For BMI, see *Notes on labs and assessments*.

INTUBATION AND AIRWAY (E.G., C-SPINE STABILITY)

C-SPINE STABILITY

Patients with C-spine instability risk spinal cord compression and/or the need for emergent airway protection during surgery.

Risk factors: C-spine trauma, RA, Down syndrome

Thromboembolic risk (prior deep vein thrombosis, thrombophilia)

Risk factors: older than 40; malignancy; immobilization; varicose veins; major vascular injury; cardiopulmonary disease (see *cardiopulmonary risk*, above); history of stroke, DVT, or thrombophilia; paralysis or spinal cord injury; hyperviscosity (due to malignancy or polycythemia vera); presence of current symptoms (leg pain, limb edema, calf tenderness)

Investigations: CBC, PT/INR, aPTT, platelets

Medication-related risk (e.g., prednisone, immunosuppressants)

PREDNISONE

Patients who regularly take prednisone or other steroids (e.g., to treat autoimmune and inflammatory diseases) are at higher postoperative risk of infection (e.g., pneumonia, peritonitis, UTI), delayed wound healing, hyperglycemia, hypertension, and neuropsychiatric conditions. They may require stress-dose steroids at the time of surgery to reduce the risk of adrenal suppression by exogenous steroid use.

IMMUNOSUPPRESSANTS

Patients taking immunosuppressants are at higher postoperative risk of sepsis, infections, and delayed wound healing.

ANTIREJECTION DRUGS

Investigations: renal function, liver function, metabolic assessment, CBC, acid-base fluid status, electrolytes, PT/INR, aPTT, platelets, plasma fibrinogen, 12-lead ECG, chest x-ray, echocardiogram, pulmonary function testing

CHEMOTHERAPY

Investigations: CBC, electrolytes, liver function, PT/INR, aPTT, platelets, plasma fibrinogen

ANTICOAGULANTS

Perioperative management of patients taking warfarin (see the perioperative management pointer) depends on evaluation of the risk of thrombotic events versus the risk of bleeding events.

HIGH RISK OF THROMBOSIS

Risk factors: mitral valve or mechanical aortic valve (cage-ball or tilting-disk type); thromboembolism within last 3 months; history of thromboembolism on stopping warfarin; severe thrombophilia

INTERMEDIATE RISK OF THROMBOSIS

Risk factors: bileaflet-mechanical or bioprosthetic aortic valve; AF plus major risk factors for stroke (history of stroke, hypertension, diabetes, left ventricular condition, or older than 75)

LOW RISK OF THROMBOSIS

Patients have no major risk factors for stroke, and no thromboembolism for > 12 months.

Keys to patient encounter

Key concerns

Assess perioperative issues.

Recommend strategies to minimize perioperative morbidity and mortality.

History

CURRENT HEALTH STATUS

Ask about the patient's current health concerns. Listen for symptoms consistent with undiagnosed diabetes (polydipsia, weight loss, fatigue); undiagnosed obstructive sleep apnea (e.g., snoring, daytime fatigue, nighttime apnea observed by others); current thrombosis (leg pain, limb edema, calf tenderness); and current cardiopulmonary disorder (e.g., chest pain, shortness of breath, syncope).

CURRENT FUNCTIONAL CAPACITY

Ask how many blocks the patient can walk without stopping.

PAST MEDICAL HISTORY

Ask about heart disease, diabetes, lung disease, renal problems, hypertension, dyslipidemia, and thrombotic risk factors (e.g., stroke, DVT, malignancy); and for risk factors associated with anesthetic (obstructive sleep apnea), intubation (RA, Down syndrome), and postoperative infection (e.g., asthma). Ask about a history of spinal trauma (this is relevant for intubation).

ANESTHETICS

Ask about the patient's history with anesthetics and about a family history of problems with anesthetics.

MEDICATIONS

Obtain a full medication list, including OTC medications. Ask specifically about steroids (e.g., prednisone), immunosuppressants, and anticoagulants.

REVISED CARDIAC RISK INDEX SCORE

Determine the patient's risk for cardiovascular complications with the Revised Cardiac Risk Index (RCRI) (see the pointer on perioperative scoring instruments).

Physical exam

Vital signs

Cardiovascular

Respiratory

Mouth and throat: Assess for a Mallampati score (see the pointer on perioperative scoring instruments).

Investigations

Routine surgeries on healthy patients do not necessarily require blood work or x-rays.

Fasting glucose or HbA_{1c} in suspected undiagnosed diabetes

HbA_{1c} in patients with diagnosed diabetes

NT-proBNP in patients with a higher risk of cardiovascular complications (patients 65 years or older, or with an RCRI score greater than 1, or age 45 to 64 with significant cardiovascular disease)

Creatinine in patients with renal disease

C-spine x-ray in patients with RA

Other specific tests to evaluate the current status of preexisting conditions (e.g., cardiac disease, respiratory disease, endocrine disease)

Perioperative management

Communicate the risks of surgery to the patient and optimize care for existing conditions (see the pointer).

POINTER

Perioperative scoring instruments

REVISED CARDIAC RISK INDEX

This 6-point system predicts the risk of cardiac complications in noncardiac surgeries. It rates the risk of the type of surgery, and the risks from prior ischemic heart disease, CHF, cerebrovascular disease, and from existing diabetes and kidney disease.

MALLAMPATI SCORE

This 4-point system predicts ease of intubation based on how many of the following structures are visible when the patient opens their mouth and sticks out their tongue: tonsillar pillars, soft palate, and uvula. The more structures that are visible, the better the score for intubation.

POINTER

Perioperative management of key conditions

CONDITION	MANAGEMENT
Cardiac condition	Counsel smoking cessation. Optimize therapy prior to surgery. This may include beta-blockers (do not start within 24 hours before surgery), statins, and surveillance.
Diabetes	Be alert to undiagnosed diabetes. Optimize glycemic control. This may include medication compliance or adjustments, and smoking cessation; and will include proper monitoring, appropriate diet, and adequate exercise.
Chronic obstructive pulmonary disease	Treat this aggressively. Treatment includes bronchodilators; smoking cessation; antibiotics and systemic steroids, as required, in suboptimal management despite therapy; and chest physical therapy.
Patients at risk of postoperative pulmonary infection	Counsel smoking cessation. Optimize asthma control, which may include medication adjustments or compliance, and avoiding triggers (e.g., environmental allergens, secondhand smoke).
Obstructive sleep apnea (OSA)	Be alert to undiagnosed OSA. Perioperative management involves nighttime continuous positive airway pressure with a ventilator.
Thrombosis	Provide prophylactic anticoagulants, especially in asymptomatic, high-risk patients scheduled for major or orthopedic surgery. Note that postoperative management for patients at risk of thrombosis includes early ambulation, graduated compression stockings, intermittent pneumatic compression devices, and resumption of oral anticoagulants.

(*Continued on next page*)

CONDITION	MANAGEMENT
Patients taking prednisone	Patients on high-dose steroids require supplemental perioperative doses of corticosteroids to reduce the risk of adrenal crisis (hypotension, cardiovascular collapse). This should be given for 24 hours for moderate surgery, and for 48 to 72 hours for major surgery.
Patients taking antirejection drugs	Continue immunosuppressive therapy. Monitor blood levels of the immunosuppressive drug (e.g., tacrolimus or cyclosporine) daily.
Patients taking chemotherapy	Treat anemia and thrombocytopenia, as necessary. Optimize the patient's nutrition.
Patients taking anticoagulants	**High risk of thrombosis** Initiate bridging therapy (replace warfarin with injected short-acting anticoagulants 4 to 5 days before surgery; stop all anticoagulants 4 to 6 hours before surgery; resume warfarin immediately after surgery). Note that INR monitoring (aPTT) is required during bridging therapy if it uses IV unfractionated heparin.
	Intermediate risk of thrombosis Initiate bridging therapy on a case-by-case basis (e.g., initiate for surgeries or procedures with a high risk of bleeding events: neurologic, cardiac, major vascular, or major urologic surgery; joint replacement; lung resection; pacemaker or defibrillator insertion; intestinal anastomosis; kidney, prostate, or cervical cone biopsy; pericardiocentesis; colon polypectomy).
	Low risk of thrombosis Continue existing warfarin therapy.

PO

PRURITUS

Pruritus

Differential diagnosis

SKIN LESIONS

Primary skin disease

BLISTERS (E.G., DERMATITIS HERPETIFORMIS)

DERMATITIS HERPETIFORMIS

Signs and symptoms: rash (bumps, blisters) that is extremely itchy and bilaterally symmetrical; located on the elbows, knees, back, buttocks (common); sensitivity to gluten

Investigations: skin biopsy; tTG antibodies (to rule out celiac disease)

RASH (E.G., PSORIASIS, LICHEN PLANUS)

PSORIASIS (GUTTATE PSORIASIS)

Note that chronic plaque psoriasis is another form of psoriasis, but it is usually not itchy.

Signs and symptoms: numerous, small pink papules and plaques 2–15 mm in diameter with fine overlying scale; URTI 2 to 3 weeks before the appearance of symptoms; located on the trunk and proximal extremities, or on the scalp, hands, feet, nails

LICHEN PLANUS

This is a common, chronic inflammatory condition of the skin (common locations: inner wrists, forearms, lower legs, lower back) and/or mucous membranes (locations: mouth, vagina).

Signs and symptoms (skin): acute lesions that are planar, purple, polygonal, pruritic, papules (mnemonic: **5 Ps**); lesion diameter of 2–4 mm; Wickham striae on lesions (lacy white lines, particularly visible on mucous membranes) (often)

Investigations: biopsy

Parasitosis (e.g., scabies, pediculosis)

SCABIES

Signs and symptoms: thin, grayish, reddish-brownish threadlike elevated lines in the superficial epidermis, 2–15 mm long (from female mites burrowing under the skin)

Location in adults: sides of fingers and webbed spaces between fingers; inside surfaces of the wrists, elbows;

armpits; belt line; feet; scrotum; areolae (women); **not** the head

Location in children: the palms, soles, head

Location in the elderly: the back (appearing as excoriations)

PEDICULOSIS

Finding nits and lice confirms the diagnosis.

Signs and symptoms: itchy skin with excoriations

Head lice: on the scalp; persistent pyoderma around the neck or ears

Body lice: on the shoulders, buttocks, abdomen; small red spiky spots; excoriations on the trunk and neck; urticaria; superficial bacterial infection

Pubic lice: on the lower abdomen, proximal thighs, buttocks

Allergy (e.g., eczema, allergic dermatitis, urticaria)

ECZEMA (ATOPIC DERMATITIS)

Signs and symptoms: chronic symptoms that flare and subside; onset before age 5 years (usual); scaly, itchy rash; family or personal history of asthma, allergies

Location (most common): hands; feet; ankles; wrists; neck; upper chest; eyelids; inside the elbows and knees; face, scalp (infants)

ALLERGIC DERMATITIS

This is a type of contact dermatitis. Examples of allergens include nickel (e.g., jewelry), hair dye, topical antibiotics, and perfumes.

Signs and symptoms: red, sore, or inflamed skin; severely itchy; history of direct contact of symptomatic skin with a substance (no reaction occurs on first exposure; reaction occurs 24 to 48 hours after subsequent exposures, but may occur after months of exposure); personal or family history of allergies or specific allergic reactions

Investigations: patch testing to detect allergens

URTICARIA (HIVES)

Common causes include infections (viral, bacterial, parasitic), allergic reactions (medications, insect bites, latex, foods), and contact with radio-contrast agents.

Signs and symptoms: rash that is itchy, painless; lesions that are circumscribed, raised (round, oval, or with wavy margins; < 1 cm to several cm in diameter); plaques with central pallor; located anywhere on the body

Duration: < 6 weeks (acute); > 6 weeks, recurrent (chronic)

Investigations: allergy tests for specifically suspected allergens (otherwise, lab tests are not helpful)

Arthropod bites

Signs and symptoms: red, sore bump at site of a bite; mild pain and itching; swelling, burning, numbness, or tingling

Risk for complications: personal or family history of allergies; type of arthropod

Factitious dermatitis

Signs and symptoms: red bumps, blisters, or dry, cracked lesions; located on the face, lower extremities, hands, forearms, torso (common)

History: low health-related quality of life; perception of skin condition; possible psychosocial stressor; substance abuse; psychiatric disorder (e.g., somatic symptom disorder)

Investigations: skin biopsy to rule out underlying pathologies

NO SKIN LESIONS

Dry skin

Signs and symptoms: older age; frequent washing or bathing

Drugs or food

MEDICATIONS AND DRUGS

Causes include opiates with intrathecal or epidural administration, and anticancer agents (EGF inhibitors, tyrosine kinase inhibitors, BRAF inhibitors, MEK inhibitors).

Recreational drugs: opioids, cocaine, amphetamines

Signs and symptoms: itch without skin manifestations (skin lesions from scratching and rubbing are present: lichenified plaques, excoriations, prurigo nodules)

FOOD (ALLERGY)

Signs and symptoms: personal or family history of allergies

Obstructive biliary disease

Causes of blocked bile ducts include cysts or tumors; inflammation or scarring within the bile ducts; and gallstones.

Signs and symptoms: history of liver disease, gallstones; itching that affects the whole body; normal-looking skin, except for excoriations; abdominal pain; nausea; pale stools; dark urine; jaundice; fever

Investigations: increased bilirubin and liver enzymes (these can indicate biliary distress); imaging to detect blocked bile ducts

Uremia or kidney injury

UREMIC PRURITUS

Pruritus is common in patients with end-stage renal disease.

Signs and symptoms: itching whose duration ranges from a few minutes per day to continuous; xerosis

> Worse: at night (leading to sleep disruption); in hot temperatures; when sweating excessively; during stress
>
> Better: in cool temperatures; with physical activity
>
> Location: first, the back; then, the arms, head, abdomen (common)

Investigations: blood tests (GFR, BUN, creatinine, potassium, phosphate, calcium, sodium); 24-hour urine collection; nuclear medicine radioisotope (iothalamate) clearance (this is the best test, but it is expensive), or eGFR using the Modification of Diet in Renal Disease (MDRD) formula or Cockcroft-Gault formula

Hematological (anemia, leukemia)

ANEMIA

Signs and symptoms: itch with dry or rough skin (no skin lesions); fatigue; weakness; headache; irritability; exercise intolerance

Investigations: see *Anemia* (under *Hematological concerns*)

LEUKEMIA

Signs and symptoms: fever; chills; persistent fatigue and weakness; frequent or severe infections; weight loss; pallor; swollen lymph nodes; enlarged liver or spleen; easy bleeding and bruising; recurrent nosebleeds; petechiae; excessive sweating; bone pain or tenderness

Investigations: CBC; peripheral blood smear; flow cytometry; bone marrow aspiration and biopsy

Carcinoma or carcinoid syndrome

Carcinoid tumor most commonly occurs in the GI tract or lungs and is generally discovered incidentally.

Carcinoid syndrome results from secretions into the blood by advanced tumors.

Signs and symptoms (carcinoid syndrome): skin flushing on the face and upper chest; facial lesions; diarrhea; breathing difficulty; tachycardia

Investigations: blood and urine tests to detect specific molecules such as serotonin and 5-HIAA respectively; CT scan or MRI of chest or abdomen

Endocrine disorder (diabetes, thyroid disease)

DIABETES

Pruritus occurs in diabetic patients who have associated disorders; otherwise, itching does not occur at a higher rate in diabetic patients.

Examples of causes include dermatophyte infections; xerosis; pruritus in the lower extremities, scalp, or trunk due to diabetic neuropathy; anogenital pruritus due to *Candida* infections; and pruritus vulvae due to poorly controlled diabetes.

THYROID DISEASE

HYPERTHYROIDISM

Signs and symptoms: changes in menstrual patterns, enlarged thyroid, tachycardia, palpitations, diarrhea, muscle weakness, tremor, hyperactive reflexes, weight loss, sweating

Skin: itching; warm skin; sweating; onycholysis and softening of the nails; hyperpigmentation; hair loss

Investigations: decreased thyrotropin (TSH)

HYPOTHYROIDISM

Signs and symptoms: cold intolerance, decreased reflexes, weight gain, impaired cognition

Skin: dry, itchy, pale skin; decreased sweating; skin discoloration (yellowish tinge or hyperpigmentation); coarse hair; brittle nails; hair loss; nonpitting edema

Investigations: elevated thyrotropin (TSH)

PSYCHIATRIC OR EMOTIONAL DISORDERS

In psychogenic excoriation, patients excessively pick and scratch normal skin.

Signs and symptoms: personal or family history of mental health disorders; recent psychological stress (e.g., death of a friend or family member; divorce; job loss); scattered, linear, crusted skin lesions on the extremities or anywhere the patient can reach to scratch

Keys to patient encounter

Key concerns

Differentiate excoriations due to scratching from skin lesions.

Identify any skin lesions.

If no skin lesions are present, identify the underlying cause of pruritus.

History

HISTORY OF PRESENT ILLNESS

Ask when the itching started and what skin symptoms the patient has noticed. Listen for acute versus slow or recurrent onset (acute onset suggests acute stress or an exposure as a cause); and for the presence and location of skin lesions (this information focuses the differential diagnosis considerably).

PAST MEDICAL HISTORY

Ask about celiac disease, liver disease, kidney disease, anemia, leukemia, cancer, diabetes, thyroid disease, and psychiatric disorders.

MEDICATIONS AND DRUGS

Ask about recent changes in medications, and about topical antibiotics and opiates, anticancer drugs, recreational drugs (opioids, cocaine, amphetamines), and OTC drugs.

ALLERGIES

Ask about a personal or family history of allergies.

SOCIAL HISTORY

Ask about occupations and living situations with exposure risks for lice and scabies (e.g., day-care worker; parent with children in day care; social worker; institutionalized people; people living without shelter).

Physical exam

The main purpose of the physical exam is to differentiate pruritus associated with skin lesions from that without skin lesions. If skin lesions are present, determine their character and distribution.

Investigations

If the patient has no skin lesions, order investigations to diagnose systemic disorders (see the differential diagnosis).

Management

Identification and removal or modification of the underlying cause is the first line of management.

Local pruritus is treated with topical corticosteroids. If these are ineffective or cannot be used, consider calcineurin inhibitors (tacrolimus or pimecrolimus). Alternatively, consider topical anesthetics, capsaicin cream, or doxepin cream.

For larger areas of skin or for generalized pruritus, prescribe oral antihistamines. Alternatives include SSRIs or TCAs.

In the case of CKD, a low protein diet and antihypertensive medications are used. If the patient is diabetic, blood sugars must be controlled.

PSYCHIATRIC PRESENTATIONS

Anxiety

Differential diagnosis

ANXIETY DISORDERS IN GENERAL

Signs and symptoms: symptoms with significant impact on day-to-day life (e.g., significant distress, significant impaired functioning); symptoms that last for weeks or months (as opposed to a few days)

GENERALIZED ANXIETY DISORDER[1(p222)]

Signs and symptoms: excessive anxiety across a number of contexts (e.g., work, school); anxiety that is difficult to control; presence of symptoms for most of the time for ≥ 6 months; **no** evidence of anxiety effects from drugs or medications (e.g., caffeine, alcohol, cannabis, phencyclidine, opioid, amphetamine, cocaine), or medical conditions (e.g., hyperthyroidism, Cushing syndrome)

Risk factors: female; family history of anxiety

POSTTRAUMATIC STRESS DISORDER[1(pp271–272)]

Signs and symptoms in adults: symptoms that begin after a traumatic event and last ≥ 1 month; intrusive symptoms (e.g., flashbacks, recurrent memories, recurrent dreams) about the event; negative changes to mood or perceptions (e.g., exaggerated negative beliefs about self, others, or the world; loss of interest in usual activities); marked changes in arousal or reactions (e.g., verbal or physical aggression with little provocation; self-destructive behavior; hypervigilance)

Traumatic events: exposure to death, threat of death, serious injury, or sexual violence through direct experience, witnessing, or repeated exposure (e.g., in the case of first responders), or learning of traumatic events involving close family or friends; **not** exposure via images (e.g., television, movies), unless this occurs through work

SEPARATION ANXIETY DISORDER[1(pp190–191)]

Signs and symptoms: excessive anxiety (e.g., distress, worry, nightmares) about separation from a particular person; physical symptoms provoked by anxiety (e.g., headaches, stomach aches)

Children and adolescents: presence of symptoms for ≥ 4 weeks

Adults: presence of symptoms for ≥ 6 months (usual)

PHOBIA[1(p197)]

Specific phobia

Signs and symptoms: excessive anxiety about an object or situation (e.g., insects, receiving an injection); presence of symptoms for ≥ 6 months

PANIC DISORDER[1(pp208–209)]

Signs and symptoms: recurrent unexpected panic attacks; anxiety about future panic attacks; behaviors to avoid attacks for ≥ 1 month; **no** evidence of anxiety effects from drugs or medications (e.g., caffeine, alcohol, cannabis, phencyclidine, opioid, amphetamine, cocaine), or medical conditions (e.g., hyperthyroidism, cardiopulmonary disorders)

Panic attack: symptoms that peak within minutes; symptoms that can include palpitations, accelerated heart rate, shortness of breath, chest pain, dizziness, numbness or tingling, fear of losing control, fear of dying

ADJUSTMENT DISORDER[1(pp286–287)]

Signs and symptoms: excessive anxiety in response to an identifiable stressor and within 3 months of the stressor; symptoms with significant impact on day-to-day life; abatement of symptoms within 6 months of cessation of stressor

Keys to patient encounter

History

HISTORY OF PRESENT ILLNESS

Ask about the patient's symptoms. Listen for evidence that:

- distinguishes true anxiety disorders from situational stress (see the pointer)
- is consistent with particular anxiety entities (e.g., persistent anxiety across many contexts with fatigue and muscle tension in generalized anxiety disorder)
- is consistent with hyperthyroidism (weight loss, tremor, weakness, diarrhea)

Ask about a personal or family history of mental illness.

Assess the patient for risk factors for self-harm: ask about substance addiction and abuse, and suicidal ideation.

MEDICATIONS AND DRUGS

Ask about caffeine, alcohol, and recreational drugs (to rule these out as a source of the symptoms).

SOCIAL HISTORY

Ask about recent life stressors (e.g., job loss, divorce).

Physical exam

Vital signs: Look for tachycardia (relevant for hyperthyroidism) and hypertension (relevant for Cushing syndrome).

Signs of hyperthyroidism: These include enlarged thyroid, hyperpigmentation, hair loss, and hyperactive reflexes.

Signs of Cushing syndrome: These include round, red face; pronounced

POINTER

Anxiety disorders versus situational stress

Anxiety disorders have the following characteristics, compared to situational stress:

- They involve severe symptoms that significantly disrupt daily life.
- They can involve specific triggers (e.g., phobic objects in specific phobia).
- They have features of persistence: they occur in a variety of contexts and for longer periods of time.

abdominal weight; hump on the upper back; thin arms and legs; stretch marks; and acne.

Investigations

Investigations are generally not needed.

Thyrotropin (TSH) in suspected hyperthyroidism

Serum cortisol or dexamethasone suppression test in suspected Cushing syndrome

Management

Ensure the immediate safety of the patient. A patient with specific and immediate plans for suicide requires admission to hospital for psychiatric assessment and monitoring. In patients not at immediate risk, consider referral to a psychiatrist. Treat any underlying or comorbid illness. Initiate treatment with pharmacological and/or psychological therapy, and ensure adequate follow-up.

REFERENCE

1. American Psychiatric Association. Diagnostic and statistical manual of mental disorders. 5th ed. Arlington, VA: American Psychiatric Association; 2013. 991 p.

PSYCHIATRIC PRESENTATIONS

Depressed mood

Differential diagnosis

MAJOR DEPRESSIVE DISORDER[1(pp160–161)]

Major depressive disorder is characterized by a persistent "down" mood, with no manic or hypomanic episodes (the presence of these episodes indicates bipolar disorder, by definition—see *bipolar disorder*, below).

Signs and symptoms: symptoms that are present most of the time for ≥ 2 weeks; symptoms with significant impact on day-to-day life

Key symptoms: depressed mood and/or loss of interest in usual activities

Other symptoms: significant weight change; sleep disturbance; slowed or agitated mental processes; loss of concentration; recurrent thoughts of death or suicide

Risk factors: family history of mental health disorders (depression, anxiety, suicide); personal history of other mental health disorders; substance abuse; chronic illness (e.g., cancer, stroke, chronic pain)

BIPOLAR DISORDER (TYPE I, TYPE II)[1(pp123–134)]

BIPOLAR DISORDER IN GENERAL

Bipolar I disorder **always** involves at least 1 manic episode, and **may** involve hypomanic and/or major depressive episodes.

Bipolar II disorder **never** involves manic episodes, and **always** involves swings between hypomanic and major depressive episodes.

Family history of bipolar disorder is a risk factor for bipolar disorder.

Manic episode

Signs and symptoms: symptoms that are present most of the time for ≥ 1 week; symptoms with significant impact on day-to-day life, and that may pose a risk of harm to self and others

Key symptoms: abnormally elevated (and/or irritable) mood and goal-directed activity

Other symptoms: increased self-importance, increased talking, racing thoughts, decreased need for sleep, risky pursuits (e.g., that could damage finances or relationships), psychosis (e.g., delusions, hallucinations)

Hypomanic episode

Signs and symptoms: symptoms resembling a manic episode in presentation and duration, except:

No significant impact on day-to-day life

No risk of harm to self or others

No psychosis (e.g., delusions, hallucinations)

Major depressive episode

Signs and symptoms: symptoms that are present most of the time for ≥ 2 weeks; symptoms with significant impact on day-to-day life

Key symptoms: depressed mood and/or loss of interest in usual activities

Other symptoms: significant weight change; sleep disturbance; slowed or agitated mental processes; loss of concentration; recurrent thoughts of death or suicide

PERSISTENT DEPRESSIVE DISORDER (DYSTHYMIA)[1(p168)]

Signs and symptoms: symptoms with significant impact on day-to-day life; presence of symptoms for most of the time for ≥ 2 years (children and adolescents: ≥ 1 year), with no break from symptoms for ≥ 2 months; **no** manic or hypomanic episodes

Key symptoms: depressed mood (or, possibly, irritability in children and adolescents)

Other symptoms: change in eating and sleeping routines; fatigue; low self-esteem; loss of concentration; feelings of hopelessness

CYCLOTHYMIC DISORDER[1(pp139–140)]

Cyclothymic disorder resembles bipolar II disorder, but the mood swings are not as severe.

Signs and symptoms: mood swings, with symptoms that **do not** represent hypomanic or major depressive episodes (see *bipolar disorder*, above); symptoms with significant impact on day-to-day life; presence of symptoms for most of the time for ≥ 2 years (children and adolescents: ≥ 1 year), with no break from symptoms for ≥ 2 months

Risk factors: family history of cyclothymic disorder, substance abuse disorders, bipolar disorders

NORMAL GRIEF[1(pp125–126)]

Signs and symptoms: history of a significant personal loss (e.g., death of a family member or friend, financial ruin, serious medical diagnosis); symptoms that resemble a major depressive episode **except**:

Positive feelings or humor often occur.

Symptoms become less intense over time.

Symptoms are triggered by specific reminders of the personal loss.

SUBSTANCE-INDUCED MOOD DISORDER

Examples of drugs that can provoke mood disturbances include stimulants, steroids, levodopa, antibiotics, CNS drugs, dermatological agents, chemotherapeutic drugs, immunological agents, and OCs.

MOOD DISORDER DUE TO A MEDICAL CONDITION

Examples of medical conditions that can provoke mood disturbances include Parkinson disease, Huntington disease, stroke, brain injury from trauma, Cushing disease, hypothyroidism, and MS.

ADJUSTMENT DISORDER[1(pp286–287)]

Signs and symptoms: onset of emotional or behavioral symptoms in response to an identifiable stressor and within 3 months of the stressor; distress out of proportion to the stressor; symptoms with significant impact on day-to-day life; abatement of symptoms within 6 months of cessation of stressor

Keys to patient encounter

Key concern

Assess suicide risk and the potential need for urgent care.

History

HISTORY OF PRESENT ILLNESS

Ask about the patient's symptoms and their impact on routines and relationships. Listen for significant impairment and/or distress (this is the hallmark of a mental health disorder), and for characteristic symptoms (e.g., cycling up and down moods in bipolar II disorder; enduring symptoms in persistent depressive disorder and cyclothymic disorder).

PAST MEDICAL HISTORY

Ask about the patient's psychiatric history, and about Parkinson disease, Huntington disease, stroke, head trauma, Cushing disease, hypothyroidism, and MS.

FAMILY HISTORY

Ask about mental health disorders.

MEDICATIONS AND DRUGS

Ask about the patient's medications and recreational drug use, looking for substances that can provoke mood disorders (e.g., stimulants, steroids, antibiotics, dermatological agents, chemotherapeutic drugs, immunological agents, OCs).

SOCIAL HISTORY

Ask about current stressors in the patient's life.

Risk assessment

Assess the patient's risk of suicide (see the pointer). Ask if they have specific suicidal plans and intent, and if they have the means to carry out their suicide plan. Ask about previous suicide attempts.

Physical exam

Physical exam is unlikely to provide information useful to diagnosis or management.

Investigations

Thyrotropin (TSH)

Urine drug screen if substance abuse cannot be ruled out

POINTER

Indicators of suicide risk

Patients are at risk of suicide if they have suicidal thoughts, a plan, and intent.

The following additional factors put them at high risk of suicide:

- a history of suicide attempts
- access to firearms
- a psychiatric disorder or disorders (e.g., depression; bipolar disorder; schizophrenia; alcohol or substance abuse; personality disorder; anxiety disorder)
- current substance abuse
- male
- lack of social support (e.g., they live alone)
- for children and adolescents: exposure to abuse, violence, victimization, or bullying; family history of suicide; member of a minority in sexual orientation

Management

A patient with specific and immediate plans for suicide requires admission to hospital for psychiatric assessment and monitoring. If a patient at risk of suicide refuses admission, consider involuntary admission. The regulations for involuntary admission vary by jurisdiction, but generally require a written order by 2 physicians.

If the patient is not at immediate risk, consider referring the patient to a psychiatrist. Start pharmacotherapy in the case of major depressive disorder (with an antidepressant) or bipolar disorder (with a mood-stabilizing agent such as lithium carbonate or valproic acid). Consider the need for patient and/or family support resources.

REFERENCE

1. American Psychiatric Association. Diagnostic and statistical manual of mental disorders. 5th ed. Arlington, VA: American Psychiatric Association; 2013. 59–60. 991 p.

PSYCHIATRIC PRESENTATIONS

Mania or hypomania

Differential diagnosis

BIPOLAR DISORDER (TYPE I, TYPE II)[1(pp123–134)]

BIPOLAR DISORDER IN GENERAL

Bipolar I disorder **always** involves at least 1 manic episode, and **may** involve hypomanic and/or major depressive episodes.

Bipolar II disorder **never** involves manic episodes, and **always** involves swings between hypomanic and major depressive episodes.

Family history of bipolar disorder is a risk factor for bipolar disorder.

Manic episode

Signs and symptoms: symptoms that are present most of the time for ≥ 1 week; symptoms with significant impact on day-to-day life, and that may pose a risk of harm to self and others

Key symptoms: abnormally elevated (and/or irritable) mood and goal-directed activity

Other symptoms: increased self-importance, increased talking, racing thoughts, decreased need for sleep, risky pursuits (e.g., that could damage finances or relationships), psychosis (e.g., delusions, hallucinations)

Hypomanic episode

Signs and symptoms: symptoms resembling a manic episode in presentation and duration, except:

No significant impact on day-to-day life

No risk of harm to self or others

No psychosis (e.g., delusions, hallucinations)

Major depressive episode

Signs and symptoms: symptoms that are present most of the time for ≥ 2 weeks; symptoms with significant impact on day-to-day life

Key symptoms: depressed mood and/or loss of interest in usual activities

Other symptoms: significant weight change; sleep disturbance; slowed or agitated mental processes; loss of concentration; recurrent thoughts of death or suicide

SUBSTANCE-INDUCED MOOD DISORDER

Examples of drugs that can provoke mood disturbances include stimulants, steroids, levodopa, antibiotics, CNS drugs, dermatological agents, chemotherapeutic drugs, immunological agents, and OCs.

MOOD DISORDER DUE TO A MEDICAL CONDITION

Examples of medical conditions that can provoke mood disturbances include Parkinson disease, Huntington disease, stroke, brain injury from trauma, Cushing disease, hypothyroidism, and MS.

CYCLOTHYMIC DISORDER[1(pp139–140)]

Cyclothymic disorder resembles bipolar II disorder, but the mood swings are not as severe.

Signs and symptoms: mood swings, with symptoms that **do not** represent hypomanic or major depressive episodes (see *bipolar disorder*, above); symptoms with significant impact on day-to-day life; presence of symptoms for most of the time for ≥ 2 years (children and adolescents: ≥ 1 year), with no break from symptoms for ≥ 2 months

Risk factors: family history of cyclothymic disorder, substance abuse disorders, bipolar disorder

Keys to patient encounter

Key concern

Identify patients in potential need of urgent care.

History

Obtain collateral information on the patient's behavior (e.g., from an accompanying caregiver), if possible.

HISTORY OF CURRENT ILLNESS

Ask about the patient's symptoms. Listen for features consistent with particular entities (e.g., delusions, hallucinations, homicidal ideation in bipolar I disorder; cycling up and down moods in bipolar II disorder; enduring symptoms in cyclothymic disorder).

PAST MEDICAL HISTORY

Ask about Parkinson disease, Huntington disease, and other entities associated with mood disorder (e.g., stroke, head trauma, MS).

MEDICATIONS AND DRUGS

Ask about the patient's medications and recreational drug use, looking for substances that can provoke mood disorders (e.g., stimulants, steroids, antibiotics, dermatological agents, chemotherapeutic drugs, immunological agents, OCs).

FAMILY HISTORY

Ask about a family history of mental illness.

Physical exam

Mental status: Perform a mental status exam to assess the patient's capacity, and to identify risk factors for self-harm or harming others (see the pointer).

Investigations

Thyrotropin (TSH)

Urine drug screen if drug abuse cannot be ruled out

Management

Ensure the immediate safety of the patient and others.

A patient with specific and immediate plans for suicide or

POINTER

Mental status exams

Mental status exams use both observation and direct questioning to make assessments. Generally, they assess:

- general appearance and behavior
- mood
- speech: rate, tone, volume
- thought content: obsessions, preoccupations, hallucinations, delusions, suicidal ideation, homicidal ideation
- thought process: circumstantial, tangential, flight of ideas, loosening of associations
- orientation to time and place
- attention and concentration
- patient insight into their present condition

---

homicide requires admission to hospital for psychiatric assessment and monitoring. If a patient at risk of committing suicide or homicide refuses admission, consider involuntary admission. The regulations for involuntary admission vary by jurisdiction, but generally require a written order by 2 physicians.

If the patient is not at immediate risk, consider referring the patient to a psychiatrist. In patients experiencing a manic phase of bipolar disorder, start pharmacotherapy with an antipsychotic medication. Consider the need for patient and/or family support resources.

REFERENCE

1. American Psychiatric Association. Diagnostic and statistical manual of mental disorders. 5th ed. Arlington, VA: American Psychiatric Association; 2013. 991 p.

PSYCHIATRIC PRESENTATIONS

Obsessive-compulsive and related disorders

PQ

Differential diagnosis

OCD AND RELATED DISORDERS IN GENERAL

DSM-5 identifies OCD and related disorders as a group of disorders characterized by obsessions and repetitive behaviors. This group includes OCD, body-dysmorphic disorder, hoarding disorder, trichotillomania, and excoriation disorder. OCD often occurs with other psychiatric disorders.

ADVERSE CHILDHOOD EXPERIENCES

These include abuse (physical, sexual, emotional); neglect (physical, emotional); exposure to domestic violence; and family dysfunction due to divorce (or separation), substance abuse, mental illness, or imprisonment.

GENETIC NEUROLOGICAL DYSFUNCTION

A family history of OCD is a risk factor for developing OCD.

OTHER PSYCHIATRIC DISORDERS (E.G., TIC DISORDER, ANXIETY DISORDERS, DEPRESSION, SUBSTANCE USE DISORDER)

Tic disorder

Signs and symptoms: symptom onset in childhood or adolescence; motor and/or vocal tics (examples of motor tics: eye blinking, facial grimacing, head jerking; examples of vocal tics: grunting, repeating what others say, repeating particular words or phrases)

> Tourette syndrome: presence of both motor and vocal tics (not necessarily concurrently); presence of tics for ≥ 1 year; presence of tics before age 12 (common)
>
> Chronic tic disorder: presence of either motor or vocal tics; presence of tics for ≥ 1 year
>
> Provisional tic disorder: presence of motor and/or vocal tics; presence of tics for < 1 year

Risk factors: male (3 to 4 times more common); family history of tic disorder

Anxiety disorders[1(pp189–234)]

Examples of anxiety disorders in *DSM-5* include generalized anxiety disorder, panic disorder, separation anxiety disorder, social anxiety disorder, and specific phobia.

Signs and symptoms: anxiety about anticipated events; panic attacks (possible); symptoms with significant impact on day-to-day life

> Generalized anxiety disorder: excessive worry about a number of contexts (e.g., work, school); presence of other symptoms, such as fatigue, irritability, loss of concentration, muscle tension, sleep disturbance; family history of anxiety disorders; presence of symptoms for most of the time for ≥ 6 months
>
> Separation anxiety disorder: excessive anxiety (e.g., distress, worry, nightmares) about separation from a particular person; physical symptoms provoked by anxiety (e.g., headaches, stomach aches); presence of symptoms for ≥ 6 months (in adults)
>
> Social anxiety disorder: excessive anxiety about scrutiny by others and being negatively judged; avoidance of social situations; presence of symptoms for ≥ 6 months (typical, in adults)

Specific phobia: excessive anxiety about an object or situation (e.g., insects, receiving an injection); presence of symptoms for ≥ 6 months

Panic disorder: recurrent unexpected panic attacks (surges of intense fear or discomfort that peak within minutes); worry and/or avoidance behaviors regarding future panic attacks for ≥ 1 month

Major depressive disorder[1(pp160–161)]

Signs and symptoms: symptoms that are present most of the time for ≥ 2 weeks; symptoms with significant impact on day-to-day life

Key symptoms: depressed mood and/or loss of interest in usual activities

Other symptoms: significant weight change; sleep disturbance; slowed or agitated mental processes; loss of concentration; recurrent thoughts of death or suicide

Risk factors: family history of mental health disorders (depression, anxiety, suicide); personal history of other mental health disorders; substance abuse; chronic illness (e.g., cancer, stroke, chronic pain)

Substance use disorder[1(p483)]

Signs and symptoms: using a substance for longer or in larger quantities than intended; unsuccessful attempts to quit using it; substantial time spent in acquiring the substance and/or recovering from its use; increasing need for the substance; maintaining the substance use despite negative consequences (e.g., financial trouble, jeopardized relationships) and known dangers to physical and/or mental health; withdrawal symptoms on attempts to quit

OTHER MEDICAL CONDITIONS (E.G., INFECTIONS)

Pediatric autoimmune neuropsychiatric disorders associated with streptococcal infections (PANDAS)

This is an autoimmune disorder that damages the basal ganglia (which help control movement and behavior) following a group A streptococcal infection.

It is a controversial diagnosis, in part because a causal link between group A streptococcal infection and OCD remains uncertain.

Signs and symptoms: OCD symptoms following a streptococcal infection (e.g., strep throat), which may or may not have been diagnosed

Strep throat: sudden-onset fever and sore throat; enlarged lymph nodes in the neck; swollen tonsils, possibly with white spots or pus; palatal petechiae

Keys to patient encounter

Key concern

Identify the possible etiology and coexisting conditions.

History

HISTORY OF PRESENT ILLNESS

Ask about the patient's symptoms and how they affect daily life. Listen for evidence consistent with OCD and related disorders (e.g., obsessive thoughts, repetitive behaviors, tics, phobias, panic attacks, sleep disturbance, loss of concentration, anxiety); and for significant impact of the symptoms on the patient's relationships, employment, and/or education.

PSYCHOSOCIAL HISTORY

Ask about childhood experiences, and current and past stressors.

Physical exam

Full physical: Pay particular attention to the neurological and dermatological exams.

Investigations

Urine drug screen

Specific testing for infectious agents (e.g., *Streptococcus*) if indicated

Head CT or MRI if indicated

Management

Consider referring the patient to a psychiatrist or psychologist. Consider the psychosocial impact of the patient's symptoms and assess the need for family counseling. Initiate treatment with an SSRI.

REFERENCE

1. American Psychiatric Association. Diagnostic and statistical manual of mental disorders. 5th ed. Arlington, VA: American Psychiatric Association; 2013. 991 p.

PSYCHIATRIC PRESENTATIONS

Personality disorders

Differential diagnosis

GENERAL PERSONALITY DISORDER[1(pp646–647)]

Signs and symptoms: an enduring, inflexible pattern of behavior that significantly deviates from cultural expectations, and has significant impact on day-to-day life; symptom onset no later than early adulthood; presence of symptoms across many contexts

Key symptoms: deviations in perceptions, emotional response (e.g., range, intensity), interpersonal functioning, impulse control

Personality disorder types[1(pp645–684)]

CLUSTER A PERSONALITY DISORDERS

General pattern: odd, eccentric behaviors

Paranoid personality disorder: distrust, suspiciousness

Schizoid personality disorder: detachment from social relationships; restricted emotional range

Schizotypal personality disorder: discomfort with close relationships; cognitive and perceptual distortions (e.g., about causal events or the meaning of events); eccentric behaviors

CLUSTER B PERSONALITY DISORDERS

General pattern: dramatic, emotional, and erratic behavior; marked difficulty with impulse control and emotional regulation

Antisocial personality disorder: disregard for others, violating others' rights

Borderline personality disorder: instability in interpersonal relationships and self-image; impulsivity; suicidal behavior

Histrionic personality disorder: excessive emotions, attention seeking

Narcissistic personality disorder: grandiosity, need for admiration, lack of empathy

CLUSTER C PERSONALITY DISORDERS

General pattern: anxiety, fearfulness

Avoidant personality disorder: social inhibition, feelings of inadequacy, hypersensitivity to criticism

Dependent personality disorder: submissive behavior to satisfy an excessive need to be taken care of

Obsessive-compulsive personality disorder: preoccupation with orderliness, perfection, control

Coexisting psychiatric conditions (e.g., mood disorder)

MAJOR DEPRESSIVE DISORDER[1(pp160–161)]

Signs and symptoms: symptoms that are present most of the time for ≥ 2 weeks; symptoms with significant impact on day-to-day life

Key symptoms: depressed mood and/or loss of interest in usual activities

Other symptoms: significant weight change; sleep disturbance; slowed or agitated mental processes; loss of concentration; recurrent thoughts of death or suicide

Risk factors: family history of mental health disorders (depression, anxiety, suicide); personal history of other mental health disorders; substance abuse; chronic illness (e.g., cancer, stroke, chronic pain)

BIPOLAR DISORDER (TYPES I AND II)[1(pp123–134)]

Bipolar I disorder **always** involves at least 1 manic episode, and **may** involve hypomanic and/or major depressive episodes.

Bipolar II disorder **never** involves manic episodes, and **always** involves swings between hypomanic and major depressive episodes.

Family history of bipolar disorder is a risk factor for bipolar disorder.

MANIC EPISODE

Signs and symptoms: symptoms that are present most of the time for ≥ 1 week; symptoms with significant impact on day-to-day life, and that may pose a risk of harm to self and others

Key symptoms: abnormally elevated (and/or irritable) mood and goal-directed activity

Other symptoms: increased self-importance, increased talking, racing thoughts, decreased need for sleep, risky pursuits (e.g., that could damage finances or relationships), psychosis (e.g., delusions, hallucinations)

HYPOMANIC EPISODE

Signs and symptoms: symptoms resembling a manic episode in presentation and duration, except:

No significant impact on day-to-day life

No risk of harm to self or others

No psychosis (e.g., delusions, hallucinations)

MAJOR DEPRESSIVE EPISODE

Signs and symptoms: symptoms that are present most of the time for ≥ 2 weeks; symptoms with significant impact on day-to-day life

Key symptoms: depressed mood and/or loss of interest in usual activities

Other symptoms: significant weight change; sleep disturbance; slowed or agitated mental processes; loss of concentration; recurrent thoughts of death or suicide

Keys to patient encounter

Key concerns

Differentiate between personality disorders and other mental illness.

Recognize the high prevalence of comorbidities.

Formulate a management plan.

History

HISTORY OF PRESENT ILLNESS

Ask what problems the patient is having with mental health and for how long. Listen for details that point to a diagnosis of personality disorder and/or a comorbid condition. In particular, note that personality disorders involve long-standing and enduring symptoms (inflexible behaviors); mood disorders involve episodic symptoms.

Note symptoms unique to particular disorders (e.g., inappropriate perceptions and emotional responses in personality disorders; loss of interest and fatigue in major depressive disorder; hallucinations in bipolar I disorder; alternating "up" and "down" moods in bipolar II disorder).

POINTER

Mental status exams

Mental status exams use both observation and direct questioning to make assessments. Generally, they assess:

- general appearance and behavior
- mood
- speech: rate, tone, volume
- thought content: obsessions, preoccupations, hallucinations, delusions, suicidal ideation, homicidal ideation
- thought process: circumstantial, tangential, flight of ideas, loosening of associations
- orientation to time and place
- attention and concentration
- patient insight into their present condition

Note the patient's insight into their condition. Ask about their interest in changing their situation.

PAST MEDICAL HISTORY

Ask about previous psychiatric diagnoses.

SOCIAL HISTORY

Ask about alcohol and recreational drug use.

Physical exam

Mental status: Perform a mental status exam (see the pointer).

Investigations

Urine drug screen if drug abuse cannot be ruled out

POINTER

Personality disorders and pharmacotherapy

Personality disorders are not treatable by pharmacotherapy. Prescribe pharmacotherapy only in the context of coexisting psychiatric disorders.

Remember that pharmacotherapy involves the risk of abuse and overdose. In particular, prescriptions for sedative-hypnotics run the risk of diversion or abuse, and all psychotropic medications run the risk of overdose. These risks can be reduced by dispensing small quantities of medication (e.g., 1 week at a time) and arranging frequent follow-up with the patient.

Management

Initiate treatment for concurrent psychiatric illness (see the pointer). Consider referral to a psychiatrist or a clinical psychologist for cognitive behavioral therapy. Discuss a plan to treat any coexistent substance abuse.

REFERENCE

1. American Psychiatric Association. Diagnostic and statistical manual of mental disorders. 5th ed. Arlington, VA: American Psychiatric Association; 2013. 991 p.

PSYCHIATRIC PRESENTATIONS

Psychosis

Differential diagnosis

PSYCHOTIC DISORDERS (E.G., SCHIZOPHRENIA, SCHIZOAFFECTIVE DISORDER)

Schizophrenia[1(p99)]

Schizophrenia is the most common primary disorder associated with psychosis.

Signs and symptoms: presence of active symptoms for ≥ 1 month, and continuous presence of symptoms (active, and prodromal and/or residual) for ≥ 6 months

- Key symptoms: delusions, hallucinations, and/or disorganized speech
- Other symptoms: disorganized or catatonic behavior; negative symptoms (e.g., reduced emotional response)

Schizoaffective disorder[1(p105)]

Signs and symptoms: manic or major depressive episode that occurs at the same time as delusions, hallucinations, and/or disorganized speech; presence of delusions or hallucinations for ≥ 2 weeks over the total duration of the illness, during times when a manic or major depressive episode is not present

MANIC EPISODE[1(pp123–134)]

Signs and symptoms: symptoms that are present most of the time for ≥ 1 week; symptoms with significant impact on day-to-day life, and that may pose a risk of harm to self and others

- Key symptoms: abnormally elevated (and/or irritable) mood and goal-directed activity
- Other symptoms: increased self-importance, increased talking, racing thoughts, decreased need for sleep, risky pursuits (e.g., that could damage finances or relationships), psychosis (e.g., delusions, hallucinations)

MAJOR DEPRESSIVE EPISODE[1(123–134)]

Signs and symptoms: symptoms that are present most of the time for ≥ 2 weeks; symptoms with significant impact on day-to-day life

- Key symptoms: depressed mood and/or loss of interest in usual activities

Other symptoms: significant weight change; sleep disturbance; slowed or agitated mental processes; loss of concentration; recurrent thoughts of death or suicide

PSYCHOTIC DISORDER DUE TO A MEDICAL CONDITION (E.G., SEIZURE DISORDERS, CENTRAL NERVOUS SYSTEM TUMORS)

Seizure disorders

Signs and symptoms: history of seizures; behavioral or other abnormalities; history of complications during gestation (e.g., toxin exposure such as alcohol) and/or delivery; neurologic abnormalities; growth abnormalities; dysmorphic features; hypothyroidism; exposure to lead

Central nervous system tumor

Signs and symptoms: headache that gets worse over time (common symptom: 50% of cases); vision impairment; balance problems; personality or behavior changes; seizures; drowsiness

Risk factors: exposure to radiation (e.g., to treat leukemia in childhood); family history (rare); neurofibromatosis type 1 or type 2; tuberous sclerosis; Von Hippel-Lindau disease; Li-Fraumeni syndrome; immune system disorders

SUBSTANCE-INDUCED PSYCHOTIC DISORDER (E.G., CORTICOSTEROIDS, COCAINE)

Corticosteroids

These are used to treat inflammatory diseases (e.g., rheumatologic diseases).

Psychiatric symptoms occur in 1 out of every 2 to 3 patients. They typically develop 3 to 4 days after beginning therapy. Symptoms with features of hypomania, mania, and psychosis are the most common.

Abuse of cocaine or amphetamine

Signs and symptoms: persecutory delusions (typical); visual, auditory, tactile hallucinations; physical evidence of drug abuse such as nasal septum perforation (from long-term cocaine use), track marks on the arms

Alcohol withdrawal

This is the most common cause of substance-induced psychosis.

Symptoms: agitation; irritability; confusion; delirium; fatigue; restlessness; body tremors; sensitivity to light, sound, or touch; seizures; hallucinations

Keys to patient encounter

Key concern

In acute psychosis, differentiate a primary psychotic disorder from delirium, psychosis due to a medical condition, and substance-induced psychosis.

History

Obtain collateral information (e.g., from an accompanying caregiver), if possible.

HISTORY OF PRESENT ILLNESS

Ask about features consistent with delirium (e.g., sudden-onset changes in level of consciousness following recent surgery or substance withdrawal) and CNS tumor (headaches; vision impairment; balance problems; personality or behavior changes; seizures; drowsiness).

PAST MEDICAL HISTORY

Ask about psychotic disorders, seizure disorder, and inflammatory diseases.

MEDICATIONS

Ask about corticosteroids.

SOCIAL HISTORY

Ask about cocaine, amphetamines, and alcohol.

Physical exam

Mental status: Perform a mental status exam to assess the patient's capacity, and to identify risk factors for self-harm or harming others (see the pointer).

Management

Ensure the immediate safety of the patient and others.

A patient with specific and immediate plans for suicide or homicide requires admission to hospital for psychiatric assessment and monitoring. If a patient at risk of committing suicide or homicide refuses admission, consider involuntary admission. The regulations for involuntary admission vary by jurisdiction, but generally require a written order by 2 physicians.

If the patient is not at immediate risk, refer the patient to a psychiatrist. Provide antipsychotic pharmacotherapy for the patient's acute symptoms and for maintenance therapy. Treat any underlying comorbidity. Ensure the patient has monitoring and regular follow-up to assess their capacity and possible need for a substitute decision maker. Involve the patient's family members, or friends, as appropriate, and consider referring the patient, and family and friends, for counseling about psychosis and support.

POINTER

Mental status exams

Mental status exams use both observation and direct questioning to make assessments. Generally, they assess:

- general appearance and behavior
- mood
- speech: rate, tone, volume
- thought content: obsessions, preoccupations, hallucinations, delusions, suicidal ideation, homicidal ideation
- thought process: circumstantial, tangential, flight of ideas, loosening of associations
- orientation to time and place
- attention and concentration
- patient insight into their present condition

REFERENCE

1. American Psychiatric Association. Diagnostic and statistical manual of mental disorders. 5th ed. Arlington, VA: American Psychiatric Association; 2013. 991 p.

PSYCHIATRIC PRESENTATIONS

Suicidal behavior

Differential diagnosis

PSYCHIATRIC DISORDER (E.G., DEPRESSION, SCHIZOPHRENIA)

Major depressive disorder[1(pp160–161)]

Signs and symptoms: symptoms that are present most of the time for ≥ 2 weeks; symptoms with significant impact on day-to-day life

> Key symptoms: depressed mood and/or loss of interest in usual activities
>
> Other symptoms: significant weight change; sleep disturbance; slowed or agitated mental processes; loss of concentration; recurrent thoughts of death or suicide

Risk factors: family history of mental health disorders (depression, anxiety, suicide); personal history of other mental health disorders; substance abuse; chronic illness (e.g., cancer, stroke, chronic pain)

Schizophrenia[1(p99)]

Schizophrenia is the most common primary disorder associated with psychosis.

Signs and symptoms: presence of active symptoms for ≥ 1 month, and continuous presence of symptoms (active, and prodromal and/or residual) for ≥ 6 months

> Key symptoms: delusions, hallucinations, and/or disorganized speech
>
> Other symptoms: disorganized or catatonic behavior; negative symptoms (e.g., reduced emotional response)

PSYCHOSOCIAL STRESSORS (E.G., DIVORCE, ADVERSE CHILDHOOD EXPERIENCE)

Examples of psychosocial stressors include recent divorce, job loss, financial ruin, death of a friend or family member, and serious medical diagnoses.

Adverse childhood experiences include abuse (physical, sexual, emotional); neglect (physical, emotional); exposure to domestic violence; and family dysfunction due to divorce (or separation), substance abuse, mental illness, or imprisonment.

SUBSTANCE USE

Signs and symptoms: family or personal history of substance abuse; physical signs of substance abuse (track marks on the arms; nasal septum perforation, which indicates long-term cocaine use); tachycardia; tremor and/or sweating

OTHER (E.G., SERIOUS CHRONIC DISEASE)

Examples of serious chronic disease include heart disease, MS, Parkinson disease, and chronic pain.

Keys to patient encounter

Key concerns

Determine the degree of risk.

Provide appropriate management.

Risk assessment

Assess the patient for imminent risk of suicide (see the pointer). Ask if they have specific suicidal plans and intent, and if they have the means to carry out their suicide plan. Ask about previous psychiatric history and previous suicide attempts. Ask about recent life stresses and life events.

Physical exam

Assess the patient for obvious signs of intoxication and/or drug impairment.

Management

A patient with specific and immediate plans for suicide requires admission to hospital

POINTER

Indicators of suicide risk

Patients are at risk of suicide if they have suicidal thoughts, a plan, and intent.

The following additional factors put them at high risk of suicide:

- a history of suicide attempts
- access to firearms
- a psychiatric disorder or disorders (e.g., depression; bipolar disorder; schizophrenia; alcohol or substance abuse; personality disorder; anxiety disorder)
- current substance abuse
- male
- lack of social support (e.g., they live alone)
- for children and adolescents: exposure to abuse, violence, victimization, or bullying; family history of suicide; member of a minority in sexual orientation

for psychiatric assessment and monitoring. If a patient at risk of suicide refuses admission, consider involuntary admission. The regulations for involuntary admission vary by jurisdiction, but generally require a written order by 2 physicians.

If the patient is not at immediate risk, initiate management of the underlying problems—for example, treat depression with an SSRI, or refer the patient for counseling about psychosocial stressors. Involve family members as appropriate. Ensure the patient has monitoring and regular follow-up (especially if the patient's life, work, or social situation changes) and a psychiatric referral.

REFERENCE

1. American Psychiatric Association. Diagnostic and statistical manual of mental disorders. 5th ed. Arlington, VA: American Psychiatric Association; 2013. 991 p.

RESPIRATORY PRESENTATIONS

Cough

Differential diagnosis

ACUTE COUGH

Infectious cough

PNEUMONIA

This is the key concern with infectious cough.

Signs and symptoms: shortness of breath; cough; purulent sputum; chest pain on coughing or deep breaths; fatigue; tachypnea; tachycardia; decreased oxygen saturation; lung crackles on auscultation; lung dullness on percussion

Children: fever

Elderly: confusion, low body temperature

Risk factors: very old, very young, smoking, immune compromise (e.g., due to chronic illness), hospitalization

Investigations: chest x-ray to detect consolidation

COVID-19

Signs and symptoms: highly variable symptoms that may include: fever and chills; cough; shortness of breath or difficulty breathing; fatigue; body aches; headache; loss of sense of taste or smell; sore throat; nasal congestion; runny nose; nausea, vomiting; diarrhea

Risk factors: contact with COVID-19 cases, older age (> 50 years), unvaccinated, chronic lung disease, heart disease, immunosuppression, obesity, pregnancy

Investigations: swab for COVID-19

Irritant-induced cough

Common irritants include tobacco smoke, pollen, dust, and animal dander.

Signs and symptoms: history of environmental allergies or asthma; runny nose or postnasal drip; exposure to known allergens

Other condition (e.g., cardiac condition)

CARDIAC CONDITION

Signs and symptoms: chest pain (often); shortness of breath; personal or family history of cardiac disease (e.g., MI, pericarditis, CHF); abnormal heart sounds; lung rales

CHF: increased JVP, dependent edema

Pericarditis: autoimmune disease, uremia

Investigations: elevated cardiac enzymes (e.g., troponin) (this suggests MI); ECG; chest x-ray to detect possible pulmonary edema

CHRONIC COUGH (LASTING 3 WEEKS OR LONGER)

Upper respiratory condition

Signs and symptoms: postnasal drip; frequent throat clearing; sinus pain on palpation (this suggests sinusitis); mucous in the oropharynx and/or cobblestone appearance to the mucosa; normal lung sounds

Pulmonary condition

CHRONIC BRONCHITIS

Signs and symptoms: frequent exposure to irritants (e.g., workplace exposure; firsthand or secondhand smoke), wheezing

Investigations: reduced capacity on pulmonary function testing

COUGH-VARIANT ASTHMA

Signs and symptoms: worse symptoms after exercise and/or on exposure to irritants (e.g., workplace exposure; firsthand or secondhand smoke), wheezing

Investigations: lung hyperinflation on chest x-ray

BRONCHOGENIC CARCINOMA

Signs and symptoms: history of smoking (usual); constitutional symptoms (fever, weight loss, night sweats, fatigue); enlarged lymph nodes in the neck and axilla

Investigations: chest x-ray to detect mass

INTERSTITIAL LUNG DISEASE

Investigations: prominent interstitium on CT scan of the lungs; reduced capacity on pulmonary function testing

CHRONIC INFECTION

TUBERCULOSIS

Signs and symptoms: fever; night sweats; cough; hemoptysis; exposure to infected persons; poor, crowded living conditions; immunosuppression (including HIV)

Investigations: purified protein derivative skin test, sputum culture

ASPERGILLOSIS

Signs and symptoms: fever, cough, hemoptysis, fatigue, shortness of breath

Risk factors: CF, asthma or other underlying lung diseases; immunosuppression

ENDEMIC FUNGAL DISEASES (E.G. COCCIDIOIDES, HISTOPLASMA, BLASTOMYCES, PARACOCCIDIOIDES, SPOROTHRIX*)*

Signs and symptoms: nonspecific symptoms (often); possible symptoms: cough, fever, skin lesions, lymphadenopathy

Risk factors: living in an endemic area; farming or other exposure to soil; immunosuppression

Gastrointestinal condition (e.g., gastroesophageal reflux)

GASTROESOPHAGEAL REFLUX DISEASE

Signs and symptoms: burning chest pain radiating into the throat (often with a bitter taste in the mouth or regurgitation of food into the mouth; often worse with lying down; often better with standing up or taking antacids; worse with spicy food, coffee, alcohol, fatty foods, peppermint), acid damage to teeth

Risk factors: obesity, pregnancy

Cardiac condition—see above

Other condition (e.g., drug-induced condition, work-related exposure)

DRUG-INDUCED CONDITION

Examples of drugs include ACE inhibitors and oxymetazoline (Afrin).

WORK-RELATED EXPOSURE

Examples of exposures are dust (e.g., farming, demolition), particulates (e.g., metal work), smoke (e.g., firefighting), and chemicals (e.g., laboratory work, construction).

Signs and symptoms: cough that occurs or worsens at work

Keys to patient encounter

Key concern

Distinguish benign from serious causes that require full investigation and further management.

History

HISTORY OF PRESENT ILLNESS

Ask how long the patient has had the cough, what triggers it, and what other symptoms the patient has. The duration defines the cough as acute (less than 3 weeks), subacute (3 to 8 weeks), or chronic (more than 8 weeks). Listen for triggers such as smoke (including smoking), occupational or recreational exposures, exertion, and cold air; and for symptoms consistent with particular entities. Examples of characteristic associated symptoms include:

GERD: heart burn

Pneumonia: shortness of breath

Cardiac conditions: chest pain

Ask about the presence and quality of sputum. Ask about constitutional symptoms (fever, fatigue, night sweats, weight loss). Ask about recent colds.

Ask about COVID-19 vaccination status and possible infectious contacts.

PAST MEDICAL HISTORY

Ask about asthma, GERD, environmental allergies, cancer, TB, and AIDS.

MEDICATIONS

Ask about ACE inhibitors and beta-blockers.

FAMILY HISTORY

Ask about environmental allergies and asthma.

SOCIAL HISTORY

Ask about the patient's occupation, recreational pursuits, and smoking history, including exposure to secondhand smoke. Ask about exposure to TB and endemic fungal diseases. Take a travel history.

Physical exam

Head, ears, nose, throat:

- Look for obstructions and discharge in the nose.
- Examine the throat and oropharynx.
- Examine the external acoustic meatus and the tympanic membranes.

Cardiovascular: Auscultate the heart.

Respiratory: Auscultate the lungs.

Investigations

Chest x-ray in coughs lasting more than 2 weeks

Pulmonary function testing in suspected asthma

IN SUSPECTED INFECTIOUS CAUSES

Sputum for microscopic analysis and culture

Tissue histopathology
Antigen assays
Antibody assays

Management

Management depends on the specific cause identified. Remember that the 3 most common causes are rhinosinusitis (e.g., allergies), asthma, and GERD. Treatment for asthma includes inhaled glucocorticoids and bronchodilators. Treatment for GERD includes PPIs, or H_2 blockers. Treatments for postnasal drip include antihistamines, glucocorticoids, and decongestants. For cough without a specific cause, consider the use of cough suppressants.

RESPIRATORY PRESENTATIONS

Pediatric respiratory distress

Differential diagnosis

UPPER AIRWAY PROBLEM

Croup

This is due to swelling around the larynx, trachea, and bronchi in infants and children.

The common cause is viruses. Severe cases may be caused by bacteria.

Signs and symptoms: difficulty breathing; "barking" cough; stridor; hoarseness; fever; inflamed nasal mucous membranes; chest wall in-drawing; cyanotic nose and mouth

Foreign body aspiration

Signs and symptoms of airway obstruction (immediate intervention is required): no audible speech or cough, possibly with gagging or choking (this indicates complete upper airway obstruction; partial obstruction allows some phonation and breath sounds)

Laryngeal disorder

LARYNGEAL TUMOR

Signs and symptoms: hoarseness, breathy voice, shortness of breath, difficulty swallowing, otalgia, hemoptysis

Investigations: biopsy

LARYNGOCELE

Signs and symptoms: hoarseness; airway obstruction; mass on the neck (if the laryngocele is external)

Investigations: CT scan (finding: smooth, ovoid, low-density mass)

Epiglottitis

This is a potentially life-threatening condition from inflammation or swelling of the epiglottis that blocks airflow to the lungs. The typical causes include infection or injury to the throat. The *H. influenzae* type B (Hib) vaccine has made it less common in Canada.

Signs and symptoms (these may develop within hours): fever; throat soreness or pain; difficulty breathing or stridor

Investigations: blood or throat culture to detect infection; CBC; x-ray of the neck or chest

Retropharyngeal abscess

This is a deep neck infection arising from a URTI. It is rare. The mean age of incidence is 3 to 5 years.

The cause is often polymicrobial: group A streptococci, *S. aureus*, methicillin-resistant *S. aureus*, and/or respiratory anaerobes (*Fusobacteria*, *Prevotella*, *Veillonella*).

Signs and symptoms: moderate fever for several days; difficulty swallowing, pain on swallowing, or drooling; unwillingness to extend the neck; voice changes; stridor; tachypnea; neck swelling, mass, or lymphadenopathy

Investigations: increased WBCs; throat culture; blood culture (this is rarely positive); CT scan with contrast of the neck (this is the best imaging modality in this context) (findings: an area in the deep spaces of the neck with low attenuation, a surrounding enhanced ring, and possible central lucency)

Choanal atresia

This is a congenital obstruction (either partial or complete obstruction) of the nasal airway by tissue. It is the most common nasal abnormality in newborns and occurs twice as often in females.

Signs and symptoms: nasal obstruction on physical exam

Investigations: nasal endoscopy; CT scan to visualize abnormalities; sinus x-ray to detect structural deformities

LOWER AIRWAY, PULMONARY DISORDER

Bacterial tracheitis

This is relatively rare and usually affects children younger than 6 years. It can result in severe respiratory distress, which requires immediate intubation.

Signs and symptoms: symptom onset during fall and winter (common); 3 days of URTI (rhinorrhea, cough, fever) followed by respiratory distress, stridor, nonpainful cough, shortness of breath, fever, toxic appearance

Investigations: endoscopy (in severe respiratory distress); Gram stain of endoscopy exudates (findings: neutrophils and bacterial morphologies); x-ray of soft tissues in the lateral neck to detect severe airway obstruction (findings: narrowing of the subglottic trachea, tracheal edema, and sloughing of tracheal mucosa)

Viral infections

BRONCHIOLITIS

This is most commonly caused by RSV. RSV usually causes mild illness, but can cause severe illness, especially in children younger than 1 year.

Signs and symptoms: URTI for the first few days (rhinorrhea, cough, fever) followed by lower respiratory tract infection (wheezing and/or crackles; increased respiratory rate; chest retractions, nasal flaring; tachypnea); symptoms that resolve in 5 days (usual); cough that resolves in 2 weeks (usual)

Investigations: swab for RSV; ABG, chest x-ray (consider these)

INFLUENZA

This commonly occurs in the context of seasonal influenza outbreaks.

Signs and symptoms: rapid onset of high fever; body aches; headache; cough (often severe); fatigue; possible GI symptoms (e.g., nausea, vomiting, and diarrhea)

COVID-19

This is often asymptomatic in children, but may be severe, especially in children with underlying medical conditions such as obesity, diabetes, and cardiac, lung, and neurologic disorders.

Investigations: swab for COVID-19

Pneumonia, atelectasis

PNEUMONIA

Signs and symptoms: fever, cough, and tachypnea that do not resolve

Newborns: poor feeding; irritability, restlessness; tachypnea; hypoxemia

Infants: cough, tachypnea, chest retractions, hypoxemia, fever, irritability, decreased feeding

Adolescents: symptoms similar to younger children; possible constitutional symptoms (headache, pleuritic chest pain, vague abdominal pain)

Risk factors: poverty; crowded living conditions; secondhand smoke; recent URTI; cardiopulmonary disorders; other medical conditions (CHD, bronchopulmonary dysplasia, CF, asthma, sickle cell disease, neuromuscular disorders)

Investigations: chest x-ray where there is clinical evidence for pneumonia

ATELECTASIS

This generally presents with few findings on physical exam, unless larger areas of the lung are atelectatic. It is sometimes incidentally found on US. Mucus plugging is the most common cause of atelectasis in children.

Signs and symptoms (when larger areas of the lung are atelectatic): localized decreased breath sounds; dullness with percussion; wheezing, rales on auscultation; **no** fever; grunting on expiration; neuromuscular weakness (atelectasis is common in these patients)

Investigations: x-ray to detect areas of pulmonary opacity, and assess mediastinal shift and extent of volume loss

Asthma, bronchospasm

Signs and symptoms (in general): recurrent wheezing; recurrent dry or productive cough; symptoms triggered by URTI (often), allergens, exercise

Asthma: shortness of breath; chest tightness, pain; disturbed sleep from symptoms

Risk factors (asthma): family history of asthma; secondhand smoke; exposure to air pollution; other allergic conditions (e.g., atopic dermatitis)

Investigations: pulmonary function testing; chest x-ray to detect specific inflation or structure abnormalities

Respiratory distress syndrome of the neonate

This is common in premature neonates due to deficiency of pulmonary surfactant.

Signs and symptoms: tachypnea; grunting; chest retractions; nasal flaring; cyanosis; apnea

Investigations: chest x-ray to detect ground-glass appearance, air bronchograms, low lung volume, absence of thymus

Tracheoesophageal fistula

This is a common, life-threatening congenital abnormality. It is diagnosed shortly after birth or in infancy.

Signs and symptoms: drooling; white frothy bubbles in the mouth and nose; choking; respiratory distress; inability to feed; abdominal distention; maternal polyhydramnios

Investigations: catheter insertion into stomach (this stops at 10–15 cm), with chest x-ray (this detects the catheter curled in the upper esophageal pouch); lateral chest x-ray to detect gas in the GI tract

PLEURAL DISORDER

Pleural effusion, empyema

Signs and symptoms (in general): chest pain, (sharp, stabbing pain that worsens on inspiration), especially if exudative effusion is present; pain that radiates to the shoulder (due to diaphragmatic irritation from pneumonic condition); fever; localized decreased breath sounds; tactile fremitus; dullness on percussion

Investigations: anterior-posterior and lateral chest x-rays to distinguish pulmonary from cardiac etiologies for pleural fluid; pulmonary US to detect pleural effusion

Pneumothorax

SPONTANEOUS PNEUMOTHORAX

This occurs in the absence of any identified trauma.

Signs and symptoms: generally asymptomatic if the pneumothorax is small; adolescent male (more common); tall, thin body; family history of spontaneous pneumothorax; sudden-onset shortness of breath; chest pain (sharp, stabbing pain after a popping sensation); hyperresonance on percussion; decreased breath sounds in the affected lung; decreased chest excursion; **no** tactile fremitus

Investigations: ABG (in cases of respiratory distress)

SECONDARY PNEUMOTHORAX

Causes include use of inhaled drugs, undiagnosed asthma, foreign body aspiration, respiratory tract infection, and connective tissue disease.

Investigations: chest x-ray

Findings for infants (large pneumothorax): hyperlucency

Findings for children (take x-rays in the upright position): pleural line; hyperlucency; attenuation of vascular and lung markings

NEUROLOGIC DISORDER (E.G., DRUGS)

Drugs

Examples include accidental or intentional drug overdose (especially from opiate and sedative medications).

Toxins (e.g., botulism) can also cause neurologic disorders with respiratory distress.

CARDIAC DISORDER

Congestive heart failure (left-to-right shunt, left ventricular failure)

Signs and symptoms: excessive sweating, persistent tachypnea, tachycardia

Investigations: echocardiogram

Cardiac tamponade

Signs and symptoms: sharp chest pain, possibly worse on deep inhalation or coughing; difficulty breathing; palpitations; Beck triad (hypotension, high JVP, muffled heart sounds)

Investigations: echocardiogram

Keys to patient encounter

Key concerns

Consider respiratory rate in the context of the age of the child.

Differentiate cardiac causes from infectious, pulmonary, neuromuscular, and other causes.

Airway and hemodynamic status

Check the patient's ABCs. Check for tachypnea (see the pointer). Provide emergency care to any patient with unstable vital signs.

POINTER

Pediatric tachypnea

Many guidelines on pediatric respiration rates exist, with a variety of age breakdowns and ranges. As a reference point, consider the following examples of pronounced tachypnea:

0–3 years	> 60 breaths/minute
4–10 years	> 40 breaths/minute
11–18 years	> 30 breaths/minute

History

HISTORY OF PRESENT ILLNESS

Ask when the patient started having difficulty breathing. Listen for evidence of sudden onset versus recurrent symptoms (sudden onset is consistent with entities such as epiglottitis and pneumothorax; recurrent symptoms are consistent with asthma). Ask about suspected triggers for onset (e.g., trauma, URTI, allergies). Ask about symptoms consistent with cardiac disorders (excessive sweating, tachycardia, chest pain, palpitations); and for symptoms consistent with particular disorders (e.g., barking cough in croup; fever in infectious entities; difficulty swallowing in laryngeal tumor and retropharyngeal abscess). Ask about infectious contacts, including contacts with COVID-19. Ask about vaccination status, including COVID-19 and influenza vaccines.

PAST MEDICAL HISTORY

Ask about asthma and a history of immunosuppression.

FAMILY HISTORY

Ask about asthma.

Physical exam

Vital signs: Measure oxygen saturation.
General inspection: Look for cyanosis.
Cardiovascular: Auscultate the heart.
Respiratory: Auscultate the lungs.

Investigations

CBC

ABG

Chest x-ray

Respiratory viruses to assess for COVID-19, RSV, and influenza, as appropriate

- Tests for respiratory viruses are often available as a panel.

Management

Provide supplemental oxygen. Admit the patient to hospital and consult a pediatrician. Treat the underlying etiology. Bacterial pneumonia is treated with antibiotics. Antiviral medications may be indicated for certain viral infections (e.g., influenza, COVID-19).

RESPIRATORY PRESENTATIONS

Pleural effusion

Differential diagnosis

TRANSUDATIVE (E.G., CONGESTIVE HEART FAILURE, NEPHROTIC SYNDROME, CIRRHOSIS)

TRANSUDATIVE PLEURAL EFFUSION IN GENERAL

This is caused by a combination of increased hydrostatic pressure and decreased plasma oncotic pressure.

Asymptomatic transudates require no treatment. Symptomatic transudates require thoracentesis, chest tube drainage, pleurodesis, pleurectomy, or a combination.

Signs and symptoms: **no** agreement with Light criteria (see *exudative*, below)

Risk factors: CHF; cirrhosis with ascites; hypoalbuminemia due to nephrotic syndrome

Congestive heart failure

Signs and symptoms: history of heart disease (or risk factors for heart disease: diabetes, hypertension, hyperlipidemia, and smoking) or hepatic vein thrombosis (Budd-Chiari syndrome); severe shortness of breath; elevated JVP; edema in the abdomen and legs; pink phlegm; heart murmurs and extra cardiac sounds

Investigations: chest x-ray to detect pulmonary edema; NT-proBNP; echocardiogram to distinguish forms of HF; cardiac stress testing, either with exercise or pharmacological agent

Nephrotic syndrome

Signs and symptoms: progressive lower extremity edema (ankles and feet); swelling around the eyes; weight gain (from water retention); foamy urine

Risk factors: conditions that damage the kidneys (e.g., diabetes, SLE, amyloidosis); use of NSAIDs, antibiotics; HIV, HBV, HCV, malaria

Investigations: urine (proteinuria, spot urine protein:creatinine ratio, lipuria); hyponatremia with low fractional sodium excretion; low serum albumin; high total cholesterol (hyperlipidemia); elevated BUN

Cirrhosis

Signs and symptoms: jaundice; easy bruising, bleeding; itching; ascites; spiderlike blood vessels on the skin; systemic symptoms (anorexia, weight loss, weakness, fatigue)

> History of chronic alcohol abuse; chronic HBV, HCV; hemochromatosis; nonalcoholic fatty liver disease
>
> HBV and HCV risk factors: autoimmune conditions, unprotected sex, IV drug abuse, blood transfusions, tattoos, body piercings, imprisonment, workplace exposure to body fluids

Investigations: liver function tests

EXUDATIVE

EXUDATIVE PLEURAL EFFUSION IN GENERAL

Signs and symptoms: symptoms that meet Light criteria

> Light criteria: ratio of pleural fluid protein to serum protein > 0.5; and/or ratio of pleural fluid LDH to serum LDH > 0.6; and/or pleural fluid LDH > 0.6 times ULN of a lab's serum LDH (labs define this differently)

Risk factors: pneumonia, malignancy, PE, viral infection, TB

Infectious/inflammatory causes (e.g., parapneumonic effusion, empyema, rheumatoid arthritis)

PARAPNEUMONIC EFFUSION

Signs and symptoms: cough; fever; pleuritic chest pain; shortness of breath and/or sputum production

UNCOMPLICATED PARAPNEUMONIC EFFUSION

Symptoms resolve with resolution of pneumonia.

Signs and symptoms: exudative, neutrophilic effusions (these result from inflammation associated with pneumonia); fluid that is sterile, and slightly cloudy or clear

COMPLICATED PARAPNEUMONIC EFFUSION

This requires drainage for resolution.

Signs and symptoms: fluid that is often sterile (false negative), but cloudy, with putrid odor

Investigations: increased neutrophils; pleural fluid acidosis; decreased glucose; increased LDH (> 1000 IU/L [16.7 µkat/L]); anaerobic infection on Gram stain

EMPYEMA

Causes include complications of pneumonia, thoracotomy, abscesses (lung, liver, or subdiaphragmatic), and penetrating trauma with secondary infection.

Signs and symptoms: fever for several days (> 48 hours); malaise; frank pus in the pleural space (observed when drained by thoracentesis); pleural fluid that is thick, viscous, and opaque

> History of recent URTI; bronchitis; pneumonia; recurrent aspiration (e.g., due to poor oral hygiene, alcoholism)

RHEUMATOID ARTHRITIS

RA is among a group of systemic, inflammatory, autoimmune diseases that also includes SLE, scleroderma, temporal arteritis, and interstitial lung disease.

Signs and symptoms: fatigue, muscle weakness, fever, body aches, joint pain, skin rash

> Lung signs and symptoms: generally asymptomatic; small volume of pleural fluid, which is usually unilateral (left side) with high titers of rheumatoid factor and low glucose levels (< 25 mg/dL [1.4 mmol/L])

Neoplasm (e.g., primary, metastatic, mesothelioma)

Malignant pleural effusion is diagnosed with thoracentesis.

The pleura is more commonly involved in metastatic disease or advanced-stage tumors (lung, breast, lymphoma); mesothelioma; large primary tumors; and adenocarcinoma.

Malignant cells may be identified in cytologic examination of pleural fluid.

Signs and symptoms: shortness of breath, chest pain, malaise, dry cough

Pulmonary embolus

Signs and symptoms: sharp chest pain; shortness of breath; cough (possibly with blood); hypoxia; possible unilateral swelling of the lower limbs (this indicates DVT); elevated pulse and respiratory rate; arrhythmias; lung rales on auscultation; lower-lung dullness on percussion; motor or sensory deficits

Risk factors: HF; cancer; surgery; prolonged immobility (e.g., long plane trips); smoking; estrogen replacement therapy; OCs; current pregnancy; previous DVT, embolism, or stroke; family history of embolism

Investigations: elevated d-dimer level; area of reduced pulmonary perfusion on V/Q scan; CT angiography to detect blocked vessel

Gastrointestinal condition (e.g., ruptured esophagus, pancreatitis, chylothorax)

RUPTURED ESOPHAGUS (BOERHAAVE SYNDROME)

This is a life-threatening emergency (watch out for atypical presentations).

Signs and symptoms: male, middle-aged (common); recent severe vomiting or trauma; lower anterior chest or upper abdominal pain (other pain locations: the neck, back); subcutaneous emphysema; difficulty swallowing; shortness of breath; hematemesis; dark, tarry stools; history of dietary overindulgence, overconsumption of alcohol

> Mackler triad (classic presentation): chest pain, vomiting, subcutaneous emphysema
>
> Atypical presentation: shoulder pain, facial swelling, hoarseness, voice changes

Investigations: thoracentesis for pleural fluid (fluid has food fragments, pH < 6, elevated salivary amylase, leukocytosis); thoracic, cervical x-ray; contrast esophagram

PANCREATITIS

Pleural effusion is a complication in one-third of acute pancreatitis cases.

Signs and symptoms: constant upper abdominal pain that radiates to the back (sitting up and leaning forward may reduce the pain; pain occurs with coughing, vigorous movement, deep breathing); shortness of breath; nausea, vomiting; hypotension; fever; jaundice; abdominal tenderness

> History of gallstones or chronic alcoholism (usual); hyperlipidemia; hypercalcemia; change of medication

Investigations: serum amylase and lipase (levels are ≥ 3 times ULN; elevated lipase indicates pancreatic damage); possible elevated calcium; possible elevated cholesterol; possible elevated ALT (this indicates associated liver inflammation); chest x-ray (this may show left-sided or bilateral pleural effusion; atelectasis); abdominal x-ray (this may show calcifications within pancreatic ducts; calcified gallstones; or localized ileus of a segment of small intestine); US

CHYLOTHORAX

Signs and symptoms: unilateral pleural effusion, right hemithorax involvement (often); decreased breath sounds; dullness to percussion

> Traumatic chylothorax: postoperative, cardiothoracic surgery (most common); pleural effusion on serial x-rays, or

persistent drainage of pleural fluid from a preexisting chest tube

Nontraumatic chylothorax: malignancy (e.g., lymphoma, chronic lymphocytic leukemia, metastatic cancer); gradual onset of symptoms; decreased exercise tolerance; shortness of breath; heavy feeling in the chest; fatigue; rarely fever or chest pain

Investigations: thoracentesis for pleural fluid (fluid is milky or opaque; triglyceride > 110 mg/dL [1.2 mmol/L]) confirms chylothorax; chylomicrons are present on electrophoresis, predominately lymphocytes); chest x-ray to detect the side of the chest with effusion; CT scan of the thorax and abdomen to identify site of thoracic duct rupture

Keys to patient encounter

Key concern

Identify the underlying etiology of pleural effusion based on pleural fluid analysis.

History

Ask about the patient's medical history, occupation, and current health status. Listen for a history of conditions that cause edema (e.g., HF); infectious disease, or symptoms consistent with infectious disease (e.g., fever); neoplastic disease; and high-risk occupations for asbestos exposure (e.g., asbestos mining, construction, firefighting, industrial work).

When you identify a probable underlying condition, concentrate on the history of the condition and the seriousness of the symptoms the patient is experiencing.

Physical exam

Cardiovascular: Auscultate the heart.

Respiratory: Auscultate and percuss the lungs.

Other signs: Perform a focused exam based on the probable diagnosis identified from the history.

Investigations

Chest X-ray

Thoracentesis as indicated (for diagnosis and/or symptom relief)

R

INTERPRETATION OF THORACENTESIS ANALYSIS

CAUSES OF PLEURAL EFFUSION	PLEURAL FLUID ANALYSIS
Exudative	Cloudy; pH 7.3–7.45; positive Light criteria
Transudative	Clear; absolute total protein < 3.0 g/dL (30 g/L); pH 7.4–7.55
PE	Exudate
RA	Exudate; low glucose (< 25 mg/dL [1.4 mmol/L])
Ruptured esophagus	Exudate; amylase that exceeds ULN serum amylase; pleural fluid/serum amylase ratio > 1.0; low pH; ingested food fragments in fluid; low glucose (< 60 mg/dL [3.3 mmol/L]) or a pleural fluid/serum glucose ratio < 0.5
Pancreatitis	Exudate; amylase that exceeds ULN serum amylase; pleural fluid/serum amylase ratio > 1.0; > 10 000 nucleated cells/µL (10×10^9/L)
Chylothorax	Exudate; milky to opaque; triglycerides > 110 mg/dL (1.2 mmol/L); chylomicrons; lymphocytosis
Parapneumonic effusion	Exudate; cloudy or clear; low glucose (< 60 mg/dL [3.3 mmol/L]) or a pleural fluid/serum glucose ratio < 0.5; > 50 000 nucleated cells/µL (50×10^9/L) (neutrophilic)
Empyema	Exudate; fluid that has pus and putrid odor; thick, viscous, opaque; positive culture; LDH > 1000 IU/L (16.7 µkat/L); very low glucose (sometimes undetectable) or a pleural fluid/serum glucose ratio < 0.5; > 50 000 nucleated cells/µL (50×10^9/L)
Malignancy/ neoplasm (primary, metastatic, mesothelioma)	Exudate; positive cytology; sometimes LDH > 1000 IU/L (16.7 µkat/L); low glucose (30–50 mg/dL [1.7–2.8 mmol/L]) or a pleural fluid/serum glucose ratio < 0.5; elevated levels of soluble mesothelin-related peptides or mesothelial cells in mesothelioma
CHF	Transudate; serum-to-pleural-fluid albumin gradient > 1.2 g/dL (12 g/L); elevated blood NT-proBNP when Light criteria yield results in exudative range
Nephrotic syndrome	Transudate
Cirrhosis	Transudate; < 250 polymorphonuclear leukocyte cells/µL (0.25 cells $\times 10^9$/L); low protein (< 2.5 g/dL [25 g/L]); low albumin; pleural fluid/LDH ratio < 0.6; pleural fluid/serum bilirubin ratio < 0.6; pH > 7.4

Management

Specific management depends on the identified cause. Consider the need for referral to an internist or surgeon.

SCROTAL PRESENTATIONS

Scrotal mass

Differential diagnosis

CYSTIC MASS (E.G., HYDROCELE)

Hydrocele

Causes include injury or infection (filariasis from *W. bancrofti* infection) of the scrotum. (In infants, the cause is an unsealed opening between the abdomen and the scrotum, which resolves by age 1 year.)

Signs and symptoms: painless (often) swelling of the scrotum; scrotal pain or discomfort; heavy or full feeling of the scrotum; swelling and irritation of the skin around the scrotum

Investigations: light test to detect solid masses in the sac; or US to detect fluid collection surrounding the testis, which are avascular on Doppler

SOLID MASS

Benign (e.g., hematoma)

HEMATOMA

This is common after a vasectomy or other trauma. It usually resolves on its own within 4 to 8 weeks.

Signs and symptoms: asymptomatic (small hematoma); scrotal swelling, bruising, pain (large hematoma)

Investigations: lack of color on Doppler flow US, isoechoic/hyperechoic region in the affected testicle

Malignant (e.g., seminoma)

SEMINOMA

This is a testicular germ cell tumor that is treatable and curable if discovered in early stages.

It is the most common malignancy in males age 15 to 35.

Signs and symptoms: Caucasian (more common); painless testicular mass (noticeable from days to months)

Investigations: abnormal semen findings (possible subfertility); scrotal US (homogenous intratesticular mass; lower echogenicity than normal testicle; well-defined, oval, without invasion; usually confined to tunica albuginea); AFP (if elevated, it is not seminoma)

Inflammatory or infectious (e.g., orchitis, scrotal abscess)

ORCHITIS

The common cause is mumps (more common in children).

Signs and symptoms: acute symptoms that resolve in 3 to 10 days (usual); enlarged, firm, tender testis; enlarged epididymis; red scrotal skin; prostatitis; fever; chills; nausea; headache; fatigue; myalgias

SCROTAL ABSCESS

For superficial abscesses, common causes include infected hair follicles, infections of scrotal lacerations, and minor scrotal surgeries (confined to scrotal wall).

For intrascrotal abscesses, common causes include bacterial epididymitis and tuberculous infection in the epididymis.

Signs and symptoms (superficial, intrascrotal): penile discharge; frequent urination and urge to urinate; difficult or painful urination; red, swollen, tender scrotum

Keys to patient encounter

Key concern

Differentiate malignant testicular tumors from other types of scrotal masses.

History

Ask when and how the patient found the mass, what characterizes it, and what other symptoms the patient has. Listen for details consistent with malignancy (slow onset, no pain, no fever). Ask about recent scrotal trauma or surgery. Ask about risk factors for infection (prolonged travel in the tropics, which is relevant for lymphatic filariasis; lapsed immunizations, which is relevant for mumps; exposure to TB).

Physical exam

Vital signs: Look for fever.

Scrotum: Look for masses, tenderness, swelling, and redness.

Inguinal lymph nodes: Look for enlargement.

Investigations

Scrotal US with Doppler to assess blood flow

—and/or—

CT scan

Management

Consider referring the patient to a urologist.

POINTER

Diagnostic features of varicocele

Varicocele is usually unilateral (sometimes bilateral) and, if unilateral, is almost always on the left side. Unilateral right-side varicocele is rare and may indicate a retroperitoneal mass.

SCROTAL PRESENTATIONS

Scrotal pain

Differential diagnosis

TESTICULAR TORSION

This is common in boys age 12 to 16 years (but it can occur at any age, including neonates).

Testicular torsion requires emergency surgery to save the testicle and preserve future fertility. Surgery within 6 hours of pain onset has a high success rate (up to 100%); surgery after 12 hours has a ≤ 50% success rate.

Signs and symptoms: sudden severe pain with swelling in the scrotum; a testicle that is higher than normal or at an abnormal angle; swollen, tender, firm, erythematous testicle; nausea, vomiting

Investigations: scrotal US

INFLAMMATION (E.G., ACUTE EPIDIDYMITIS, ORCHITIS, TRAUMA)

Acute epididymitis

This is the most common cause of scrotal pain in adults.

It is most commonly due to STI (chlamydia, gonorrhea) in men younger than 35.

Signs and symptoms: symptoms lasting < 6 weeks (acute condition); testicular swelling, pain, tenderness, firmness

Orchitis

The common cause is mumps (more common in children).

Signs and symptoms: acute symptoms that resolve in 3 to 10 days (usual); enlarged, firm, tender testis; enlarged epididymis; red scrotal skin; prostatitis; fever; chills; nausea; headache; fatigue; myalgia

Trauma

Examples of trauma include scrotal avulsion; blunt and penetrating trauma; and injury to scrotal contents. Causes include animal attacks, car accidents, self-mutilation, assaults, and machinery-related accidents.

Signs and symptoms: age 10 to 13 years (most common group); acute scrotal pain, swelling, bruising, associated skin loss; injured right testicle (more common than left)

Investigations: US to detect intratesticular and extratesticular hematomas (consider testicular torsion in cases of minor injuries with nonperfusion of testis on US and extensive scrotal pain, swelling, and bruising)

INCARCERATED HERNIA

Signs and symptoms: palpable mass or swelling in the abdomen, groin, or upper thigh; rapid-onset acute pain at the site of the mass or swelling; nausea, vomiting; constipation; history of abdominal surgery (this is common in ventral hernias)

Risk factor (ventral hernia): obesity

Investigations: US or CT scan

HEMORRHAGE INTO TESTICULAR TUMOR

Testicular tumors can hemorrhage to produce swelling and pain. The tumors themselves are often painless lumps or swellings on either testicle.

Some men have acute pain secondary to bleeding into the testis from extravasation of tumor vessels.

Keys to patient encounter

Key concern

Sudden-onset pain requires emergent investigation for testicular torsion.

History

HISTORY OF PRESENT ILLNESS

Establish the age of the patient (this helps point to a diagnosis). Ask when the pain started and how quickly it developed. Listen for sudden versus gradual onset (sudden onset suggests testicular torsion or incarcerated hernia). Ask about enlarged, tender unilateral or bilateral salivary glands (this suggests mumps), masses or lumps (this suggests tumor or hernia), and constipation (this suggests hernia). Ask whether the patient's immunizations are up to date (lapsed immunizations are a risk factor for mumps).

SURGICAL HISTORY

Ask about abdominal surgery (this a risk factor for ventral hernia).

SOCIAL HISTORY

If the patient is sexually active, ask about risk factors for STIs (unprotected sex, multiple sexual partners).

Physical exam

Vital signs: Look for fever.

Scrotum: Look for abnormalities (e.g., masses, swelling, redness, tenderness, abnormal position of the testes).

Abdominal: Look for masses and tenderness.

Investigations

Emergent US of the testes in suspected testicular torsion

Urinalysis

Scrotal US

STI testing

Management

Testicular torsion is a medical emergency that requires immediate surgical assessment.

Treat any infection identified (including STI). Consider referral to a urologist.

SEXUALLY CONCERNED PATIENT

Sexually concerned patient

Differential diagnosis

SEXUAL DYSFUNCTION

SEXUAL DYSFUNCTION IN GENERAL

Signs and symptoms: in men, erectile dysfunction (see the presentation: *Erectile dysfunction*); in women, recurring reduced sexual desire or response, anorgasmia, and/or pain with intercourse

Psychological or emotional condition (e.g., depression, abuse)

MAJOR DEPRESSIVE DISORDER[1(pp160–161)]

Signs and symptoms: symptoms that are present most of the time for ≥ 2 weeks; symptoms with significant impact on day-to-day life

Key symptoms: depressed mood and/or loss of interest in usual activities

Other symptoms: significant weight change; sleep disturbance; slowed or agitated mental processes; loss of concentration; recurrent thoughts of death or suicide

Risk factors: family history of mental health disorders (depression, anxiety, suicide); personal history of other mental health disorders; substance abuse; chronic illness (e.g., cancer, stroke, chronic pain)

INTIMATE PARTNER ABUSE

Signs and symptoms: disclosed abuse (physical; psychological or emotional; sexual; economic; social isolation); bruising, scars, healed fractures; recurrent symptoms or injuries; resistance by the partner to having the patient interviewed alone (usual)

Note: victims do not always disclose abuse.

Risk factors: pregnancy; threat to leave; partner's history of violence or substance abuse

Hormonal condition (e.g., menopause)

MENOPAUSE

Menopause has occurred when 12 months have passed since a woman's last menstrual period. This can occur naturally (usually around age 50); or because of surgical removal of the ovaries, or chemotherapy or radiation therapy.

Signs and symptoms: dry, inelastic vaginal tissue, which leads to difficult or painful intercourse; hot flashes; irritability; weight gain

Neurologic dysfunction

Common causes include spinal cord injury, brain injury, stroke, and MS.

Vascular insufficiency (e.g., diabetes mellitus)

DIABETES

Signs and symptoms: personal or family history of diabetes; history of diabetic complications and/or inadequate monitoring; polydipsia, polyuria, and/or weight loss

Investigations: fasting glucose or HbA_{1c}

Drug side effects (e.g., beta-blockers)

Trauma (e.g., episiotomy)

PARAPHILIAS (E.G., PEDOPHILIA)

Pedophilic disorder[1(p697)]

Signs and symptoms: age 16 or older; symptoms that are present ≥ 6 months; recurrent fantasies or urges about sexual activity with children (at least 5 years younger than the individual); symptoms with significant impact on day-to-day life, including acting on the urges or fantasies

GENDER IDENTITY DISORDERS

Gender dysphoria in adolescents and adults[1(pp452–453)]

Signs and symptoms: incongruence between the expressed gender and the assigned gender of an individual (e.g., rejection of the sex characteristics of the assigned gender; desire for the sex characteristics of the expressed gender; desire to be treated as a member of the expressed gender); symptoms that are present ≥ 6 months; symptoms with significant impact on day-to-day life

SPECIAL POPULATIONS

People with disabilities

Possible issues include personal and social acceptance of the sexuality of people with disabilities; depression, anxiety due to lack of acceptance; appropriate contraception (e.g., women with reduced mobility have higher risk of thrombosis from OCs); genetic concerns, if the disability is congenital; and adaptive practices (e.g., use of sex aids).

LGBT and other Queer populations

Possible issues include personal and social acceptance of sexual and/or gender identity; depression, anxiety due to lack of acceptance; violence and bullying due to sexual and/or gender identity; risks associated with sexual behavior and/or sexual network (e.g., men who have sex with men may be at higher risk of STIs—HIV, hepatitis, HPV, HSV, gonorrhea, chlamydia, syphilis—because of a combination of community and behavioral factors).

Children and adolescents

Possible issues include sexual identity, consent, sexual abuse, bullying, contraception, and safe sex.

Elderly people

Possible issues include sexual dysfunction from declining general health; depression; erectile dysfunction; urogenital atrophy causing difficult or painful intercourse (women); and institutionalization, resulting in a lack of privacy with partners.

Keys to patient encounter

Key concerns

Provide acceptance and appropriate care for patients of all gender identities.

Set the patient at ease.

History

Ask what problems the patient has been having, which will quickly establish the nature of the patient's issue.

Where appropriate (for example, if the patient expresses concerns about sexual orientation or identity), establish the patient's sexual development (socially and physically), sexual orientation, and comfort with their orientation. For example, ask: How long have you had these concerns? What brought the concerns to

---

POINTER

Setting patients at ease

Patients can be embarrassed or reluctant to discuss their concerns. Some general strategies for setting them at ease include:

- maintaining eye contact
- remaining calm and respectful
- expressing support for the patient's decision to seek your help
- expressing confidence in your ability to provide help
- assuring the patient that you will listen and provide care without judging the patient

---

the surface? What has been your experience with your physical sexual maturation? What has been your experience with sexual relationships? How have your experiences affected your relationships with family and friends? How do you regard your sexual orientation?

In male erectile dysfunction, concentrate on identifying treatable causes (e.g., diabetes, hypertension; see the clinical presentation: *Erectile dysfunction*).

Physical exam

Physical exam is indicated in erectile dysfunction (see the clinical presentation: *Erectile dysfunction*).

Investigations

HBA_{1c} if indicated

Management

Manage treatable causes. Counsel and educate the patient. Consider psychological support and referral.

REFERENCE

1. American Psychiatric Association. Diagnostic and statistical manual of mental disorders. 5th ed. Arlington, VA: American Psychiatric Association; 2013. 991 p.

SKIN RASHES, TUMORS, AND ULCERS

Skin rashes, tumors, and ulcers

S

Differential diagnosis

RASHES

Macules

MACULES IN GENERAL

These are flat, abnormally colored lesions.

VIRALLY CAUSED MACULES

Causes include measles, rubella, and EBV.

Signs and symptoms: small, pink-red spots or patches (typical) that appear in 1 area and can spread to others (e.g., they can appear on the trunk and then spread to the arms and legs); viral symptoms (e.g., fever, headache)

PHOTO-DISTRIBUTED MACULES

Drugs that commonly cause photosensitivity include phenothiazines and TCAs (psychiatrics); tetracyclines and sulfonamides (antibiotics); methotrexate (chemotherapy); sulfonylureas (antihyperglycemics); and chlorothiazide (diuretic).

Signs and symptoms: dermatitis-like rash with red macules (more common), or areas of gray-blue hyperpigmentation (less common), on sun-exposed skin

TINEA VERSICOLOR

This is a fungal overgrowth infection.

Signs and symptoms: white, pink, red, or brown spots that spread slowly and do not tan (they become more noticeable on tanning); dry, scaly (possibly); itchy (possibly); located on the trunk and shoulders (common; also on the back, chest, neck, upper arms)

VITILIGO

This involves the death or dysfunction of melanocytes. It is often associated with autoimmune disease processes.

Signs and symptoms: segmental or localized discolored patches; located anywhere on the body

Papules

PAPULES IN GENERAL

These are raised lesions that may be isolated with distinct borders (e.g., keratoacanthoma) or involved in eruptions (e.g., acne).

KERATOACANTHOMA

These are noncancerous skin growths associated with sun exposure.

Signs and symptoms: round, firm lesions located on sun-exposed skin (face, lips, ears, scalp, neck, back of hands, forearms) that contain characteristic central keratinous material

ACNE VULGARIS

Signs and symptoms: erythema; telangiectasia; presence of whiteheads, blackheads, pustules, nodules, cystic lesions; located on the face, neck, chest, back, shoulders, scalp (usual)

Vesiculobullous

VARICELLA-ZOSTER INFECTION

This causes chickenpox (this is generally a childhood disease, which has become less common because of immunization) and, in adults, shingles. Chickenpox is generally diagnosed clinically.

Signs and symptoms: itchy, red fluid-filled lesions that start on the scalp or trunk (typical) and spread; fever (often)

Investigations: culture of blisters (in suspected shingles)

HERPES SIMPLEX INFECTION

HSV-1 causes oral herpes. HSV-2 causes genital herpes.

Signs and symptoms: burning, sore, or itchy skin for 1 or 2 days before the appearance of the rash; rash composed of ≥ 1 painful, fluid-filled sores that break open, ooze, and form crusts

> Oral herpes: sores on the lips and around the mouth (common); also on the face or tongue
>
> Genital herpes: sores on the penis, vagina, buttocks, and/or anus

CONTACT DERMATITIS

Signs and symptoms: red rash with macules, dry scaly skin, and blisters at the site(s) of allergen contact (e.g., hands)

STEVENS-JOHNSON SYNDROME

This is a rare reaction to medications and/or infections. The most common causes include antigout medications, anticonvulsants, antipsychotics, sulfonamides, nevirapine, and analgesics.

Less than 10% of body surface is affected in Stevens-Johnson syndrome; if > 30% is affected, the condition is toxic epidermal necrolysis by definition.

Signs and symptoms: first, blisters on the skin and the mucous membranes of the mouth, nose, eyes, and genitals; then, painful red or purplish rash

Pustular

IMPETIGO

This is generally diagnosed clinically.

Signs and symptoms: red sores around the mouth and nose (common) that rupture, ooze, and crust over; mild itching and soreness

Risk factors: age 2 to 5 years (more common); attendance at school or day care (common); summer (more common)

FOLLICULITIS

Causes include bacterial infection (e.g., *S. aureus*, *Pseudomonas*) and yeast infection (*Pityrosporum*).

Signs and symptoms: small, raised red- or white-headed lesions around hair follicles that are itchy, burning, and/or tender

Pseudomonas folliculitis ("hot-tub folliculitis"): onset of symptoms 1 to 2 days after exposure to bacteria in a hot tub or swimming pool (common)

Plaques

INFECTIONS (E.G., FUNGAL, LYME DISEASE)

Infectious plaques grow if left untreated.

Signs and symptoms (in general): raised red patches; circular or ring-shaped; no scales

ACANTHOSIS NIGRICANS

This is caused by a systemic condition and typically occurs in obese or diabetic individuals.

Signs and symptoms: slow-developing dark, thick, "velvety" skin; located in folds and creases (e.g., armpits, groin, and neck folds)

ECZEMA, PSORIASIS

Signs and symptoms (in general): raised, red skin lesions or patches (abundant or few); scaly (sometimes: scales are silvery if present); located anywhere on the body

TUMORS

Benign

EPIDERMAL INCLUSION CYST

This is the most common cutaneous cyst. It is usually diagnosed clinically.

Signs and symptoms: age 30 to 40 (more common); male (more common); skin-colored dermal cyst or nodule; visible central punctum; asymptomatic (usually); freely mobile on palpation; located on the face, neck, trunk (common)

If infected: larger, erythematous, painful

Investigations: histology

Premalignant

ACTINIC KERATOSIS

This may progress to invasive squamous cell carcinoma.

Signs and symptoms: adult male (more common); fair skin, older age (common); solitary or multiple lesions; erythematous, scaly macules or papules, or plaques; ≤ 2 cm in diameter; located on sun-exposed skin (balding scalp; neck; backs of hands; top sides of forearms; lower extremities for women); sun damage on surrounding skin (yellow or pale; spotted hyperpigmentation; telangiectasia; xerosis)

Risk factors: chronic sun exposure

Investigations: biopsy to distinguish between actinic keratosis and squamous cell carcinoma

Malignant (e.g., melanoma)

MELANOMA

Signs and symptoms (mnemonic: **ABCDE**): **a**symmetry; **b**order irregularities; **c**olor variation in the same region (deep colored: red-purple-blue-brown-black variations); **d**iameter > 6 mm; **e**volution or enlargement of symptoms over time

Location: sun-exposed skin (common: face, back, arms, legs), but possible anywhere on the body

Risk factors: personal or family history of melanoma; moles (nevi) that are atypical and numerous; sun or UV exposure, especially at a young age; sun-sensitive individuals (light skin; fair hair; high-density freckles; green, blue, or hazel eyes)

Investigations: biopsy

ULCERS

Vascular cause

ARTERIAL INSUFFICIENCY

Signs and symptoms: ischemic ulcers on the feet and ankles; intermittent claudication and atypical pain in the affected muscles

Ischemic ulcers: minor wounds that do not heal (due to lack of blood supply)

Risk factors: male; African descent; age 70 or older; smoking; diabetes; arteriosclerosis; hypertension; hyperlipidemia

Infectious cause

BACTERIAL INFECTION

Signs and symptoms: erythema; warmth; tenderness; swelling; pus or foul smelling discharge at ulcer site

Autoimmune disorder

VASCULITIS

Signs and symptoms: ulcers that are symmetrically distributed; asymptomatic, or associated with pruritus, burning sensations, pain

Vasculitis of small dermal vessels: superficial ulcers with regular borders, palpable purpura, hemorrhagic bullae

Vasculitis of muscular arteries (medium-sized vessels): irregularly shaped, deep ulcers or gangrene; painful red nodules

RA (patients with this condition have chronic ulcers due to vasculitis): deep ulcers on the lower legs (medium-sized vessels vasculitis); nail-fold lesions; palpable purpura; digital ischemic lesions and gangrene; rheumatoid nodules

Investigations: skin biopsy; immunofluorescence on the most recent lesions of the ulcers (< 48 hours) to detect inflammation in vessels

Pressure ulceration

This commonly occurs in residents of nursing homes, and bed- or wheelchair-bound individuals.

The cause is soft tissue compression, usually between a bony prominence and the overlying skin.

Signs and symptoms: nonblanchable erythema of intact skin, or deep ulcers down to the bone; muscle that is resistant and necrotic before the skin breaks; chronic pain (exacerbated by ulcer exam)

Risk factors: immobility, malnutrition, sensory loss, reduced perfusion

Tumors

INVASIVE CUTANEOUS SQUAMOUS CELL CARCINOMA (SCC)

Signs and symptoms: skin ulcers with papules, plaques, or nodules on the head and neck (common; possible anywhere on the body)

Oral SCC: ulcers (or indurated plaques) in the oral cavity (common: floor of the mouth and lateral/ventral tongue); history of tobacco or alcohol use

SCC of the lip: ulcers (or nodules, or indurated white plaques) on the lower lip

Investigations: biopsy

Toxic

SPIDER BITES

Spider bites that become problematic are rare.

Signs and symptoms: ulcer (or papule, pustule, welt, plaque, or ecchymotic plaque at site of bite); mild pain, itching; swelling, burning, numbness, or tingling

Keys to patient encounter

Key concern

Determine whether a condition is benign, malignant, or associated with an underlying condition.

History

HISTORY OF PRESENT ILLNESS

Ask about the location and characteristics of the lesions, and how they have changed. Listen for details of location (e.g., location on sun-exposed skin suggests malignancy or actinic keratosis); pain, itching, and/or discharge (these suggest ulcer or infection); and growth of an individual mole (looking for features of melanoma).

Ask about risk factors for melanoma (sun exposure, family history, fair complexion).

PAST MEDICAL HISTORY

Ask about diabetes, hypertension, hyperlipidemia, and RA (relevant for ulcers).

MEDICATIONS

Ask about drugs that can cause photosensitivity (phenothiazines, TCAs, tetracyclines, sulfonamides, methotrexate, sulfonylureas, chlorothiazide); and recent changes in medication (relevant for possible drug eruptions).

Physical exam

Vital signs: Pursue this if indicated by the history, looking for fever (this suggests viral infection) and hypertension (this is relevant for vascular causes).

Dermatological: Determine the morphology and distribution of the lesions (this will considerably narrow the possible entities: see the differential diagnosis).

Investigations

As appropriate, based on the history and physical exam, consider:

Bacterial, fungal, and viral cultures

Investigations for underlying disease as indicated

IF THE DIAGNOSIS IS IN DOUBT

Skin biopsy

Management

Depending on the specific diagnosis, consider topical or systemic therapy, patient education, and changes to the patient's workplace environment or recreation routine. Consider referral to a dermatologist.

SLEEP-WAKE DISORDERS

Sleep-wake disorders

Differential diagnosis

EXTERNAL FACTORS (E.G., SLEEP DISRUPTION DUE TO POOR SLEEP ENVIRONMENT)

Poor sleep environment

Poor sleep environments may have too much light, too much noise, uncomfortable temperatures (too hot or cold), or cosleepers with sleep disorders (e.g., snoring).

INTRINSIC SLEEP DISORDERS (E.G., CIRCADIAN RHYTHM DISORDERS, INSOMNIA, SLEEP-DISORDERED BREATHING)

Circadian rhythm sleep-wake disorders

Signs and symptoms: symptoms that last > 3 months; chronic or recurrent pattern of insomnia and/or excessive sleepiness; associated daytime distress or impairment

Delayed sleep-wake disorder: adolescents and young adults (high incidence); late bedtime (2 am or later) and late wake time (e.g., 3 pm); undisturbed sleep once initiated; daytime sleepiness and impaired performance when early rising is required (e.g., for school or work)

Advanced sleep-wake disorder: older person (high incidence); early bedtime (6 pm to 9 pm) and early wake time (1 am to 5 am); insomnia; sleepiness in the late afternoon to early evening

Irregular sleep-wake disorder: children with developmental disorders (common); adults with Alzheimer, Parkinson, or Huntington disease (common); no clearly defined circadian rhythm of sleeping and waking

Non-24 hour sleep-wake rhythm disorder: blind patients (common); reduced sleep time; poor sleep quality at night; sleepiness during the daytime

Insomnia

Signs and symptoms: impaired daytime function (difficulty with paying attention, concentration, memory); daytime sleepiness; difficulty falling asleep; difficulty staying asleep; earlier than desired wake time

Short-term insomnia: symptoms that last < 3 months; symptoms related to stressors such as pain, grief, medications, illness, altered sleep environment; resolution of symptoms on cessation of stressor or patient adaptation to stressor

Chronic insomnia: symptoms that last > 3 months and occur ≥ 3 times/week; symptoms related to depression, chronic stress, chronic pain, chronic illness, some medications; in children and young adults, sleep latency or wake periods of > 20 minutes; in adults: sleep latency or wake periods of > 30 minutes

Other insomnia: symptoms of insomnia without meeting the criteria for short-term or chronic insomnia

Risk factors: female (more common); older age; mental health disorder or medical condition; high stress

Sleep-disordered breathing

A common cause is obstructive sleep apnea.

Signs and symptoms: abnormal respiration (apneas or hypopneas); disrupted sleep with snoring, restlessness, resuscitative snorts; difficulty breathing during sleep (during sleep, breathing stops for ≥ 10 seconds despite inspiration efforts); excessive daytime sleepiness, fatigue, poor concentration; nocturnal hypoxemia; morning headache; poorly controlled hypertension

Risk factors (these increase with age): obesity; male; craniofacial and upper airway abnormalities

Investigations: sleep study (polysomnography)

COMORBID CONDITIONS (E.G., PSYCHIATRIC DISORDERS, NEUROLOGIC DISORDERS, SUBSTANCE ABUSE, DYSPNEA)

Psychiatric disorders often present with sleep disruption (e.g., depression, anxiety).

Neurologic disorders (e.g., Alzheimer disease, Parkinson disease, disorders with chronic pain) can present with insomnia associated with physical limitations, reduced social participation, and fatigue.

Substance abuse can cause sleep disruption: insomnia in alcohol abuse; reduction in sleep latency in cannabis use; difficulty falling asleep in cannabis withdrawal; increased sleep latency in cocaine use; and poor sleep efficiency and reduced sleep time in opioid use. Dyspnea is a sign and symptom of comorbid insomnia.

Keys to patient encounter

History

HISTORY OF PRESENT ILLNESS

Ask about the problems the patient has been having with sleep. Listen for evidence of external factors (shift work, sleep environment) and intrinsic factors (pain, illness, emotional stress, dysfunctional circadian rhythms, obstructive sleep apnea).

Ask if the patient has a sleep log or diary with them. If so, ask to review it. If not, obtain a sleep history: ask what time the patient usually goes to bed, what time they usually wake, how well they usually sleep, and what they usually do before going to bed.

Obtain collateral information on the patient's sleep routine, if possible.

PAST MEDICAL HISTORY

Ask about psychiatric conditions and neurological conditions.

SOCIAL HISTORY

Ask about recreational drugs and substance abuse.

Physical exam

Vital signs: Look for hypertension.

Height and weight: Calculate the patient's BMI (see *Notes on labs and assessments*).

Investigations

Polysomnography if the diagnosis is in doubt

Management

Screen the patient for safety concerns (e.g., excessive work-time somnolence).

Counsel the patient on managing their sleep disorder. Treat comorbidities (e.g., substance abuse, obesity).

SORE THROAT AND/OR RHINORRHEA

Sore throat and/or rhinorrhea

Differential diagnosis

INFECTION (E.G., VIRAL, BACTERIAL, CANDIDAL)

Viral infection

Examples include the common cold, influenza, and mononucleosis.

Signs and symptoms: sore throat; rhinorrhea; sneezing; cough; fatigue; myalgia; symptoms that last < 2 weeks (average: 1 week), followed by continued coughing and fatigue

> Influenza: fever, chills, headache, myalgias
>
> Mononucleosis (classic triad): fever, sore throat, lymphadenopathy (usually posterior cervical)

Investigations (mononucleosis): CBC to detect lymphocytosis ($> 50\%$); peripheral blood smear to detect atypical lymphocytes; heterophile antibody test (e.g., Monospot); EBV-specific serology testing (definitive)

Bacterial infection

Examples include group A streptococci and bacterial rhinosinusitis.

Signs and symptoms: sudden-onset sore throat; fever; rhinorrhea; symptoms that last > 10 days or that continue to become worse after 1 week

Investigations: rapid antigen test to detect group A streptococci

Candida (yeast) infection

This is common in healthy infants; immunocompromised patients; patients using antibiotics or inhaled glucocorticoids, or undergoing chemotherapy or radiation.

Signs and symptoms: sore throat; white plaques on the tongue, buccal mucosa, oropharynx, or palate

ALLERGIC CONDITION (E.G., CHRONIC ALLERGIC RHINOSINUSITIS)

Chronic allergic rhinosinusitis

Patients may develop hypersensitivity to allergens over time (sensitivity to low levels of allergens). They often do not seek medical attention until symptoms are severe.

Signs and symptoms: sudden attacks of sneezing; clear rhinorrhea; nasal itching; postnasal drip; cough; irritability; fatigue; **no** fever; **no** myalgia

Perennial allergies (more common) are caused by indoor allergens: dust mites, mold spores, animal dander, and insects.

Seasonal allergies are caused by outdoor allergens: pollens from trees, grasses, and weeds.

OTHER (E.G., TRAUMA, NEOPLASM, FOREIGN BODY)

Trauma

Trauma can cause cerebrospinal-fluid rhinorrhea, which is due to nasal or skull fractures.

Signs and symptoms: clear nasal discharge (unilateral or bilateral) without mucosal inflammation

Neoplasm

Signs and symptoms: chronic sinus congestion; recurrent nasal obstruction; nasal discharge; nosebleeds; unilateral symptoms (**unlike** rhinitis, chronic sinusitis, or nasal polyps, which have similar presentations)

Foreign body

Patients are often young children and those with intellectual disabilities. Foreign bodies can be lodged high in the nasal cavities or paranasal sinuses.

Signs and symptoms: unilateral symptoms (acute or chronic); history of foreign nasal body insertion; sometimes bloody or foul-smelling discharge

Keys to patient encounter

History

Ask when the symptoms started and how often the symptoms are present. Recurrent sore throat and rhinorrhea suggests chronic allergy; sudden onset suggests infection. Ask about symptoms of infection (fever, myalgia, sudden onset); and unilateral versus bilateral rhinorrhea.

Ask whether symptoms are more frequent or less frequent depending on the season.

Physical exam

Vital signs: Look for fever.

Nose and oropharynx: Inspect for inflammation (this suggests infection) and plaques (yeast infection).

Neck: Look for cervical lymphadenopathy (this suggests mononucleosis).

Respiratory: Auscultate the lungs (congestion suggests infection).

Investigations

Based on the history and physical exam, consider:

Group A streptococci swab for culture or rapid antigen test

Heterophile antibodies (e.g., Monospot)

Other specific tests for nonallergy causes of rhinorrhea

Management

Bacterial and fungal infections require treatment, but most viral infections do not. First-line treatment for allergic rhinitis is intranasal steroids or antihistamines.

STRABISMUS AND/OR AMBLYOPIA

Strabismus and/or amblyopia

Differential diagnosis

STRABISMUS AND AMBLYOPIA IN GENERAL

Risk factors: premature birth; low birth weight; family history of strabismus or amblyopia; developmental disability (e.g., Down syndrome, cerebral palsy); head injury

Investigations: cover test; light reflex test

ESOTROPIA (CONVERGENT, INTERNAL, CROSS-EYE): CONGENITAL AND ACQUIRED

Congenital

Signs and symptoms: present at birth; variable angle of deviation (the angle can exceed 50%)

S

Acquired

Signs and symptoms: onset at age 2 to 5 years (usual); relatively small angle of deviation

TRANSIENT (E.G., PRESENT AT YOUNGER THAN 4 MONTHS OF AGE)

Signs and symptoms: strabismus that resolves in early infancy (age 4 months)

> If no resolution by 4 months: test for strabismus (early treatment can prevent permanent disorder)
>
> Pseudostrabismus: some babies have broad epicanthal folds in 1 or both eyes at the inner corner of the eyelids. These reduce the sclera visible toward the nose and make the baby appear cross-eyed.

IDIOPATHIC (ESOTROPIA AND EXOTROPIA)

NEUROGENIC STRABISMUS (E.G., CRANIAL NERVE PARESIS)

Cranial nerve paresis

Impairment of cranial nerves III, IV, and VI can cause the eyes to turn away from the respective muscle. Causes in children include trauma (e.g., birth trauma; head or neck injury); neoplasm; infection (e.g., abscess, VZV, meningitis, CMV); vascular disorder (e.g., diabetes); intracranial disorders (e.g., aneurysm); and neurologic disorder (e.g., pseudotumor cerebri).

Signs and symptoms: strabismus, double vision, drooping eyelid(s), papilledema, history of possible cause (see the previous paragraph)

Investigations: neuroimaging

MYOGENIC STRABISMUS (E.G., MECHANICAL RESTRICTION; NEUROMUSCULAR JUNCTION DEFECT; MUSCLE DISEASE OR INFLAMMATION)

Mechanical restriction

Causes include congenital muscle fibrosis, muscle fibrosis from thyroid disorders (this usually affects adults), and blowout fracture.

Signs and symptoms: compensatory head turning

Neuromuscular junction defect

MYASTHENIA GRAVIS

Signs and symptoms: ocular weakness (usually just this) with drooping eyelid(s), blurred vision, or double vision; oropharyngeal weakness (difficulty speaking; hoarseness; chewing and swallowing difficulty); limb weakness with difficulty climbing stairs, working with elevated arms; fluctuating weakness that is asymmetrical and worse with sustained exercise

Investigations: single fiber electromyography; serum anti-acetylcholine receptor antibody

Muscle disease or inflammation

INHERITED MUSCLE DISEASE

Signs and symptoms: family history of muscle disease (e.g., oculopharyngeal muscular dystrophy, congenital myopathy)

> Oculopharyngeal muscular dystrophy: onset at age 40 to 60; drooping eyelid(s); difficulty swallowing; ocular dysfunction including strabismus
>
> Congenital myopathy: onset during infancy (sometimes); strabismus; drooping eyelid(s); hypotonia; facial weakness; weak sucking and crying; respiratory distress; dysmorphic features

ORBITAL MYOSITIS

Signs and symptoms: sudden onset of symptoms; periocular pain; swollen, red eyelids; restricted eye movement; strabismus

Investigations: CT scan or MRI to detect inflammation of the extraocular muscles

SENSORY STRABISMUS (LOSS OF VISION DUE TO ORGANIC OCULAR ANOMALIES CAUSING STRABISMUS)

Signs and symptoms: unilateral cataract (this is the most common cause; the cataract can be congenital or due to trauma)

> Adolescents or adults: exotropia (usual)
>
> Children (relatively uncommon): onset age 0 to 5 years; esotropia (usual)

S

AMBLYOPIA WITHOUT STRABISMUS

The usual cause is untreated impaired vision in 1 eye in early life, which leads to the brain's reduced reliance on the impaired eye for vision, and altered nerve pathways between the retina and the brain.

Keys to patient encounter

Key concern

Determine the type of strabismus and the necessary urgency of treatment to prevent severe amblyopia.

History

Ask when the strabismus was identified and by whom. Ask about risk factors for strabismus: premature birth; low birth weight; family history of strabismus or amblyopia; developmental disability (e.g., Down syndrome, cerebral palsy); and head injury.

Physical exam

Cover test: Cover 1 eye and wait 1 to 2 seconds; while this eye remains covered, observe the uncovered eye for any shift in fixation.

Light reflex test: Shine a light in the patient's eyes and observe where the light reflects off the corneas (in normal ocular alignment, the light reflects symmetrically from both corneas; within each cornea, the reflection is slightly off-center, toward the nose).

OLDER CHILDREN AND ADULTS

Visual acuity

Cranial nerves

Management

Refer patients with strabismus to an ophthalmologist for immediate management.

SUBSTANCE ABUSE

Substance-related or addictive condition

Differential diagnosis

ADDICTION IN GENERAL

Signs and symptoms: need to use a substance, or engage in a behavior, every day; increasing need for the substance or behavior; maintaining the substance use or behavior despite negative consequences (e.g., financial trouble, jeopardized relationships); taking risks because of the substance use or behavior (e.g., driving under the influence; unprotected sex; bankruptcy); unsuccessful attempts to quit; experiencing withdrawal symptoms on attempts to quit

SUBSTANCE USE

Stimulants

Examples of stimulants include cocaine, amphetamines, and methamphetamine.

Signs and symptoms: increased alertness, energy; restlessness; aggression; irritability; paranoia; rapid speech; insomnia; anorexia or weight loss; hypertension; pupillary dilation; feeling of excess confidence and exhilaration; depression as the effects of the drug wear off

Withdrawal: dysphoria; excessive sleep; hunger; severe psychomotor retardation; **no** effect on vital functions

Depressants

Examples of depressants include sedative hypnotics (e.g., barbiturates, benzodiazepines).

Patients with chronic pain are at a higher risk of overdose.

Signs and symptoms: drowsiness; dizziness; ataxia; euphoria or an exaggerated feeling of well-being; slurred speech; lack of coordination; impaired concentration and memory; nystagmus; low BP; slowed breathing; depression

Withdrawal (symptoms start 2 to 10 days after abrupt discontinuation): psychomotor and autonomic dysfunction; other symptoms that resemble alcohol withdrawal (see below)

S

Other substances

OPIOIDS

Signs and symptoms: low respiratory rate; pinpoint pupils; feeling of euphoria; drowsiness; psychomotor retardation; slurred speech; impaired memory, concentration, judgment; skin abrasions from scratching (track marks or pock marks if the opioid is injected); possible avoidance of physical exam, lab tests, treatment referrals

Withdrawal: rhinorrhea, sneezing, yawning, tears, abdominal and leg cramping, goose bumps, nausea, vomiting, diarrhea, dilated pupils

ALCOHOL

Signs and symptoms: tremor in the hands or tongue; unexplained trauma; signs of malnutrition (delayed wound healing, frequent severe infections, wasting, cachexia); cirrhosis; liver disease; oral cancer; gynecomastia in men

Mild withdrawal (symptoms start within 24 hours of last alcoholic drink): tremulousness, insomnia, anxiety, hyperreflexia, sweating, GI upset, mild autonomic hyperactivity

Moderate withdrawal (symptoms start within 24 to 48 hours of last drink): tremors, insomnia, intense anxiety, excessive adrenergic symptoms

Severe withdrawal (symptoms start > 48 hours after last drink): disorientation, agitation, hallucinations, tremulousness, tachycardia, tachypnea, hyperthermia, sweating

NICOTINE

Signs and symptoms: smoking > 20 cigarettes/day or smoking the first cigarette within 30 minutes of waking up; giving up activities (e.g., visiting nonsmoking family or friends) because of smoking

Withdrawal: increased appetite; anxiety; irritability; impaired concentration; depressed mood; insomnia; constipation or diarrhea

Risk factors for relapse: other smokers in the household; other substance use or alcohol use; depression or other psychiatric disorder; high levels of stress

CANNABIS

Signs and symptoms: heightened sense of visual, auditory, and taste perception; hypertension and tachycardia; red eyes; dry mouth; decreased coordination and reaction time; impaired memory and concentration; increased appetite; paranoia

Withdrawal: mood changes (depressed mood, irritability, anxiety); changes in sleep patterns; changes in appetite; nausea; stomach pain

PROCESS (BEHAVIORAL) ADDICTIONS (E.G., GAMBLING)

Gambling disorder[1(p585)]

Signs and symptoms: symptoms that are present for ≥ 1 year; symptoms that can include gambling with increasing amounts of money, unsuccessful attempts to quit gambling, continuing to gamble despite negative consequences (e.g., jeopardized relationships, work), reliance on others for money because of gambling, irritability (or edginess) on attempts to quit

FACTORS IN ADDICTION

Adverse childhood or traumatic experiences

These include abuse (physical, sexual, emotional); neglect (physical, emotional); exposure to domestic violence; and family dysfunction due to divorce (or separation), substance abuse, mental illness, or imprisonment.

Epigenetic changes

Drug-specific epigenetic changes occur mainly in the nucleus accumbens of the brain.

Substances that cause epigenetic changes include cocaine (with chronic use and addiction); opioids and methadone; and alcohol (with acute and chronic use).

Comorbid illness (e.g., mental illness, chronic disease states, trauma)

Patients may abuse substances to manage the symptoms of comorbid illnesses.

Patients with chronic disease and/or chronic pain can require opioids to manage their symptoms, and are at risk of opioid addiction. They may also use illicit drugs and alcohol to manage associated depression and anxiety.

Psychosocial stressors (e.g., unemployment, social isolation)

S

Keys to patient encounter

Key concerns

Identify the issue.

Identify potential consequences.

Provide immediate and continuing support and intervention.

History

HISTORY OF PRESENT ILLNESS

Seek collateral information (e.g., from an accompanying caregiver) if the patient is unable to answer or if you suspect the answers may not be accurate.

Assess the patient's risk of addiction (see the pointer on the CAGE questionnaire).

In suspected addiction, assess the risk of harm to the patient. Ask about financial problems; problems with relationships; problems with work or school performance; risk-taking behaviors such as impaired driving and unprotected sex while impaired; and withdrawal symptoms on trying to quit using a substance.

PAST MEDICAL HISTORY

Ask about chronic illnesses, and a history of addictions or substance abuse.

SOCIAL HISTORY

Ask where the patient lives and with whom. Ask who is in their family and whether the family has a history of abuse (e.g., physical, sexual) or a history of substance abuse. Determine whether the patient is in a relationship, and whether the patient has children (and if so, where the children are). Ask about the patient's work, and whether the patient has been in trouble with the law or has been to prison.

Physical exam

Vital signs: Look for evidence of drug or alcohol withdrawal (tachycardia, hyperthermia).

POINTER

CAGE questionnaire for addiction screening

The CAGE questionnaire is a brief, commonly used screening tool for alcohol addiction. **CAGE** is a mnemonic for **c**ut down, **a**nnoyed, **g**uilty, **e**ye-opener. You can adapt it for drug addiction:

- Have you ever felt the need to cut down on your drinking (or substance use)?
- Have people annoyed you by criticizing your drinking (or substance use)?
- Have you ever felt guilty about drinking (or substance use)?
- Have you ever felt you needed an eye-opener first thing in the morning (take a drink or use a substance)?

Investigations

Liver function in suspected alcohol abuse (see *Notes on labs and assessments*)

HIV and hepatitis in suspected IV drug use

Management

In suspected addiction, refer the patient to an addiction program, and to family counseling and mental health services. Provide specific treatment for substance withdrawal, if needed (see the pointer on treating withdrawal syndromes).

Administer antidotes in the event of acute intoxication (e.g., naloxone for opioids, flumazenil for benzodiazepines).

POINTER

Treatment for withdrawal syndromes

SYNDROME	TREATMENT
Alcohol withdrawal syndrome	Treat with sedative-hypnotic drugs (benzodiazepines, barbiturates, propofol). Moderate-to-severe withdrawal requires inpatient treatment with admission to ICU. Mild withdrawal can be treated on an outpatient basis.
Sedative-hypnotic withdrawal syndrome	Treat with long-acting benzodiazepine or phenobarbital. Provide a maintenance dose for a few days followed by decreasing doses over 2 to 3 weeks.
Opioid withdrawal syndrome	Treat with a long-acting opioid agonist (20–35 mg/d methadone or 4–16 mg/d buprenorphine, followed by tapering over days to weeks). A dose of 0.1–0.2 mg every 4 to 8 hours decreases the severity of symptoms. Long-acting benzodiazepines can be added to control insomnia and muscle cramps.
Stimulant withdrawal syndrome	There are no specific medications to treat this syndrome. Observe the patient.

S

REFERENCE

1. American Psychiatric Association. Diagnostic and statistical manual of mental disorders. 5th ed. Arlington, VA: American Psychiatric Association; 2013. 991 p.

SUBSTANCE ABUSE

Substance withdrawal

Differential diagnosis

CHEMICAL DEPENDENCIES AND WITHDRAWAL SYMPTOMS (E.G., ALCOHOL, ILLICIT DRUGS, TOBACCO, PRESCRIPTION DRUGS)

Alcohol

Withdrawal symptoms:

Mild withdrawal (symptoms start within 24 hours of last alcoholic drink): tremulousness, insomnia, anxiety, hyperreflexia, sweating, GI upset, mild autonomic hyperactivity

Moderate withdrawal (symptoms start within 24 to 48 hours of last drink): tremors, insomnia, intense anxiety, excessive adrenergic symptoms

Severe withdrawal (symptoms start > 48 hours after last drink): disorientation, agitation, hallucinations, tremulousness, tachycardia, tachypnea, hyperthermia, sweating

Illicit drugs

COCAINE, METHAMPHETAMINE

Withdrawal symptoms: dysphoria; excessive sleep; hunger; severe psychomotor retardation; **no** effect on vital functions

CANNABIS

Withdrawal symptoms: irritability, anxiety, insomnia, bad dreams, weight loss, depressed mood, at least 1 physical symptom (abdominal pain; tremors or shakiness; sweating; fever; chills; headache)

Tobacco

Withdrawal symptoms: increased appetite; anxiety; irritability; impaired concentration; depressed mood; insomnia; constipation or diarrhea

Risk factors for relapse: other smokers in the household; alcohol use or other substance use; depression or other psychiatric disorder; high levels of stress

Prescription drugs (and heroin)

OPIOIDS

Withdrawal symptoms: rhinorrhea, sneezing, yawning, tears, abdominal and leg cramping, goose bumps, nausea, vomiting, diarrhea, dilated pupils

Heroin: peak symptoms at 36 to 72 hours; symptom duration 7 to 10 days

Methadone: peak symptoms at 72 to 96 hours; symptom duration 2 weeks

Keys to patient encounter

Key objective

Provide immediate and continuing support and intervention.

Airway and hemodynamic status

Check the patient's ABCs. Provide emergency supportive measures (airway, fluid resuscitation, pain management), as needed.

History

HISTORY OF PRESENT ILLNESS

Seek collateral information (e.g., from an accompanying caregiver) if the patient is unable to answer or if you suspect the answers may not be accurate.

Ask what substance the patient is using, how often, and for how long. Determine the last time the patient used the substance. In the case of drugs, determine whether the drugs are street or prescription drugs.

Perform a mental status exam to assess for agitation and disorientation (see the pointer).

SOCIAL HISTORY

Ask where the patient lives and with whom. Ask who is in their family and whether the family has a history of abuse (e.g., physical, sexual) or a history of substance abuse. Determine whether the patient is in a relationship, and whether the patient has children (and if so, where the children are). Ask about the patient's work, and whether the patient has been in trouble with the law or has been to prison.

Physical exam

Focus the physical exam on identifying signs of withdrawal.

Vital signs: Look for rapid pulse, high BP.

General inspection: Look for dilated pupils, sweating, and confusion.

Balance and gait: Assess for tremulousness and ataxia.

Investigations

Urine drug screen to confirm which classes of drugs are being used

Management

Identify the type of withdrawal syndrome based on patient history and symptoms (see the differential diagnosis). Ensure a safe environment (hospital, recovery center). Provide specific treatment based on the withdrawal syndrome (see the pointer on treating withdrawal syndromes). If appropriate, refer the patient to an addiction program, and to family counseling and mental health services.

POINTER

Mental status exams

Mental status exams use both observation and direct questioning to make assessments. Generally, they assess:

- general appearance and behavior
- mood
- speech: rate, tone, volume
- thought content: obsessions, preoccupations, hallucinations, delusions, suicidal ideation, homicidal ideation
- thought process: circumstantial, tangential, flight of ideas, loosening of associations
- orientation to time and place
- attention and concentration
- patient insight into their present condition

POINTER

Treatment for withdrawal syndromes

SYNDROME	TREATMENT
Alcohol withdrawal syndrome	Treat with sedative-hypnotic drugs (benzodiazepines, barbiturates, propofol). Moderate-to-severe withdrawal requires inpatient treatment with admission to ICU. Mild withdrawal can be treated on an outpatient basis.

(*Continued on next page*)

SYNDROME	TREATMENT
Sedative-hypnotic withdrawal syndrome	Treat with long-acting benzodiazepine or phenobarbital. Provide a maintenance dose for a few days followed by decreasing doses over 2 to 3 weeks.
Opioid withdrawal syndrome	Treat with a long-acting opioid agonist (20–35 mg/d methadone or 4–16 mg/d buprenorphine, followed by tapering over days to weeks). A dose of 0.1–0.2 mg every 4 to 8 hours decreases the severity of symptoms. Long-acting benzodiazepines can be added to control insomnia and muscle cramps.
Stimulant withdrawal syndrome	There are no specific medications to treat this syndrome. Observe the patient.

SYNCOPE AND PRESYNCOPE

Syncope and presyncope

Differential diagnosis

CARDIOVASCULAR CONDITION

Cardiac arrhythmia

Signs and symptoms: light-headedness or fainting; shortness of breath; tachycardia or bradycardia; hypotension

Investigations: ECG

Reduced cardiac output (e.g., aortic stenosis, myocardial infarction)

AORTIC STENOSIS

Signs and symptoms: chest pain; feeling faint, fainting with exertion; shortness of breath, especially on exertion; fatigue, especially during and after exertion; palpitations

Risk factors: bicuspid aortic valve; older age; history of rheumatic fever

Investigations: echocardiogram; chest x-ray; coronary angiography; CT scan; MRI; ECG to measure electrical impulses from the heart muscle; exercise testing

MYOCARDIAL INFARCTION

Presyncope signs and symptoms: symptom onset over hours to weeks; fatigue; palpitations; sleep disturbance; chest discomfort

Other symptoms: shortness of breath; nausea, vomiting; weakness; sweating; chest pain or pressure usually in substernal region radiating to the neck, jaw, left shoulder, left arm; pain on exertion (often)

Syncope signs and symptoms: sudden collapse (the patient is unresponsive to touch and sound; is not breathing or has abnormal breathing such as gasping); hypertension or hypotension; bradycardia or tachycardia (possible: vital signs are often unremarkable)

Investigations: ECG to identify type of infarction (STEMI, NSTEMI); cardiac troponin (preferred diagnostic biomarker)

Reflex or underfilling (e.g., vasovagal, orthostatic)

VASOVAGAL SYNCOPE

This is the most common type of syncope, and is common in young and healthy patients with or without cardiac or neurologic disease, and in athletes.

Signs and symptoms: triggered by emotional or orthostatic distress (fear; pain; prolonged standing; seeing or using needles) (diagnostic)

Older patients: triggered by cough, urination, defecation, swallowing (possible)

ORTHOSTATIC HYPOTENSION

This is the most common cause of syncope among the elderly. It may be idiopathic or related to Parkinson disease.

Signs and symptoms: light-headedness or dizziness on standing after sitting or lying down

BP signs: normal BP when upright; on standing after lying down for 5 minutes, ≥ 20 mmHg fall in systolic BP and ≥ 10 mmHg fall in diastolic BP within 2 to 5 minutes (diagnostic)

CEREBROVASCULAR CAUSES (E.G., CAROTID ARTERY DISEASE, TRANSIENT ISCHEMIC ATTACK)

Carotid artery disease

Signs and symptoms: dizziness; loss of balance; blurred vision or loss of vision; confusion; loss of memory or sensation; speech or language problems; weakness in the face or limbs; bruits in carotid arteries in the neck on auscultation

Investigations: serum lipids and glucose levels; US of the carotid arteries to observe the quality of blood flow; angiography to examine blood vessels in the neck and brain

Transient ischemic attack

TIAs cause no permanent damage, but 1 in 3 patients have a stroke within a year.

Signs and symptoms: symptoms that resolve within a few minutes (usual); weakness, numbness, paralysis (unilateral); slurred speech; difficulty understanding others; loss of vision in 1 or both eyes, double vision; dizziness; loss of balance and/or coordination

Embolic TIA: symptoms that last hours, or are infrequent, or that present differently (depending on the migration of the emboli)

Risk factors: family or personal history of TIA or stroke; older than 55; anemia or sickle cell disease; hypertension; high cholesterol; cardiovascular disease; diabetes; obesity; smoking; excessive alcohol intake

OTHER

Metabolic disorder (e.g., hypoglycemia)

HYPOGLYCEMIA

Metabolic disorders rarely cause syncope. Hypoglycemia is the most common metabolic cause and is usually due to diabetes treatment.

Signs and symptoms: palpitations, pallor, nightmares, fatigue, hunger

Severe: confusion, disorientation, blurred vision, seizures, coma

Investigations: low plasma glucose level (symptoms typically develop at concentrations ≤ 54 mg/dL [3.0 mmol/L])

Drugs (e.g., antihypertensive medications)

Psychiatric disorder (e.g., panic disorders)

PANIC ATTACKS[1(pp189–234)]

Panic attacks can arise from anxiety disorders, such as generalized anxiety disorder, panic disorder, separation anxiety disorder, social anxiety disorder, and specific phobia. In panic disorder, panic attacks occur spontaneously. In other anxiety disorders, panic attacks can have specific triggers (e.g., phobic objects in specific phobia).

Signs and symptoms: history of anxiety disorder and/or symptoms consistent with a panic attack; history of social or emotional triggers for symptoms (possible); lack of evidence for other causes, including hyperthyroidism (anxiety can mimic other conditions and is therefore a diagnosis of exclusion)

Panic attack: symptoms that peak within minutes; symptoms that can include palpitations, accelerated heart rate, shortness of breath, chest pain, dizziness, numbness or tingling, fear of losing control, fear of dying

Keys to patient encounter

The differential diagnosis for this clinical presentation is challenging. It includes a common, benign entity (vasovagal syncope) and a number of life-threatening entities. Often, extensive investigations are needed to determine a cause.

Key concerns

Differentiate syncope from seizure (see the pointer).

Identify patients with syncope due to serious underlying disease.

POINTER

Differentiating syncope and seizure

SYNCOPE

This is an abrupt, transient, complete loss of consciousness that results in postural tone loss. It is followed by spontaneous recovery.

Loss of consciousness has rapid onset and short duration.

It occurs when the patient is in an upright position and resolves when the patient is supine. Tilt-table testing, which changes the patient's position from supine to upright, is useful in diagnosing syncope.

SEIZURE

Epileptic tonic-clonic seizures can induce syncope. This is characterized by a longer duration of unconsciousness than other types of syncope.

Urinary incontinence and tongue biting during an episode suggest seizure rather than syncope.

Electroencephalography confirms seizures.

History

HISTORY OF PRESENT ILLNESS

Ask about the circumstances surrounding the attack: what the patient was doing and what happened. Examples of characteristic features include:

Cardiovascular condition: chest pain

Vasovagal syncope: dizziness triggered by fear or prolonged standing

Orthostatic syncope: dizziness triggered by standing after sitting

Cerebrovascular causes: vision disturbances and slurred speech

Ask about previous similar episodes.

PAST MEDICAL HISTORY

Ask about hypertension, diabetes, heart disease, Parkinson disease, epilepsy, and mental health disorders.

FAMILY HISTORY

Ask about instances of sudden death.

MEDICATIONS

Ask about antihypertensives, antidepressants, and antiarrhythmics.

Physical exam

Vital signs: Obtain supine and standing BP (looking for orthostatic hypotension).

Cardiovascular: Auscultate the heart.

Respiratory: Auscultate the lungs.

Carotid artery: Auscultate for bruits.

Neurological: Look for focal neurological deficits.

Abdominal: Palpate for AAA.

Investigations

ECG to look for cardiac rhythm disturbances

CBC to look for anemia

Serum glucose

OTHER SPECIFIC TESTS

24-hour (Holter) ECG monitor in suspected arrhythmia

Echocardiogram in patients with a history of heart disease or abnormal ECG to look for valvular disease

Tilt-table testing in unexplained syncope to look for bradycardia or hypotension suggestive of reflex-mediated syncope

IN SUSPECTED CEREBROVASCULAR CAUSE

EEG

Carotid Doppler

CT scan or MRI of the brain

Management

Specific management depends on the probable cause identified from the history, physical

POINTER

Unexplained syncope in the elderly

In elderly patients, consider the possibility of AAA as a cause of unexplained syncope.

exam, and investigations. Refer patients with an unknown cause to an internist for further investigation.

REFERENCE

1. American Psychiatric Association. Diagnostic and statistical manual of mental disorders. 5th ed. Arlington, VA: American Psychiatric Association; 2013. 991 p.

THROMBOSIS (PREVENTION OF VENOUS THROMBOSIS)

Thrombosis (prevention of venous thrombosis)

Differential diagnosis

STASIS (E.G., HOSPITALIZATION, TRAVEL)

ENDOTHELIAL INJURY (E.G., PREVIOUS THROMBOSIS)

HYPERCOAGULABILITY (E.G., DRUGS, CANCER, INHERITED OR ACQUIRED CONDITIONS)

Drugs

Examples include chemotherapy and heparin.

Cancer

Metastatic cancer is particularly associated with hypercoagulability.

Inherited conditions

SICKLE CELL DISEASE

Signs and symptoms: family history of sickle cell disease; painful swelling of the hands and feet

Investigations: CBC to detect anemia, sickle cells; positive sickle cell screen; abnormalities on peripheral blood smear; abnormalities on hemoglobin electrophoresis

CONGENITAL CLOTTING FACTOR ABNORMALITIES

These include protein C deficiency, protein S deficiency, antithrombin III deficiency, and factor V Leiden deficiency.

Signs and symptoms: family history of thrombosis; thrombosis starting at a young age; recurrent thrombosis

Acquired conditions

Examples include hypercoagulability due to pregnancy, smoking, old age, OCs, and estrogen replacement therapy.
Investigations: positive lupus anticoagulant test, positive anticardiolipin antibody test

Keys to patient encounter

Key concerns

Identify patients who may be at risk of venous thrombosis.
Assess the risk and intervene as warranted.

History

Ask about risk factors for venous thrombosis: a personal or family history of venous thrombosis; prolonged immobilization; recent surgery; current pregnancy; use of OCs or HRT; smoking; personal history of cancer, HF, inflammatory bowel disease; and age older than 60. Check for current signs and symptoms of DVT (e.g., recent stroke or uncontrolled severe hypertension; red, painful, warm, and/or swollen calf), and PE (shortness of breath, pleuritic chest pain, tachycardia, hemoptysis). In women, ask about recurrent pregnancy loss (this is a possible sign of an inherited coagulation defect).

Physical exam

Height and weight: Calculate the patient's BMI (see *Notes on labs and assessments*).

Respiratory: Look for signs of PE: in particular, lung rales on auscultation, and lower-lung dullness on percussion.

Legs: Look for signs of DVT: in particular, a swollen calf that is erythematous, tender, and > 3 cm larger than the other calf when measured 10 cm distal to the tibial tuberosity.

Investigations

Consider investigations for underlying conditions (e.g., age-appropriate cancer screening in the case of unprovoked venous thromboembolism).

Management

In asymptomatic patients at risk of venous thrombosis, suggest lifestyle changes such as weight loss, exercise, and smoking cessation. Consider compression stockings.

Treat DVT or PE with anticoagulant therapy (in hemodynamically unstable patients with PE, treat with IV thrombolysis). Prescribe LMWH and overlap this therapy with warfarin or direct oral anticoagulants (dabigatran, rivaroxaban; there is no need to overlap in the case of apixaban or edoxaban). Treatment is continued for 3 to 6 months. Consider indefinite treatment or a change to acetylsalicylic acid in patients with an underlying coagulopathy or nonmodifiable risk factors.

TRAUMA EMERGENCY

Trauma emergency

Keys to patient encounter

Trauma emergencies can involve blunt trauma or penetrating trauma. Provide an emergency referral to a trauma team, implement the local trauma protocol, or follow the Advanced Trauma Life Support (ATLS) guidelines. Trauma protocols involve primary, secondary, and tertiary surveys to ensure all injuries are assessed.

Steps in emergency management

PRIMARY SURVEY

Perform these steps (mnemonic **ABCDE**):

Airway and cervical spine: Protect the C-spine (immobilize the patient with a collar), provide oxygen, assess the airway.

Breathing: Inspect the chest for abnormalities; assess pulse oximetry and ABG.

Circulation and hemorrhage control: Assess shock; assess tissue perfusion; control bleeding from the chest and abdomen; monitor BP.

Disability: Perform a brief neurological exam; assess the patient's level of consciousness with the GCS; check the pupils; monitor blood sugar.

Expose: Assess temperature, undress, cover.

SECONDARY SURVEY

When you have completed the primary survey, immediately start on a secondary survey, which includes:

History: Ask about the mechanism of injury to determine the likely severity of the injury and the possibility of other associated injuries. If the patient is unable to give a history, seek information from an accompanying caregiver.

Full regional physical exam: The purpose of this exam is to identify all injuries.

NEXT STEPS

Start IV access with normal saline or Ringer's lactate, and give supplemental oxygen.

Perform a tertiary survey, which is a series of complete regional physical exams to look for missed injuries, identify complications, and assess the patient's response to resuscitation.

INVESTIGATIONS

Investigations should be deferred in unstable patients.

CBC

POINTER

Glasgow Coma Scale

The GSC scores the way a patient's eyes and limbs respond to stimulus, and the patient's facility with speech.

Patients with a normal level of consciousness can open their eyes spontaneously, move appropriately in response to verbal commands, and speak cogently.

Patients whose level of consciousness is compromised may only respond to pain stimulus, and may have garbled speech or only make sounds.

Patients who are unconscious do not respond to any stimulus and do not speak.

Versions of the GCS are available online.

Blood type and screen in case the patient needs a blood transfusion

Other specific tests as indicated by the findings of the primary and secondary surveys (e.g., imaging, ECG)

TRAUMA, SPECIFIC INJURIES

Abdominal injuries

Keys to patient encounter

Causes of abdominal injuries include blunt trauma (e.g., blast injuries, deceleration injuries) and penetrating trauma (e.g., stab wounds, gunshot wounds).

Airway and hemodynamic status

Check the patient's ABCs. Begin resuscitation, as required. For serious injuries, provide an emergency referral to a trauma team, implement the local trauma protocol, or follow the Advanced Trauma Life Support (ATLS) guidelines (see *Trauma emergency*).

History

Perform a history and physical exam at the same time. If the patient is unable to give a history, seek information from an accompanying caregiver.

Ask about the mechanism of the injury to determine the likely severity of the injury and the possibility of other associated injuries. Ask about preexisting medical conditions, previous surgeries, and medications and allergies.

Physical exam

Remember that abdominal injuries commonly occur in association with other serious injuries, including thoracic and spinal injuries. Hypovolemia and/or shock are common signs of abdominal injury.

Vital signs: Look for tachycardia and hypotension.

General inspection: Look for sweating; cold, pale, or bluish skin; and altered level of consciousness.

Cardiovascular: Auscultate the heart.

Respiratory:

- Look for tachypnea.
- Auscultate the lungs.

Abdomen: Look for swelling, bruising, tenderness, and bowel sounds.

Lower limbs: Check for sensation and motor function.

Investigations

CBC to look for anemia due to intraabdominal blood loss

- Note, however, that in acute situations hemoglobin may be normal even with significant blood loss.

Blood type and screen in case the patient needs a blood transfusion

Urinalysis to look for hematuria, which may indicate injury to the bladder, kidneys, or ureter

US or CT scan without contrast of the abdomen to investigate the extent of the injury and identify associated occult injuries

Peritoneal lavage in suspected intraabdominal blood loss

Management

Establish IV access, admit the patient to hospital, and consult general surgery.

POINTER

Blunt trauma and multisystem injury

Blunt trauma typically involves a larger area of impact on the abdomen, and so has a greater risk of multisystem injury. This is especially true in events such as impact with an object, fall from a height, and motor vehicle accident.

TRAUMA, SPECIFIC INJURIES

Bone or joint injury

Differentiation of causes

HIGH ENERGY TRAUMA

Common causes include motor vehicle accidents, industrial accidents (e.g., explosions), and falls from heights. These injuries usually occur with other emergent injuries.

NONACCIDENTAL INJURY (E.G., DOMESTIC VIOLENCE, CHILD ABUSE)

Adult or intimate partner abuse

Signs and symptoms: disclosed abuse (victims do not always disclose abuse); bruising, scars, healed fractures; recurrent symptoms or injuries; resistance by the partner to having the patient interviewed alone (usual)

Risk factors: pregnancy; threat to leave; partner's history of violence or substance abuse

Child abuse

Signs and symptoms: disclosed abuse (victims do not always disclose abuse); resistance by the parent or caregiver to having the patient interviewed alone (usual); inconsistency between an injury and the explanation for the injury and/or the developmental stage of the child; other injuries (e.g., facial contusions; marks on the neck or limbs; burn marks; ligature marks on the wrists and ankles; bite marks; lash marks)

Risk factors: history of substance abuse by the parents or caregiver; unstable living situation of the parents or caregiver; dysfunctional domestic dynamics

FALLS

Examples include slipping, tripping, or loss of balance.

Causes include vertigo, gait disturbances (e.g., due to Parkinson disease), syncope, cognitive impairment, substance abuse, medications (e.g., antipsychotics, narcotics, antihypertensives), environmental factors (e.g., loose rugs), decreased vision, and urinary urgency (e.g., due to UTI).

PATHOLOGIC CONDITIONS PREDISPOSING TO INJURY (E.G., OSTEOPOROSIS, LIGAMENTOUS LAXITY, METASTATIC DISEASE)

Osteoporosis

Common sites of fracture are the hip, wrist, and spine.

Signs and symptoms: back pain, loss of height, stooped posture

Risk factors: postmenopausal patients; Caucasian or Asian descent; family history of osteoporosis; history of hyperthyroidism, eating disorders, bariatric surgery, bowel-removing surgery, celiac disease, inflammatory bowel disease, kidney disease, liver disease, cancer, SLE, multiple myeloma, RA; use of steroids or medications for seizures, GERD, cancer, transplant rejection; diet low in calcium

Investigations: bone density scan

Ligamentous laxity

Signs and symptoms: hypermobile joints (joints bend beyond the normal range of motion); family history of ligamentous laxity; chronic joint pain; frequent injuries such as sprains, dislocations

Metastatic disease

Bone lesions can arise from a primary malignancy (e.g., multiple myeloma) or metastatic malignancy (e.g., breast, prostate, lung). Common sites of fracture are the extremities and spine. The most common location is the proximal femur.

Signs and symptoms: bone pain; spontaneous fracture, or fracture with minimal trauma

Investigations: imaging (x-ray, CT scan, or MRI), bone scan, investigations for primary tumor location (if no known history of malignancy)

Keys to patient encounter

History

HISTORY OF PRESENT ILLNESS

Ask how the injury happened. Note whether minimal force was involved (this suggests bone weakened by a pathologic condition).

Ask about recurrent falls.

Ask about factors that may indicate abuse (e.g., recurrent injuries, resistance of a caregiver to having the patient interviewed alone, unexplained injuries in a child).

PAST MEDICAL HISTORY

Ask about predisposing conditions: history of cancer, osteoporosis, steroid use, and chronic disease.

In injury resulting from minimal force, ask about risk factors for osteoporosis (see the differential diagnosis) and about joint hypermobility.

IN RECURRENT FALLS OR SUSPECTED ABUSE

See:

Adult abuse, intimate partner abuse (under *Abuse, violence*)

Child abuse (under *Abuse, violence*)

Falls (under *Geriatric concerns*)

Physical exam

In addition to the injury itself, perform a targeted exam to exclude other injuries depending on the mechanism of injury.

Area of injury: Examine the area of the injury, paying particular attention to neurological and vascular status.

Spine: Rule out injury to the spine.

Investigations

X-ray or CT scan of the injured area

Management

FRACTURES

Fractures require reduction and immobilization in a cast. Refer the patient to an orthopedic surgeon for injuries that cannot be reduced or require internal fixation.

INJURY CAUSED BY PATHOLOGIC CONDITION

Treat the underlying condition. Refer the patient to an oncologist, medical specialist, and/or orthopedic surgeon as appropriate.

TRAUMA, SPECIFIC INJURIES

Chest injuries

Keys to patient encounter

Causes of chest injuries include blunt trauma (e.g., blast injuries, deceleration injuries) and penetrating trauma (e.g., stab wounds, gunshot wounds).

Key concern

Patients often present in shock or with respiratory distress: prompt resuscitation is the priority.

Airway and hemodynamic status

Check the patient's ABCs. Begin resuscitation, as required. For serious injuries, provide an emergency referral to a trauma team, implement the local trauma protocol, or follow the Advanced Trauma Life Support (ATLS) guidelines (see *Trauma emergency*).

History

Perform a history and physical exam at the same time. If the patient is unable to give a history, seek information from an accompanying caregiver.

Ask about the mechanism of the injury to determine the likely severity of the injury and the possibility of other associated injuries. Ask about preexisting medical conditions, previous surgeries, medications, and allergies.

Physical exam

Keep the most common life-threatening chest injuries in mind: aortic rupture, pericardial tamponade, tension pneumothorax, and massive hemothorax.

Chest: Examine the front and back.

Spine: Palpate for tenderness

Cardiovascular: Auscultate the heart.

Respiratory: Auscultate the lungs.

Investigations

Chest x-ray and/or CT scan
ECG

Management

Insert a chest tube for pneumothorax.
Admit the patient to hospital and consult thoracic surgery.

TRAUMA, SPECIFIC INJURIES

Drowning (near drowning)

Keys to patient encounter

Causes of near drowning include inability to swim (e.g., overestimation of capability), risk-taking behavior, boating accidents, alcohol and substance abuse (this accounts for more than 50% of adult drowning deaths), and inadequate adult supervision. Concomitant clinical difficulties include trauma, seizure, cardiovascular accident, and cardiac event.

Airway and hemodynamic status

Check the patient's ABCs. Initiate CPR if needed.

History

History taking will not be helpful in this clinical presentation, other than to establish that you are treating a victim of near drowning.

Physical exam

Monitor the patient's core body temperature. Identify any coexisting trauma (including spinal cord injury) and implement appropriate precautions.

Investigations

Conduct investigations for suspected complications as clinically indicated, including:

ECG (this is recommended)
CBC
Electrolytes (see *Notes on labs and assessments*)
ABG
Chest x-ray
PT/INR
PTT
Urinalysis
Urine drug screen
Urine myoglobin

POINTER

Priorities in near drowning

The primary focus of treatment is to recover adequate ventilation, oxygenation, and perfusion: hypoxia is the most common cause of death by drowning.

Management

Initiate additional supportive therapy: oxygen, IV fluid therapy, and correction of hypothermia. (CPR must continue until the patient's body temperature is 32–35°C.)

Recognize and manage possible complications: cerebral edema; anoxic or ischemic encephalopathy; cardiovascular collapse; cardiac dysrhythmia; ARDS; and coexisting trauma.

TRAUMA, SPECIFIC INJURIES

Facial injuries

Keys to patient encounter

Causes of facial injury include trauma (e.g., blunt, penetrating, or crush injuries) and burns.

Key concerns

Assess and control vital functions.

Make life-threatening injuries the management priority.

Airway and hemodynamic status

Check the patient's ABCs:

Airway: This may be blocked by blood, broken teeth, posterior retraction of the tongue, edema from neck damage, or foreign objects.

Breathing: Facial injury can be associated with brain injury, which can compromise breathing.

Circulation: The patient may be actively bleeding through the nose or ears, and possibly into the brain.

For serious injuries, provide an emergency referral to a trauma team, implement the local trauma protocol, or follow the Advanced Trauma Life Support (ATLS) guidelines (see *Trauma emergency*).

History

Perform a history and physical exam at the same time. If the patient is unable to give a history, seek information from an accompanying caregiver.

Ask about the mechanism of the injury to determine the likely severity of the injury and the possibility of other associated injuries. Ask about preexisting medical conditions, previous surgeries, medications, and allergies.

Physical exam

Face and head: Assess for all possible injuries.

POINTER

Glasgow Coma Scale

The GSC scores the way a patient's eyes and limbs respond to stimulus, and the patient's facility with speech.

Patients with a normal level of consciousness can open their eyes spontaneously, move appropriately in response to verbal commands, and speak cogently.

Patients whose level of consciousness is compromised may only respond to pain stimulus, and may have garbled speech or only make sounds.

Patients who are unconscious do not respond to any stimulus and do not speak.

Versions of the GCS are available online.

GCS: Assess the patient's level of consciousness (see the pointer).

Neurological:

- Neurological injury may occur if the force causing the facial injury also fractured the skull or damaged the brain.
- Assess the patient's cognitive, sensory, and motor status, and pupillary response.

Investigations

Facial x-rays and/or a CT scan of the head depending on the nature of the injury

Management

For facial fractures or significant cosmetic injuries, refer the patient for cosmetic surgery. In the case of open trauma, once the patient is stable, consider tetanus immunization.

TRAUMA, SPECIFIC INJURIES

Hand and/or wrist injuries

Differential diagnosis

DAMAGE TO TENDONS (E.G., LACERATION, TENDONITIS)

Tendon laceration

Signs and symptoms: pain, swelling, bruising, deformity in the area of the tendon; inability to fully extend joints; obvious laceration of soft tissue

Investigations: US, CT scan, MRI

Tendonitis

This is inflammation of the tendons.

Signs and symptoms: pain with palpation or tendon loading; crepitus (this is a "crackling" or "creaking" tendon on movement); observable tendon thickening for superficial tendons; inflammation in the affected area (swollen, hot, red); palpable fluid or lump in the tendon lining

Investigations: US, MRI for tendon appearance; x-ray to detect calcium deposits around tendon

DAMAGE TO NERVES (E.G., CARPAL TUNNEL SYNDROME)

Carpal tunnel syndrome

This is caused by compression or irritation of the median nerve within the carpal tunnel.

Signs and symptoms: numbness, tingling, weakness in the arm and hand

Risk factors: previous wrist injury or surgery; female; history of inflammatory conditions (e.g., RA); fluid retention from pregnancy (this resolves after delivery) or menopause; workplace factors such as working with vibrating tools, work that requires prolonged or repetitive flexing (e.g., assembly-line work), and working in cold temperatures

Investigations: x-ray (wrist, arm, or hand); EMG; nerve conduction study of the median nerve

DAMAGE TO BONES AND/OR JOINTS (E.G., FRACTURE, DISLOCATION)

Signs and symptoms (in general): pain and swelling on the dorsum of the wrist or proximal hand; dorsal tenderness over the wrist bone; limited range of wrist motion due to pain

Investigations: imaging to describe fractures including precise location, geometry (e.g., transverse, oblique, spiral, longitudinal), and comminution

- X-ray: poor sensitivity for wrist fractures
- CT scan: identification of fracture or dislocation, assessing joint surfaces (highly accurate)
- MRI: acute and chronic bony and soft tissue injuries, occult fractures, early vascular problems
- Arthrography: ligament tears

Keys to patient encounter

History

HISTORY OF PRESENT ILLNESS

In cases of trauma, determine the mechanism and timing of the injury.

For other presentations, ask about the characteristics of the patient's symptoms. Listen for evidence of constant versus sudden-onset symptoms (sudden-onset symptoms suggest fracture); alleviating or aggravating factors (e.g., pain with tendon loading in tendinitis; pain with movement in fracture or dislocation); and symptoms consistent with particular entities (e.g., tingling and numbness in nerve injuries).

SOCIAL HISTORY

Ask about the patient's occupation and recreational activities, looking for risk factors for repetitive strain injury (e.g., sports, typing, assembly-line work).

Physical exam

Neurovascular (affected hand and/or wrist):

- Assess color, temperature, and swelling.
- Palpate the medial and lateral epicondyles (common areas of tendonitis).
- Assess 2-point discrimination, light touch, and motor function.

Neurovascular (unaffected hand and/or wrist): Compare findings with the affected hand or wrist.

Investigations

X-ray in fractures and dislocations

EMG and conduction velocity studies in suspected carpal tunnel syndrome

Management

In all cases, it is important to recognize the potential for long-term impact on function.

Tendonitis is treated with pain management, antiinflammatory medication, icing, splinting, and referral to physiotherapy.

For carpal tunnel syndrome, refer the patient to a plastic surgeon.

Fractures require reduction and immobilization in a cast. Dislocations require only reduction.

In all cases, counsel the patient regarding return to work and recreational activities.

TRAUMA, SPECIFIC INJURIES

Head trauma

Differential diagnosis

HEAD TRAUMA IN GENERAL

Head trauma may result in closed or open head injury, depending on penetration and the status of the scalp.

Some brain injuries are not clinically evident and require imaging.

Signs and symptoms:

- Severe injury or complications: altered consciousness; seizures; CSF buildup; infection; blood vessel damage; nerve damage (this primarily presents as sensory problems); intellectual, emotional, or behavioral problems; communication problems
- Indications for imaging: patients with more than transiently impaired consciousness; GCS < 15; focal neurologic findings; persistent vomiting; seizures; a history of loss of consciousness; clinically suspected fractures

SKULL FRACTURE, PENETRATING INJURY

HEMORRHAGE, HEMATOMA (SUBDURAL, EPIDURAL, SUBARACHNOID)

CEREBRAL CONTUSION

EDEMA (MIDLINE SHIFT)

Keys to patient encounter

Key concerns

Determine an appropriate management plan, and select appropriate imaging and ongoing surveillance.

Airway and hemodynamic status

Check the patient's ABCs. Begin resuscitation, as required. For serious injuries, provide an emergency referral to a trauma team, implement the local trauma protocol, or follow the Advanced Trauma Life Support (ATLS) guidelines (see *Trauma emergency*).

History

Perform a history and physical exam at the same time. If the patient is unable to give a history, seek information from an accompanying caregiver.

Ask about the mechanism of injury (the most common are motor vehicle accident, falls, and assault). Ask about alcohol and drug use. Ask about the presence of headache and neck/spine pain; postinjury vomiting (this is a possible sign of increased intracranial pressure); and postinjury seizures. Ask about short-term memory deficits: does the patient remember the injury and events before and after?

POINTER

Glasgow Coma Scale

The GSC scores the way a patient's eyes and limbs respond to stimulus, and the patient's facility with speech.

Patients with a normal level of consciousness can open their eyes spontaneously, move appropriately in response to verbal commands, and speak cogently.

Patients whose level of consciousness is compromised may only respond to pain stimulus, and may have garbled speech or only make sounds.

Patients who are unconscious do not respond to any stimulus and do not speak.

Versions of the GCS are available online.

Physical exam

GCS: Document the patient's level of consciousness (see the pointer).

Neurological
Full regional physical exam: Identify any associated injuries.

Investigations

CT scan of the head in patients with significant injury, decreased level of consciousness (GCS ≤ 12), and/or neurological signs or symptoms, and/or if alcohol or drugs are involved

Urine drug screen (consider this)

Management

MILD HEAD TRAUMA (GCS >12)

Most patients with a normal neurological exam can be observed for 4 to 6 hours and discharged home with strict return precautions including: altered level of consciousness, worsening headache, and/or vomiting. Exceptions are patients with bleeding disorders, or who are taking anticoagulation or antiplatelet therapy, and patients with a history of neurosurgical procedures.

MODERATE HEAD TRAUMA (GCS 9–12)

Admit the patient to ICU and monitor. Consult neurosurgery.

SEVERE HEAD TRAUMA (GCS < 9)

Admit the patient to ICU and consult neurosurgery.

These patients often require mechanical ventilation, tracheostomy, and a feeding tube.

There is a high mortality rate and specialized care is needed to prevent secondary brain injury.

Monitor and manage intracranial pressure, airway and ventilation, BP, serum osmolality and serum sodium.

Initiate discussions about end-of-life care and organ donation as appropriate.

Recovery is often prolonged and incomplete. Consider referral to speech, occupational and physical therapy, social work, and rehabilitation medicine.

TRAUMA, SPECIFIC INJURIES

Nerve injury

Keys to patient encounter

Causes of nerve trauma include compression, stretching, contusion, and laceration.

Key concerns

Identify the peripheral nerve involved.

Identify the level and type of involvement.

History

Ask how the injury happened and when it happened.

Ask whether the patient has had loss of sensation and/or loss of motor function.

Physical exam

Neurological (affected area):

- Determine which nerve is involved.
- Assess sensory function: 2-point discrimination, light nerve tap, pinching, icing, brushing.
- Assess motor function: strength of muscle movement; reflexes; walking and balance for lower extremity nerve injuries; muscle tone; abnormal or involuntary movements.

Neurological (same area on the unaffected side): Compare findings with the affected side.

Investigations

EMG and nerve conduction velocity in chronic injury (e.g., carpal tunnel syndrome) to help classify and isolate affected nerves (consider this)

Management

Management depends on the severity of the injury.

Closed injuries with partial sensory loss and no motor loss do not require surgery. Consider managing these with analgesics, anticonvulsants, and corticosteroids.

Clean, open nerve cuts require referral to a plastic surgeon for microneural surgical repair within 7 days of injury. Note that the nature of the injury may delay needed surgery (e.g., crush nerve injuries). Nerve injuries may also show insufficient healing with time: these injuries usually require nerve grafts.

Prescribe physical therapy and/or orthotic devices as required.

TRAUMA, SPECIFIC INJURIES

Skin wounds

Keys to patient encounter

Causes of skin wounds include laceration, puncture (e.g., bites, needle sticks), crushing, avulsion, and abrasion.

Key concerns

Before closing a wound, look for damage to underlying structures (tendon, nerve, blood vessel), foreign bodies, and signs of infection.

Consider tetanus immunization (in cases of laceration).

History

Ask when and how the injury happened. Ask about tetanus vaccine status.

IN NEEDLE-STICK INJURIES

Needle-stick injuries involve sharp objects that have been in contact with blood, tissue, or other body fluids from another individual.

Ask about hollow-bore needles versus solid needles: hollow-bore needles carry a higher risk of disease transmission than solid needles, such as suture needles.

Ask whether the patient's immunizations are up to date (especially tetanus), and whether they have been immunized against HBV. Ask about the patient's current HBV, HCV, and HIV status. Ask whether the HBV, HCV, and HIV status of the other individual is known.

Physical exam

Wound site: Examine the site of the injury for signs of skin infection, foreign objects, and debris.

IN LACERATIONS TO THE HANDS

Hands are the most common site of lacerations to the extremities.

Neurovascular: Check for damage to nerves and blood vessels.

Musculoskeletal:

- Check for involvement of muscles and tendons, and damage to the nail beds.
- Check for associated fractures.
- In bite wounds, check for damage to the metacarpophalangeal joint and distal metacarpal neck.

Investigations

HBV, HCV, and HIV serology in needle-stick injuries

Management

Treat any skin infection.

IN NEEDLE-STICK INJURIES

If the wound is open and the patient is not up to date with tetanus prophylaxis, administer a tetanus vaccine.

In on-the-job needle-stick injuries involving health care providers, report injuries to the occupational health officer where the provider works, and follow the institution's protocol for antiviral prophylaxis until the HBV, HCV, and HIV status of the other individual is known.

IN OTHER INJURIES

Ensure hemostasis by applying local pressure. Order x-rays if an associated fracture is a possibility.

Irrigate the wound with saline and remove any necrotic tissue, foreign bodies, and/or debris.

Refer patients to a plastic surgeon for hand wounds with associated fractures and/or with involvement of muscles, tendons, nerves, nail beds, or blood vessels, and for bite wounds over a metacarpophalangeal joint or distal metacarpal neck. Most other wounds can be safely sutured.

Skin tears are a common presenting complaint, especially in the elderly. These are treated with moist dressings and will generally heal within several weeks. Tears not healing after 3 weeks should be referred to a wound-care specialist.

Note that nonhealing wounds may indicate undiagnosed or poorly treated diabetes.

TRAUMA, SPECIFIC INJURIES

Spinal trauma

Differential diagnosis

TRAUMATIC (FRACTURE/DISLOCATION OF VERTEBRAL COLUMN, PENETRATING INJURY)

SPINAL TRAUMA IN GENERAL

Signs and symptoms: spinal pain; head injury (this increases the possibility of spinal trauma); confusion or coma; weakness and/or loss of sensation

- High cervical cord injury: impaired breathing
- Thoracic level injury: leg symptoms
- Lumbar sacral injury: symptoms that affect 1 or both legs, and bowel and bladder control
- Emergency signs and symptoms: extreme pain or pressure in the area of the injury; weakness or paralysis in any part

of the body; numbness, tingling, loss of sensation in limbs and extremities; urinary or bowel incontinence; impaired balance, difficulty walking; difficulty breathing

ACUTE DISK RUPTURE

Signs and symptoms: pain; numbness or tingling; weakness (the location of symptoms depends on the location of the disk rupture)

Lower back disk rupture: leg symptoms

Neck disk rupture: shoulder or arm symptoms

Keys to patient encounter

Key concern

Pay particular attention to the initial immobilization of the patient, and to maintaining airway and ventilation.

Initial management

Check the patient's ABCs. Provide resuscitation as required. For serious injuries, provide an emergency referral to a trauma team, implement the local trauma protocol, or follow the Advanced Trauma Life Support (ATLS) guidelines (see *Trauma emergency*).

Ensure that the patient is properly immobilized with a cervical collar and spinal board. After immobilization, obtain IV access and catheterize the bladder.

History

Ask how and when the injury happened. Ask what symptoms the patient noticed immediately following the injury and what symptoms they have now. Listen for evidence of loss of motor function or sensation. Take a medical and medication history. Ask about allergies. Ask about the patient's history of surgery.

Physical exam

Consider the possibility of other injuries (pelvic fracture, intraabdominal injury). Patients with spinal injuries may not have symptoms typical of these other injuries.

Cardiovascular and respiratory: Examine the heart and lungs to the extent possible.

Neurological:

- Screen for motor function and sensation in the limbs and abdomen.
- Screen for function of the major cranial nerves.

Investigations

CT scan or MRI of the spine (generally deferred until the patient is stable and immobilized)

Management

Obtain an urgent neurosurgical consultation.

TRAUMA, SPECIFIC INJURIES

Urinary tract injuries

Differential diagnosis

URINARY TRACT INJURY IN GENERAL

The common cause is blunt, rather than penetrating, trauma.

Signs and symptoms: pain in the pelvis and lower abdomen with urination; abdominal or bladder distention or bloating; hematuria; difficulty with urination

KIDNEY INJURY

This is associated with posterior rib or spine fractures, and abdominal injuries.

Signs and symptoms: bruising, pain, tenderness in the abdomen or flank; gross or microscopic hematuria; shock; fever

BLADDER AND/OR URETHRA INJURY

Distal urethra (e.g., straddle injuries from bicycle riding, monkey bars)

Note that straddle injuries can cause urethral stricture, which may appear years after injury.

Proximal urethra (e.g., pelvic fracture, abdominal injuries)

Common causes include car accidents and falls from heights.

These injuries usually occur with other emergent injuries.

Car accidents usually lead to posterior urethral injuries in the case of pelvic fracture.

Abdominal injuries that cause urinary tract injury also usually cause bladder injury.

Men have a higher risk of urethral injury than women.

Signs and symptoms: penile and vaginal bleeding; hemodynamic instability; shock (hypotension, tachycardia, pallor, sweating, decreased alertness, drowsiness, coma)

Investigations: bedside US; if the patient is hemodynamically unstable, diagnostic peritoneal aspiration and x-ray

Keys to patient encounter

Key concern

Consider trauma to the bladder or posterior urethra in patients with pelvic fracture.

Airway and hemodynamic status

Check the patient's ABCs. Provide resuscitation, as required. For serious injuries, provide an emergency referral to a trauma team, implement the local trauma protocol, or follow the Advanced Trauma Life Support (ATLS) guidelines (see *Trauma emergency*).

History

Perform a history and physical exam at the same time. If the patient is unable to give a history, seek information from an accompanying caregiver.

Obtain a history of the injury. How was the patient injured and when? Ask about blood in the urine and difficulty voiding.

Physical exam

Remember that urethral injury may occur with multiple other injuries sustained in an accident.

Abdominal: Look for pain.

GU:

- Examine the urethral meatus for blood and evidence of trauma.
- Examine the perineum for swelling.

DRE (in males): Examine the prostate for injury.

Investigations

Retrograde urethrogram

Cystogram

CT scan for fractures and/or renal injury

Management

Refer the patient urgently to a urologist.

TRAUMA, SPECIFIC INJURIES

Vascular injury in limbs

Differential diagnosis

ACUTE LIMB ISCHEMIA

Signs and symptoms: variable, depending on the location of vessel occlusion and presence of prior occlusive vascular disease

Occlusive vascular disease: symptoms that develop over hours to days; new or worsening claudication; sudden paralysis of the affected limb

Vascular disease (mnemonic **6 Ps**): **p**aresthesia, **p**ain, **p**allor, **p**ulselessness, **p**oikilothermia, **p**aralysis

Risk factors: cardiovascular disorders (e.g., AF, recent MI, aortic atherosclerosis); vascular disorders (e.g., larger vessel aneurysmal disease, arterial trauma, DVT, prior lower extremity revascularization)

COMPARTMENT SYNDROME

Signs and symptoms:

Initial: burning or deep aching pain when stretched (locations include the upper and lower extremities, abdomen, buttocks); decreased peripheral sensation

Subsequent: lack of distal pulse; hypoesthesia; paresis of the injured compartment; ischemic necrosis of the affected compartment if untreated

Investigations: CK ≥ 1000–5000 U/L (16.7–83.5 μkat/L); myoglobinuria

Keys to patient encounter

Causes of vascular injury include penetrating trauma (e.g., laceration) and blunt trauma (e.g., contusion, compression, arterial spasm).

Key concern

Act quickly to ensure revascularization.

History

HISTORY OF PRESENT ILLNESS

Clarify what the patient's symptoms are (e.g., pain, paralysis, weakness in a limb).

Ask when and how the symptoms started. Listen for sudden versus gradual onset, and indications of trauma, burns, or recent extreme exercise. Ask about a history of anticoagulation medication and blood clots.

PAST MEDICAL HISTORY

Ask about diabetes, cardiovascular disease, peripheral vascular disease, and stroke. Ask about factors relevant to hypercoagulable states (e.g., cancer, smoking).

Physical exam

Focus the physical exam on the affected limb.

General inspection: Check for pulsatile bleeding, expanding hematoma, pallor, paresthesia, paralysis, and pain.

Blood vessels:

- Palpate for pulse deficits and thrills.
- Auscultate for bruits.

ABI or brachial-brachial index: A value less than 0.9 is worrisome for arterial injury.

POINTER

Red flags in vascular injury

Pulsatile bleeding
Expanding hematoma.
Pulse deficit
Vascular thrill
Vascular bruit
ABI or brachial-brachial index < 0.9

Investigations

CT arteriogram in patients with an ABI or brachial-brachial index less than 0.9, or with pallor, paresthesia, paralysis or pain but without red flags (see the pointer)

IN SUSPECTED COMPARTMENT SYNDROME

CBC

Electrolytes (see *Notes on labs and assessments*)

Creatinine

Creatine kinase

Compartment pressure

IN SUSPECTED ARTERIAL SPASM

CT scan of affected limb

Management

In a fracture or dislocation resulting in limb ischemia, prompt reduction of the fracture may restore blood flow. However, emergency referral to a surgeon (vascular, plastic, or general, depending on the location of the blockage) is needed in all acute vascular injury.

Patients with red flags (see the pointer) require urgent operative intervention. Immediately refer them to a vascular surgeon.

Peripheral artery spasm is treated with warming of the extremity. If this is unsuccessful, immediately refer patient to a vascular surgeon for further treatment.

URINARY PRESENTATIONS

Dysuria, urinary frequency and urgency, and/or pyuria

Differential diagnosis

URINARY TRACT INFECTION (E.G., CYSTITIS, PROSTATITIS, PYELONEPHRITIS)

Signs and symptoms (in general): frequent urination; painful urination; pelvic pain and/or flank pain; fever; tenderness over the bladder; history of prostatism

Investigations: urinalysis, urine culture

SEXUALLY TRANSMITTED INFECTION

Signs and symptoms: lower abdominal and pelvic pain; pain during intercourse; fever; urinary symptoms (often); vaginal or urethral discharge (anal discharge in anal sex); irregular menstruation

Risk factors: unprotected sex, multiple sexual partners

Investigations: cultures to detect gonorrhea and/or chlamydia

NONINFECTIOUS URINARY TRACT INFLAMMATION (E.G., TRAUMA, INTERSTITIAL CYSTITIS, BLADDER CARCINOMA, BLADDER STONES, URETHRAL STRICTURE)

NONINFECTIOUS URINARY TRACT INFLAMMATION IN GENERAL

Signs and symptoms: weak urine stream, dribbling; painful urination; increased urinary frequency or urgency; inability to empty bladder; nocturia; pelvic pain; abdominal pain; abdominal distention

Trauma

Examples of trauma include blunt trauma, penetrating wounds, pelvic fracture, straddle injury, and surgery.

Interstitial cystitis (painful bladder syndrome)

Signs and symptoms: chronic symptoms (≥ 6 weeks), often relapsing and remitting; bladder or pelvic discomfort or pressure, spreading to the lower abdomen and back; tenderness at affected areas; symptoms triggered by coffee, tea, alcohol, carbonated drinks, tomatoes, bananas, citrus (possible); history of UTI, autoimmune disorders, irritable bowel syndrome

Investigations: urinalysis; urine cytology; pelvic and/or abdominal imaging

Bladder carcinoma

Signs and symptoms: gross or microscopic hematuria; painless

Advanced or metastatic cancer: pain in the flank, abdomen, pelvis, bone

Investigations: cystoscopy with transurethral resection and biopsy; upper urinary tract imaging

Bladder stones

Signs and symptoms: often asymptomatic; recurrent severe pain in the lower abdomen and back; nausea, vomiting; chills; fever; hematuria; cloudy or dark urine

Investigations: urinalysis; US; x-ray; cytoscopy

Urethral stricture

This is a narrowing of the urethra due to injury, instrumentation, or infection.

Signs of injury: blood along the perineum or at the urethral meatus; high-riding prostate gland

Extreme traumas: shock (pallor, tachycardia)

Investigations: urethrogram (x-ray); cytoscopy

VULVOVAGINITIS

Vulvovaginal candidiasis (most common)

Signs and symptoms: thick, white, clumpy ("curd-like") vaginal discharge; vulvar pruritus, burning, soreness; thrush patches loosely adherent to the vulva; erythema and edema of the vestibule, labia majora, labia minora

Risk factors: diabetes; pregnancy; estrogen therapy; recent antibiotic use; contraceptive devices; immunosuppression

Investigations: normal vaginal pH (4–4.5); wet-mount test of discharge with KOH to detect yeast

Atrophic vaginitis

Signs and symptoms: postmenopausal patients (most common); vaginal pain, soreness; painful vaginal discharge; painful intercourse; vaginal bleeding, spotting

Investigations: wet mount to detect WBCs and decrease in *Lactobacillus*

Vulvar vestibulitis

Signs and symptoms: vaginal pain, soreness, burning; vulvar burning; symptoms that are aggravated by stress, exercise, tight clothing, intercourse, tampon insertion; irritating vaginal discharge; erythema around the vestibular glands

Contact dermatitis

Signs and symptoms: use of scented panty liners, pads, soaps, lotions, detergents, bubble baths; use of douches, spermicides, certain topical drugs (e.g., povidone-iodine); vaginal or vulvar pruritus, pain, burning; red, edematous skin; erosions; ulcers; necrosis

Keys to patient encounter

Key concerns

Differentiate infectious causes, such as UTI and STI, from non-infectious causes.

Differentiate UTI from other infectious causes: UTI is the most common cause of dysuria, but it needs to be differentiated from other, potentially more serious, causes (including STI, which can lead to infertility).

History

Ask when the urinary symptoms started and what other symptoms the patient has. Listen for evidence about the onset of symptoms (sudden onset is usual in infectious causes); fever or flank pain (these suggest UTI); and genital rash or other lesions (these suggest STI).

Establish whether the patient is sexually active and whether the symptoms appeared following sex (this suggests UTI or STI).

In men, ask about the symptoms of prostatism: nocturia and frequent voiding.

Physical exam

Abdominal: Palpate over the bladder looking for tenderness.

GU: Examine the urethral meatus looking for redness and other lesions (note that this exam is not necessary in straightforward UTIs).

DRE (in men): Examine the prostate for enlargement and tenderness.

Investigations

Urinalysis

Urine culture

Cultures for gonorrhea and chlamydia in suspected STI

US in recurrent UTI to determine the presence of a predisposing condition (e.g., urine stasis; presence of a stone or foreign body)

Management

Management depends on the specific diagnosis. In recurrent UTI related to sexual activity, antibiotic prophylaxis may be indicated.

URINARY PRESENTATIONS

Polyuria and/or polydipsia

Differential diagnosis

WATER DIURESIS

Excessive intake (primary polydipsia)

Signs and symptoms: symptoms of psychiatric disorder, symptoms of intracranial pathology (e.g., personality and behavior changes, headaches, neurological symptoms, apathy, somnolence, weight and appetite changes); symptoms of hyponatremia (these are highly variable, especially with hypothalamic lesions; they may include nausea, vomiting, confusion, ataxia, coma, seizures)

Risk factors: middle-aged, female; use of phenothiazine (psychiatric patients); sarcoidosis; hypothalamic lesions; autism and intellectual disabilities; psychiatric disorders (especially schizophrenia, schizoaffective disorder, bipolar disorder, and psychotic depression)

Investigations: low plasma sodium (ULN is 134–135 mEq/L [134–135 mmol/L]) with low urine osmolality (urine osmolality is less than serum osmolality)

Excessive loss (diabetes insipidus)

DIABETES INSIPIDUS IN GENERAL

Signs and symptoms: excessive urine excretion or loss (3–30 L/day)

Investigations: high-normal plasma sodium (> 142 mEq/L [142 mmol/L]); low urine specific gravity; low urine osmolality

CENTRAL DIABETES INSIPIDUS

This is caused by deficient secretion of ADH due to hypothalamic-pituitary disorders. Most cases are idiopathic. Other common causes include trauma, pituitary surgery, and hypoxic or ischemic encephalopathy.

Signs and symptoms: sudden-onset symptoms (usual in adult patients); polyuria; nocturia; polydipsia; neurologic symptoms (with underlying neurological disease); decreased bone mineral density at the lumbar spine and femoral neck

> Moderate to severe hypernatremia occurs in patients with hypodipsia because of CNS lesions (plasma sodium > 160 mEq/L [160 mmol/L]); in infants and young children who cannot freely access water; and in postoperative patients with unrecognized diabetes insipidus.

NEPHROGENIC DIABETES INSIPIDUS

This is caused by renal resistance to ADH (patients have normal ADH excretion). It is common in elderly people, those with underlying renal disease, and those with a long-term history of lithium use. In children, it is mostly caused by inherited defects: X-linked hereditary nephrogenic diabetes is due to mutations in the *AVPR2* gene encoding the ADH receptor V2; autosomal recessive and dominant nephrogenic diabetes insipidus is due to mutations in the *AQP2* gene.

Signs and symptoms: gradual onset (usual)

OSMOTIC DIURESIS

Sugar: diabetes mellitus

Signs and symptoms in addition to polydipsia, polyuria: personal or family history of diabetes; history of diabetic complications and/or inadequate monitoring; weight loss, or obesity, or current pregnancy (gestational diabetes); blurred vision; thirst; fatigue; hunger

Investigations: fasting glucose or HbA_{1c}

Urea: chronic renal disease

This is also known as CKD. It is often not reversible. It is more common in the elderly, and is associated with increased risk of cardiovascular disease, ESRD, infection, cancer, and mortality.

Definition: kidney damage (urinary albumin excretion of ≥ 30 mg/day) or decreased GFR (< 60 mL/min/1.73 m^2 for at least 3 months)

Five stages of CKD:

- Stage 1: normal or increased GFR (> 90 mL/min/1.73 m^2)
- Stage 2: mild reduction in GFR (60–89 mL/min/1.73 m^2)
- Stage 3a, 3b: moderate reduction in GFR (3a: 45–59 mL/min/1.73 m^2; 3b: 30–44 mL/min/1.73 m^2)
- Stage 4: severe reduction in GFR (12–29 mL/min/1.73 m^2)
- Stage 5 (renal failure): GFR < 15 mL/min/1.73 m^2

Signs and symptoms:

- Stages 1–3: asymptomatic
- Stages 4–5: fluid and electrolyte imbalance (volume overload, hyperkalemia, metabolic acidosis, hyperphosphatemia); hormonal or systemic dysfunction (anorexia, nausea, vomiting, fatigue, hypertension, anemia, malnutrition, hyperlipidemia, bone disease); pericarditis; pleuritis; CNS abnormalities (loss of concentration, confusion, lethargy, seizures); depression; pruritus

Salts: organic anions

Signs and symptoms: acute onset; polyuria; volume expansion due to large volumes of IV saline or to the release of bilateral urinary tract obstruction

Investigations: urine osmolality > 300 mOsm/kg (300 mmol/kg); increased total solute excretion (normal water diuresis is 600–900 mmol/day)

Keys to patient encounter

History

HISTORY OF PRESENT ILLNESS

Ask when the polyuria or polydipsia started and what other symptoms the patient has.

Examples of characteristic features include:

Central diabetes mellitus: sudden-onset symptoms, nocturia, and neurologic symptoms

Diabetes mellitus: weight loss

PAST MEDICAL HISTORY

Ask about diabetes and sarcoidosis.

MEDICATIONS

Ask about phenothiazine and lithium.

Physical exam

Vital signs

General inspection: Look for peripheral edema (this suggests CKD).

Neurological: Look for abnormalities if the symptoms suggest intracranial pathology.

Investigations

Glucose or HbA_{1c}

Urinalysis to look for proteinuria

Serum electrolytes

Serum osmolality

Urine electrolytes

Urine specific gravity

Urine osmolality

Management

Diabetic patients should be prescribed glucose-lowering medications. Patients with CKD require referral to a nephrologist. Patients with diabetes insipidus require referral to an endocrinologist.

POINTER

Polyuria versus frequent urination

It is important to distinguish true polyuria from frequent urination. The latter may be due to infection or urinary obstruction.

URINARY PRESENTATIONS

Urinary tract obstruction

Differential diagnosis

URINARY TRACT OBSTRUCTION IN GENERAL

Signs and symptoms: pain (e.g., costovertebral tenderness or abdominal tenderness from bladder distention); change in urine output; hypertension; hematuria

Investigations: elevated serum creatinine; US

INFECTION AND INFLAMMATION (E.G., CYSTITIS, PROSTATITIS)

Cystitis

Signs and symptoms: frequent urination; painful urination; pelvic pain and/or flank pain; fever; tenderness over the bladder

Investigations: urinalysis, urine culture

Prostatitis

PROSTATITIS IN GENERAL

This condition affects men of all ages.

Risk factors: young and middle-aged men; previous prostatitis; previous bladder infection or UTI; pelvic trauma (e.g., from biking or horseback riding); previous use of urinary catheter; HIV/AIDS; previous prostate biopsies

CHRONIC PROSTATITIS

This is the most common form of prostatitis.

Signs and symptoms: urinary, genital, and/or pelvic pain for ≥ 3 months of the past 6 months; pain in the perineum, lower abdomen, testicles, penis, or with ejaculation; difficulty with urination

Investigations: negative urine culture

CHRONIC BACTERIAL PROSTATITIS

This is due to chronic or recurrent UTIs that enter the prostate.

Signs and symptoms: UTI symptoms (frequent and urgent urination; difficult or painful urination; perineal discomfort; low grade fever); pain in the perineum, lower abdomen, testicles, penis, or with ejaculation; blood in the semen (sometimes)

Investigations: urine culture (if positive, it is usually *E. coli*)

ACUTE BACTERIAL PROSTATITIS

This is the least common form of bacterial prostatitis.

Signs and symptoms: fever; chills; muscle pain; malaise; urinary frequency and urgency; nocturia; pelvic and genital pain; difficult or painful urination; cloudy urine; tender prostate that is warm, firm, edematous

Investigations: CBC for peripheral leukocytosis; urinalysis and culture for pyuria, bacteriuria (*E. coli*); elevated CRP; elevated ESR

STRUCTURAL CONDITION (E.G., STONES, TUMOR, BENIGN PROSTATIC HYPERTROPHY)

Stones

Stones can occur in adults of all ages.

Signs and symptoms: severe flank pain; severe renal or ureteral colic pain (associated with obstruction due to ureteral stone); nausea, vomiting; difficult or painful urination; urinary urgency; gross hematuria

Investigations: CT scan

Tumor

Tumors can cause external compression that leads to intrarenal and urethral obstruction, and renal failure, in cancer patients.

Signs and symptoms: older adult (more common); pain if mass is present

Benign prostatic hypertrophy

A flow rate < 15 mL/second suggests obstruction.

Signs and symptoms: older male; urinary frequency, urgency, hesitancy, intermittency; nocturia; dribbling, incomplete bladder emptying; bladder distention (sometimes); nontender, enlarged prostate with rubbery consistency and lack of median furrow

Investigations: transrectal US of the prostate

MEDICAL CONDITIONS (E.G., DIABETES MELLITUS, MULTIPLE SCLEROSIS)

Diabetes

Signs and symptoms: personal or family history of diabetes; history of diabetic complications and/or inadequate monitoring; polydipsia, polyuria, and/or weight loss

Investigations: fasting glucose or HbA_{1c}

Multiple sclerosis

Signs and symptoms: variable depending on lesion location

Spinal cord: sensory or motor dysfunction; Lhermitte sign (paresthesias radiating down the extremities or trunk with neck flexion); bowel, bladder or erectile dysfunction

Brainstem: double vision; swallowing, speech difficulties; vertigo; pseudobulbar palsy

Cerebrum: cognitive impairment; depression; upper motor neuron signs; unilateral motor or sensory deficits

Cerebellum: problems with balance and coordination; vertigo

Other symptoms: tonic spasms; fatigue; pain; exercise intolerance; temperature sensitivity; painful unilateral loss of visual acuity

Risk factors: younger than 50, female

Investigations: brain and spinal cord MRI, including advanced MRI techniques, with established occurrence of multiple episodes; CSF fluid analysis

DRUGS (E.G., ANTICHOLINERGICS, OPIOIDS)

Keys to patient encounter

History

HISTORY OF PRESENT ILLNESS

Ask when the urinary symptoms started and what the symptoms involve. Listen for evidence consistent with obstruction: frequent urination or frequent urge to urinate; nighttime urination; blood in the urine; and pain with urination. If the patient indicates frequent urination, ask if the quantity voided is large or small (it is large and frequent in diabetes).

Ask about symptoms consistent with diabetes (polydipsia, weight loss, fatigue), MS (e.g., sensory or motor dysfunction; Lhermitte sign; bowel or erectile dysfunction; fatigue); and infection (fever; pelvic, bladder, or genital pain).

MEDICATIONS

Ask about anticholinergics and opioids.

Physical exam

Abdominal: Look for masses, tenderness, and a palpable bladder.

Pelvic: Look for an enlarged uterus or other masses.
DRE (men): Look for an enlarged prostate.

Investigations

Urinalysis to look for infection and blood
Creatinine

OTHER SPECIFIC TESTS

If a diagnosis is not obvious from the history, physical exam, and the above investigations, order:

Imaging of the bladder, kidneys, and pelvis (US, CT scan, or MRI) to look for sources of obstruction
PSA in males with an enlarged prostate

Management

Management depends on the specific diagnosis, but in all cases be aware of the risk of impaired renal function and consequent uremia. Patients with impaired renal function require urgent referral to a urologist.

VISION PRESENTATIONS

Diplopia

Differential diagnosis

MONOCULAR DIPLOPIA (E.G., REFRACTIVE ERROR, CATARACT)

This is double vision in only 1 eye.
Causes include dry eye, refractive error, warped cornea, cataract, macular disorders, and the wrong glasses (monocular diplopia indicates a problem with the eye itself).

BINOCULAR DIPLOPIA

Oculomotor nerve dysfunction

ISCHEMIA

Ischemia of the oculomotor nerve or of the midbrain is the most common cause of palsies that spare the pupil.

The oculomotor nerve (cranial nerve III) controls the movement of 4 of the 6 eye muscles.

Signs and symptoms: diplopia and other focusing impairments; ptosis; paresis of specific eye motions; normal pupil or partial pupil involvement

DIABETES-ASSOCIATED

CRANIAL MONONEUROPATHY III (DIABETIC TYPE)

Signs and symptoms: personal or family history of diabetes; history of diabetic complications and/or inadequate monitoring; polydipsia, polyuria, and/or weight loss

Investigations: fasting glucose or HbA_{1c}

MULTIPLE SCLEROSIS

Signs and symptoms: variable depending on lesion location

- Spinal cord: sensory or motor dysfunction; Lhermitte sign (paresthesias radiating down the extremities or trunk with neck flexion); bowel, bladder or erectile dysfunction
- Brainstem: double vision; swallowing, speech difficulties; vertigo; pseudobulbar palsy
- Cerebrum: cognitive impairment; depression; upper motor neuron signs; unilateral motor or sensory deficits
- Cerebellum: problems with balance and coordination; vertigo
- Other symptoms: tonic spasms; fatigue; pain; exercise intolerance; temperature sensitivity; painful unilateral loss of visual acuity

Risk factors: younger than 50, female

Investigations: brain and spinal cord MRI, including advanced MRI techniques, with established occurrence of multiple episodes; CSF analysis

INTRACRANIAL MASS (E.G., ANEURYSM)

ANEURYSM

Pupil involvement is a strong indication for urgent head imaging.

Signs and symptoms: typically asymptomatic if unruptured; dilated pupil that is in a "down and out" position; change in vision; pain, weakness, or numbness in the face or eye region; sudden-onset severe headache (this indicates a more serious situation)

Investigations: CSF analysis to detect blood, CT scan, MRI, CT angiography, cerebral angiography

Myasthenia gravis

Signs and symptoms: ocular weakness (usually just this) with drooping eyelid(s), and blurred vision or double vision; oropharyngeal weakness (dysarthria; hoarseness; chewing and swallowing difficulty); limb weakness with difficulty climbing stairs, working with elevated arms; fluctuating weakness that is asymmetrical and worse with sustained exercise

Investigations: single fiber electromyography, serum anti-acetylcholine receptor antibody

Graves orbitopathy

Signs and symptoms: history of thyroid disease (current or past) or symptoms of hyperthyroidism (enlarged thyroid, tachycardia, palpitations, diarrhea, muscle weakness, tremor, hyperactive reflexes, weight loss, sweating); exposure keratopathy; compressive optic neuropathy; proptosis; red eyes; retracting eyelids

Investigations: MRI of the head; decreased thyrotropin (TSH) (if undiagnosed Graves disease is suspected)

Orbital inflammation, infection, or tumor

ORBITAL CELLULITIS

This condition is an ocular emergency.

Signs and symptoms: fever; malaise; pain with eye movement; reduced vision, diplopia; red eye; swelling and/or redness of the eyelid and surrounding skin; proptosis; relative afferent pupillary defect; mucormycosis (this is a severe and destructive fungal orbital cellulitis); history of diabetes

Risk factors: preseptal cellulitis; sinus, face, or tooth infection; trauma

Investigations: leukocytosis on CBC; elevated CRP, ESR; CT scan or MRI of the head

Fracture of orbital floor or "blow out"

Signs and symptoms: history of facial trauma; facial tenderness; cervical and/or jaw tenderness

Investigations: CT scan of the head (to rule out entrapment of the eye)

Decompensation of childhood phoria (e.g., squint)

Squint (strabismus) is usually identified and treated in childhood.

Signs and symptoms: deviation in eye direction

Risk factors: premature birth; low birth weight; family history of strabismus or amblyopia; developmental disability (e.g., Down syndrome, cerebral palsy); head injury

Investigations: cover test; light reflex test

Keys to patient encounter

Key concern

Pay particular attention to whether true binocular diplopia is present (which resolves with occlusion of vision to either eye).

History

HISTORY OF PRESENT ILLNESS

Ask whether the problem involves 1 or both eyes, and how constant the problem is.

Check for red flags (see the pointer).

Examples of characteristic associated symptoms include:

Myasthenia gravis: intermittent symptoms with muscle weakness

MS: intermittent diplopia with neurologic signs such as swallowing difficulty

Orbital cellulitis: constant diplopia with fever and pain associated with eye movement

Graves orbitopathy: systemic symptoms such as palpitations and heat intolerance

PAST MEDICAL HISTORY

Ask about diabetes and thyroid disease.

Physical exam

Pay particular attention to findings that are red flags (see the pointer).

Vital signs: Look for fever.

Cranial nerves

Eyes:

- Look for bulging of 1 or both eyes.
- Check for pupillary symmetry.
- Perform an ophthalmoscopic exam looking for

POINTER

Red flags in diplopia

Any neurologic symptoms or signs besides diplopia

Pain

More than 1 cranial nerve deficit

Pupillary involvement of any degree

abnormalities of the lens (cataract, displacement) and retina (e.g., detachment).

- Measure the patient's visual acuity in each eye and both eyes together.
- Assess whether binocular diplopia is present by covering each eye and checking if the diplopia resolves.

Thyroid: Look for enlargement and tenderness.

Investigations

IN NEW ONSET DIPLOPIA

CT scan or MRI

Thyrotropin (TSH)

IN INTERMITTENT DIPLOPIA

Consider testing for myasthenia gravis and MS.

Management

Management depends on the specific entity identified. Red flags (see the pointer) should prompt urgent referral to a neurologist.

VISION PRESENTATIONS

Vision loss

Differential diagnosis

PAINLESS EYE

Vascular disorder (e.g., retinal artery occlusion, giant cell arteritis)

RETINAL ARTERY OCCLUSION

Retinal artery occlusion (RAO) is an ophthalmologic emergency: delays will lead to permanent blindness. It primarily affects the elderly.

Signs and symptoms:

Central RAO: acute, persistent, painless, complete loss of vision or blurring in 1 eye

Branch RAO: vision loss in a section of 1 eye

Risks signaled by RAO (these also need attention): systemic disease and/or stroke from carotid artery disease, diabetes, hypertension, AF, hyperlipidemia, atherosclerosis, endocarditis

Investigations: funduscopic exam

Findings immediately after RAO: afferent pupillary defect

Findings hours to days after RAO: cherry red spot, ground-glass retina, or pale optic disc

GIANT CELL ARTERITIS (TEMPORAL ARTERITIS)

This is the most common form of vasculitis.

Signs and symptoms: older than 50 (incidence increases with age); headaches; tenderness in both temples; jaw pain; acute vision loss (partial or complete); fever; fatigue; weight loss

Polymyalgia rheumatica (associated condition): shoulder, neck, torso, hip girdle pain; morning stiffness

Risk factors: Scandinavian descent, female, history of polymyalgia rheumatica

Investigations before treatment: elevated ALP, ESR, CRP

Neurologic disorder (e.g., optic neuritis)

OPTIC NEURITIS

This condition is associated with MS, neuromyelitis optica, and prior viral illness.

Signs and symptoms: eye pain on extraocular movement; change in color perception; decreased pupillary light reaction in the affected eye; contrast and brightness sensitivity; vision impairment exacerbated by heat or exercise; gradual resolution

Acute attacks: vision deficits in 1 eye (from mildly decreased visual acuity to blindness)

Retinal disorder

RETINAL DETACHMENT

This is an ophthalmologic emergency: delays may cause permanent damage. The most common form is rhegmatogenous detachment following spontaneous posterior vitreous detachment.

Signs and symptoms: perceived flashes of light and floaters in 1 eye (floaters usually have sudden onset, and number in the hundreds to thousands); visual field defect; history of recent trauma, previous ophthalmologic surgery; previous eye conditions (uveitis, vitreous hemorrhage)

DIABETIC RETINOPATHY (DR)

Signs and symptoms: asymptomatic until late stage of disease (macular edema or proliferative DR); impaired vision or vision loss; spots or dark floaters; blurred vision; fluctuating vision; impaired color vision; dark or empty areas in vision

> Nonproliferative DR (earlier disease): cotton-wool spots (nerve-fiber layer infarcts); intraretinal hemorrhages; hard exudates; intraretinal microvascular abnormalities and venous bleeding in severe cases
>
> Proliferative DR (late-stage disease): neovascularization (complications include tractional retinal detachment, vitreous hemorrhage, and vision loss if there is bleeding into the retina or if the retina is detached)

Risk factors: type 2 diabetes (more common than type 1); higher risk with more advanced diabetes

Age-related macular degeneration

This condition has 2 types: dry and wet. Dry is more common. Wet threatens vision.

Signs and symptoms: symptoms in both eyes (usual); gradual changes in vision (usual) (wet condition may present as sudden-onset central visual distortion); decreased vision, blurred vision; problems recognizing faces (if degeneration is present in both eyes)

Risk factors: older than 50; family history of macular degeneration; Caucasian (more common); obesity; history of smoking; cardiovascular disease; dietary factors

Investigations: funduscopic examination to assess presence of drusen and hemorrhages; optical coherence tomography to detect intraretinal and subretinal fluid secondary to choroidal neovascular membrane

Cataract

Signs and symptoms: blurred or dimmed vision; poor vision at night; sensitivity to glare; halos around lights; double vision in a single eye; frequent need for new prescription glasses

Risk factors: increasing age; diabetes; excessive exposure to sunlight; smoking; obesity; hypertension; previous eye injury or inflammation; prolonged use of corticosteroids; alcohol abuse

Investigations: visual acuity, slit lamp exam, retinal exam

Open-angle glaucoma

Signs and symptoms: often asymptomatic; gradual decline in peripheral vision

Investigations: visual field test; tonometry (intraocular pressure); slit-lamp exam, including dilated fundus exam, to detect glaucomatous optic nerve changes

Conversion disorder

This is a psychological disorder that affects all ages.

Signs and symptoms: onset of symptoms after trauma or a stressful event; weakness or paralysis; impaired ability to walk, swallow; tremors; loss of balance; speech dysfunction (slurred speech, inability to speak); numbness or loss of touch; vision problems (double vision, blindness); hearing impairment; seizures, convulsions, unresponsive episodes

Risk factors: family history of conversion disorder; family or personal history of mental health disorders (depression, mood disorder, anxiety disorder)

Amaurosis fugax

This may indicate an impending stroke.

Signs and symptoms: unilateral transient vision loss that is often experienced as a "curtain coming down" with resolution as a "curtain going up"; episodes that last 2 to 30 minutes

Risk factors: cardiovascular risk factors (diabetes, smoking, hypertension, hyperlipidemia); history of TIA or stroke

Investigations: cardiac risk factor identification, CBC, HBA_{1c}, Doppler US of carotid arteries to look for stenosis; ECG to look for cardiac arrhythmia

Migraine

Signs and symptoms: symptom onset in childhood or adolescence; known triggers for symptoms (e.g., light, weather changes, certain foods)

Prodrome: irritability, hyperactivity, depression, food craving

Aura: visual disturbances, vision loss, pins-and-needles sensations, aphasia, limb weakness

Attack: light-headedness; nausea, vomiting; light sensitivity; bilateral or unilateral pulsating or throbbing head pain

Intracranial pathology

Causes may include intracranial mass and MS.

Signs and symptoms: monocular or binocular vision loss; possible neurological symptoms, personality changes, headache

Investigations: neuroimaging (CT scan or MRI)

PAINFUL EYE

Acute angle-closure glaucoma

Signs and symptoms: hazy or blurred vision; rainbowlike halos around bright lights; sudden vision loss; severe eye and head pain; nausea, vomiting

Inflammatory condition (e.g., uveitis, corneal ulcer)

UVEITIS

This is eye inflammation that affects the uvea.

Signs and symptoms: sudden-onset, worsening symptoms that affect 1 or both eyes; age 20 to 50 (most common, but it may also affect children); eye redness; pain; light sensitivity; blurred vision; floaters; decreased vision

History of infection (e.g., catscratch disease, herpes zoster virus, syphilis, toxoplasmosis, TB, Lyme disease, West Nile virus), injury, autoimmune disease (e.g., sarcoidosis, ankylosing spondylitis), inflammatory disease (e.g., Crohn disease, ulcerative colitis), cancer that affects the eye (e.g., lymphoma)

Investigations: eye fluid analysis; angiography

CORNEAL ULCER

This is an open sore in the outer layer of the cornea, caused by infection, abrasions on the eye surface, or severely dry eyes.

Signs and symptoms: blurry vision; itching and discharge; photophobia

Investigations: fluorescein stain of the cornea; exam of scrapings from the ulcer; blood tests to detect inflammatory disorders

Trauma

Trauma may cause inflammation of the structures of the eye and optic nerve, or hemorrhage in the eye.

Signs and symptoms: history of trauma with sudden disturbance or loss of vision; eye pain

Investigations: imaging of the head to detect any vascular complication causing vision loss

Keys to patient encounter

History

HISTORY OF PRESENT ILLNESS

Ask when and how the vision loss began, and whether both eyes are involved. Ask about the speed of onset and whether there has been partial or complete resolution. Ask about decreased ability to read, decreased night vision, light sensitivity, double vision, and spots or loss of visual field.

Ask about associated symptoms and listen for eye pain, headaches, and neurological symptoms.

PAST MEDICAL HISTORY

Ask about eye surgery and trauma. Ask about cardiovascular disease, cardiovascular risk factors, diabetes, and stroke. Ask about a history of infection and autoimmune disease (relevant to uveitis), and mental health disorders (relevant to conversion disorder).

FAMILY HISTORY

Ask about glaucoma, and about conversion disorder and mental health disorders generally.

Physical exam

Vital signs: Look for hypertension.

Eyes:

- Look for redness, ulceration, and signs of trauma.
- In suspected infection or ulceration, examine the eyes using fluorescein dye.
- Examine the visual fields.
- Determine visual acuity in both eyes.
- Perform a funduscopic exam looking for papilledema (a sign of increased intraocular pressure) and changes to the optic disc.
- Perform a pinhole vision test (improvement in acuity indicates an undercorrected refractive error).
- Measure intraocular pressure.

Neurological: Check for deficits.

Investigations

Tonometry in suspected glaucoma

ESR in suspected giant cell arteritis (temporal arteritis)

- This is usually > 50 mm/hour in giant cell arteritis.

CT scan or MRI of the head in suspected intracranial pathology or head trauma

Eye fluid analysis in suspected uveitis

IN SUSPECTED AMAUROSIS FUGAX

See *Cerebrovascular accident and transient ischemic attack.*

IN SUSPECTED MIGRAINE

See *Headache*.

Management

ENTITIES REQUIRING URGENT MANAGEMENT

Patients with retinal artery occlusion, retinal detachment, or a history of recent eye surgery require urgent referral to an ophthalmologist.

In suspected giant cell arteritis (temporal arteritis), start the patient on high-dose oral steroids and refer them urgently for temporal artery biopsy.

In suspected amaurosis fugax, start acetylsalicylic acid therapy, and refer patients urgently to a stroke team or acute stroke unit. Aggressively manage cardiovascular risk factors.

OTHER ENTITIES

Treat corneal abrasion with topical antibiotics and patch the eye (**do not** patch the eye if a foreign body is still present, or if the abrasion is due to contact lens use).

Refer patients with intracranial pathology to a neurologist or neurosurgeon.

Refer patients with cataracts, glaucoma, and/or macular degeneration to an ophthalmologist.

MANAGEMENT OF DIABETIC RETINOPATHY

Even in the absence of symptoms, it is important to screen diabetic patients regularly for the development of retinal disease: progression can be rapid, and therapy can reduce the rate of progression.

Refer diabetic patients to an optometrist or ophthalmologist for retinal photographs and ophthalmoscopy on dilated fundi.

Screen all type 2 diabetic patients annually if retinopathy is progressing, or every 2 to 3 years following a normal eye exam by an optometrist or ophthalmologist.

Screen pregnant women with diabetes (not gestational diabetes) in the first trimester. Monitor the patient closely throughout the pregnancy and for 1 year postpartum.

Perform a comprehensive eye exam on all type 1 diabetic patients within 5 years of their diagnosis.

Strict glycemic control early in the course of type 1 and 2 diabetes, and good BP control, reduce the risk of retinopathy.
Goal for glycemic control: $HbA_{1c} \leq 7\%$
Goal for BP: < 130/80 mmHg

VOMITING AND/OR NAUSEA

Vomiting and/or nausea

Differential diagnosis

GASTROINTESTINAL SYSTEM

Esophagus, stomach, duodenum disorder (e.g., obstruction, gastroenteritis, reflux, gastroparesis, peptic ulcer disease)

GASTRIC OUTLET OBSTRUCTION

Most patients with this condition have cancer. Other causes include peptic ulcer disease, Crohn disease, pancreatitis, injuries, large gastric polyps, and TB.

Signs and symptoms: epigastric abdominal pain; postprandial vomiting, nausea; early satiety; abdominal distention and bloating; weight loss

Investigations: radiologic testing; endoscopy

GASTROENTERITIS

Signs and symptoms: abrupt-onset diarrhea; crampy abdominal pain; nausea, vomiting; fever; epigastric tenderness on abdominal examination

Risk factors: exposure to persons with similar symptoms or to large groups of people (common: most cases are viral); eating undercooked or contaminated foods, or raw fluids (these are risk factors for bacterial infection)

GASTROESOPHAGEAL REFLUX DISEASE

Signs and symptoms: burning chest pain radiating into the throat (often with a bitter taste in the mouth or regurgitation of food into the mouth; often worse with lying down; often better with standing up or taking antacids; worse with spicy food, coffee, alcohol, fatty foods, peppermint); acid damage to teeth

Risk factors: obesity, pregnancy

GASTROPARESIS

This is a gastric obstruction that is frequently associated with diabetes.

Signs and symptoms: history of diabetes (often); vomit containing food that was eaten several hours earlier; nausea, early satiety, bloating, weight loss and/or upper abdominal pain

PEPTIC ULCER DISEASE

Signs and symptoms: constant midepigastric pain, often relieved with eating or with antacids; weight loss

Investigations: *H. pylori*; endoscopy to detect ulcer or inflammation of the gastric lining

Small bowel, colon disorder (e.g., acute infectious enteritis, obstruction, inflammatory bowel disease)

ACUTE INFECTIOUS ENTERITIS

Examples include acute gastroenteritis caused by bacterial, viral, or parasitic pathogens.

Signs and symptoms: duration < 1 week; diarrhea that occurs ≥ 3 times per day (or ≥ 200 g of stool per day); nausea, vomiting; fever; abdominal pain; weight loss; fatigue

SMALL BOWEL OBSTRUCTION (ACUTE)

This condition requires emergent surgery.

Signs and symptoms: abdominal distention; abdominal tenderness and pain (every 5 minutes); nausea, vomiting; dehydration (tachycardia, orthostatic hypotension, reduced urine output)

SMALL BOWEL OBSTRUCTION (RECURRENT)

Signs and symptoms: similar to acute obstruction, but with resolution, and followed by diarrhea; asymptomatic between recurrences with normal abdominal exam

INFLAMMATORY BOWEL DISEASE

Signs and symptoms: younger than 30 (usually); family history of inflammatory bowel disease; fluctuating symptoms with periods of exacerbation and remission; diarrhea (possibly with nocturnal waking); blood in the stool; abdominal pain; weight loss; fever; fatigue; right lower quadrant and periumbilical pain; extraintestinal manifestations (e.g., uveitis, arthritis)

Crohn disease: right lower quadrant mass, uveitis, arthritis

Investigations: elevated CRP (this suggests active inflammation); fecal calprotectin; colonoscopy with biopsy (this is a standard diagnostic procedure); CT scan or MRI (findings: diagnostic structural changes associated with inflammatory bowel disease)

Hepatobiliary disease or pancreatic disease (e.g., acute hepatitis, acute pancreatitis, acute cholecystitis)

ACUTE HEPATITIS

Signs and symptoms: viral-like illness; abdominal pain; jaundice; palpable, tender liver

> History of infection with HAV, HBV, or HCV, or risk factors for these infections (autoimmune conditions, unprotected sex, IV drug abuse, blood transfusions, tattoos, body piercings, imprisonment, workplace exposure to body fluids); toxic ingestion (e.g., acetaminophen); adverse drug reaction (e.g., change of medication)
>
> HCV: often asymptomatic

Investigations: elevated AST, ALT, bilirubin; abnormal PT/INR; positive viral serologic tests (e.g., HAV, HBV, HCV)

ACUTE PANCREATITIS

Signs and symptoms: persistent, severe abdominal pain and tenderness in the right upper quadrant; pain that radiates to the back; nausea, vomiting; abdominal distention; hypoactive bowel sounds

> Severe symptoms: shortness of breath; epigastric tenderness on palpation; diffuse tenderness over the abdomen; fever; tachypnea; hypoxemia; hypotension

Investigations: elevated serum amylase, serum lipase

ACUTE CHOLECYSTITIS

Signs and symptoms: steady, severe right upper quadrant or epigastric pain (pain may radiate to the right shoulder or back); positive Murphy sign; nausea, vomiting; fever; anorexia; fatty food ingestion $\geq$ 1 hour prior to pain

Investigations: leukocytosis with increased band forms; abdominal US

Peritoneal irritation (e.g., appendicitis)

PERITONEAL IRRITATION IN GENERAL

Signs and symptoms: abdominal tenderness, bloating, pain with movement; fever; loss of appetite; nausea, vomiting; constipation and diarrhea; fatigue

Investigations: elevated WBCs due to infection or inflammation

APPENDICITIS

Signs and symptoms: child (often); periumbilical pain that migrates over several days to localize in the right lower quadrant; anorexia; fever; localized pain over the McBurney point on abdominal palpation

Investigations: elevated WBCs; US or CT scan for distended appendix

CENTRAL NERVOUS SYSTEM

Increased intracranial pressure (e.g., infection, trauma, tumor)

Examples of infections include meningitis, encephalitis, and abscesses. Examples of tumors include glioma, meningioma, and brain metastasis.

Signs and symptoms: intracranial pressure ≥ 20 mmHg; headache; depressed level of consciousness; vomiting (projectile vomiting when arising from sleep)

Vestibular nerve lesions

Examples of lesions include vestibular neuritis or labyrinthitis.

Signs and symptoms: rapid-onset severe vertigo; nausea, vomiting; gait instability; nystagmus that is unilateral, horizontal, or horizontal-torsional (this is suppressed with visual fixation); positive head thrust test

Labyrinthitis: unilateral hearing loss

Brainstem lesions

MS is an example of a condition that can cause brainstem lesions.

Signs and symptoms: impaired senses (vision, hearing, touch); speech impairments (difficulty speaking, voice change); motor impairments (gait instability); vertigo or dizziness causing nausea, vomiting; muscle weakness

Psychiatric or psychological conditions

Signs and symptoms: personal or family history of psychiatric conditions (e.g., anxiety, major depressive disorder); excessive worry; loss of interest in friends and usual activities; changes in sleep habits; hallucinations or delusions; suicidal thoughts; history of adverse experience (emotional, physical, or sexual abuse; recent stress such as death of a friend or family member), or substance abuse

Cyclic vomiting syndrome: emotional stress with recurrent nausea, vomiting, lethargy, pallor, abdominal pain, diarrhea, headache that lasts up to 10 days

OTHER CONDITION

Endocrine and/or metabolic condition (e.g., diabetes, hypercalcemia, pregnancy)

DIABETES

Diabetes can produce GI symptoms, such as vomiting and nausea, in the context of gastroparesis or diabetic ketoacidosis.

Signs and symptoms (diabetes in general): personal or family history of diabetes; history of diabetic complications and/or inadequate monitoring; polydipsia, polyuria, and/or weight loss

Investigations: fasting glucose or HbA_{1c}

HYPERCALCEMIA

Signs and symptoms: constipation, polyuria, polydipsia, dehydration, anorexia, nausea, muscle weakness, altered sensory status

History of sarcoidosis, malignancy, hyperparathyroidism, immobilization, use of diuretics (thiazide)

Investigations: blood test (hypercalcemia is total calcium ≥ 10.52 mg/dL [2.63 mmol/L] or ionized calcium ≥ 5.6 mg/dL [1.4 mmol/L]); albumin; PTH

PREGNANCY

Signs and symptoms: amenorrhea (some experience spotting); sexual activity, especially without contraception or with inconsistent use of contraception; nausea, vomiting (common early sign); breast enlargement and tenderness; increased frequency of urination without pain or difficulty; fatigue

Investigations: blood or urine β-HCG

Cancer

Cancers that commonly cause nausea and vomiting include malignant bowel obstruction and cancer that affects the brain.

Sepsis (e.g., pyelonephritis, pneumonia)

SEPSIS IN GENERAL

Definition: infection with systemic inflammatory response, dysfunction of ≥ 1 organ system

Signs and symptoms: fever or hypothermia; tachycardia; tachypnea; infection (most common: pneumonia, abdominal infection, kidney infection, bacteremia)

Severe: oliguria; mental status changes; shortness of breath; extreme hypotension, unresponsive to fluid replacement (this indicates septic shock)

Risk factors: very young, very old; compromised immune system; wounds, burns; catheterization, intubation

Investigations: CBC with differential; cultures (blood, CSF, urine) to detect causative organism; ABG to detect acidosis; elevated creatinine; chest x-ray to detect pulmonary edema

PYELONEPHRITIS

Signs and symptoms: frequent urination; painful urination; tenderness over the costovertebral angle

Investigations: urinalysis, urine culture

PNEUMONIA

Signs and symptoms: shortness of breath; cough; purulent sputum; chest pain on coughing or deep breaths; fatigue; tachypnea; tachycardia; decreased oxygen saturation; lung crackles on auscultation; lung dullness on percussion

Children: fever

Elderly: confusion, low body temperature

Risk factors: very old, very young; smoking; immune compromise (e.g., due to chronic illness); hospitalization

Investigations: chest x-ray to detect consolidation

Drugs and toxins (e.g., chemotherapy, food poisoning)

CHEMOTHERAPY

Nausea and vomiting are common side effects of chemotherapy, especially for highly emetic agents (e.g., combination of cyclophosphamide and doxorubicin in breast cancer; combination of anthracycline and cyclophosphamide in breast cancer; combination of vincristine and prednisone in non-Hodgkin lymphoma; cisplatin).

FOOD POISONING

Signs and symptoms: history of eating undercooked meat or poorly refrigerated food; symptoms that develop within 6 hours of contaminated food consumption

Keys to patient encounter

Key concern

Important causes of vomiting can arise outside the GI system: differentiate GI from non-GI causes.

History

Ask whether the vomiting began suddenly or gradually, whether it is constant or intermittent, and what makes it better and worse.

Ask about changes in appetite or weight, changes in satiety, and changes in bowel habits. Ask about associated fever.

Check for symptoms of neurological disease: headaches, personality changes, vision changes, focal neurologic symptoms, and altered gait.

Check for symptoms of cardiac ischemia: chest pain, shortness of breath, and exercise intolerance.

Ask about symptoms of relevant metabolic conditions: diabetes (polyuria, polydipsia, weight loss), hypercalcemia (constipation, polyuria, polydipsia, dehydration, anorexia, nausea, muscle weakness), and pregnancy (amenorrhea; breast enlargement and tenderness).

Physical exam

Vital signs: Look for signs of dehydration (including hypotension and tachycardia) and fever (this suggests infection or malignancy).

Dermatological: Examine the skin for tenting (from dehydration).

Abdominal: Look for tenderness (this suggests infection or blockage).

Neurological: In suspected neurological cause, examine the fundi for papilledema (this indicates increased intracranial pressure).

Investigations

Serum electrolytes

Serum creatinine

Serum calcium

Serum glucose

Serum cortisol

Other specific tests and/or imaging if the history and physical exam suggest a non-GI cause

Management

Target the underlying cause. Pay special attention to conditions requiring immediate management (dehydration, increased intracranial pressure). Note that, in some patients, no cause will be found. Where appropriate, recommend the use of common anti-nausea or antiemetic medications.

Weakness (not caused by cerebrovascular accident)

Differential diagnosis

PRIMARY MUSCLE DISEASE

Congenital (e.g., muscular dystrophy)

MUSCULAR DYSTROPHY

Common types of MD include Duchenne MD, Becker MD, facioscapulohumeral MD, and myotonic dystrophy.

Signs and symptoms: progressive muscular wasting, scoliosis, limited range of movement, muscle spasms, poor balance, waddling gait, calf deformation, walking difficulty, shortness of breath, cardiomyopathy

Investigations: muscle biopsy, increased creatine phosphokinase, EMG, genetic testing

Acquired (e.g., myositis, myasthenia gravis)

MYOSITIS

This describes a group of inflammatory diseases including dermatomyositis, inclusion body myositis, and polymyositis.

Signs and symptoms: gradual-onset muscle weakness (dermatomyositis and polymyositis: core-muscle weakness; inclusion body myositis: weakness in the thighs, wrist, and fingers); difficulty swallowing

Dermatomyositis: rash

MYASTHENIA GRAVIS

Signs and symptoms: ocular weakness (usually just this) with drooping eyelid(s), blurred vision, or double vision; oropharyngeal weakness (difficulty speaking; hoarseness; chewing and swallowing difficulty); limb weakness with difficulty climbing stairs, working with elevated arms; fluctuating weakness that is asymmetrical and worse with sustained exercise

Investigations: single fiber electromyography, serum anti–acetylcholine receptor antibody

CENTRAL NERVOUS SYSTEM

Malignancy

BRAIN TUMOR

Types of brain tumor include meningioma, astrocytoma, oligodendroglioma, glioblastoma, and Schwannoma.

Signs and symptoms: acute-onset headaches; older than 50; change in chronic headache pattern; increasing intensity and frequency of headaches; headaches that disturb sleep; unilateral headache pain, always on the same side; position-evoked crescendo headache; impaired vision; light-headedness

Other symptoms: focal seizures, confusion, memory loss, personality change, loss of coordination, muscle weakness

Investigations: imaging for intracranial masses (MRI with contrast enhancement is best for tumors and abscesses); biopsy

SPINAL CORD TUMOR

Signs and symptoms: back pain; bilateral numbness and/or weakness in the arms or legs; loss of bladder and/or bowel control

Investigations: spinal MRI or CT scan; biopsy

Infection (e.g., encephalitis)

ENCEPHALITIS

Viral infection is the most common cause: HSV-1, HSV-2; EBV; VZV; Enteroviruses (e.g., Coxsackievirus); and insect-borne viruses (e.g., West Nile disease, Lyme disease).

Signs and symptoms: seizures, altered mental status (e.g., decreased level of consciousness, lethargy, personality change, behavior change), fever, headache, nausea, vomiting

Infants and neonates: poor feeding, irritability, lethargy

Children and adolescents: irritability, movement disorder, ataxia, stupor, coma, hemiparesis, cranial nerve defect, status epilepticus (severe symptom)

Adults: motor or sensory deficits; speech or movement impairment; flaccid paralysis

Investigations: blood tests (CBC, differential, platelets, electrolytes, glucose, BUN, creatinine, aminotransferases, coagulation); MRI (to detect brain edema; inflammation of the cerebral cortex, gray-white matter junction, thalamus, basal ganglia); CSF tests (perform LP after results of MRI; order CSF protein, glucose, cell count, differential, Gram stain, bacterial culture); EEG (usually abnormal) to differentiate from nonconvulsive seizure activity

Degenerative

DIABETIC NEUROPATHY

Signs and symptoms: polydipsia, polyuria, and/or weight loss; autonomic neuropathy effects (indigestion, nausea, diarrhea, constipation, dizziness upon standing, urinating difficulty, erectile dysfunction, vaginal dryness)

HUNTINGTON DISEASE

Signs and symptoms: family history of Huntington disease; abnormal eye movements; tics (uncontrolled movement in the fingers, feet, face, trunk); myoclonus; chorea (progressive chorea in late-onset Huntington disease; older than 50); psychiatric symptoms (depression; apathy; anxiety; obsessions, compulsions; irritability; psychosis; paranoid and acoustic hallucinations; hypersexuality); cognitive symptoms (impaired executive function; loss of mental flexibility, concentration, judgment, memory, awareness); motor symptoms (bradykinesia, dystonia, muscle weakness); profuse sweating from autonomic disturbance

Investigations: DNA analysis (PCR or Southern blot); neuroimaging (MRI, CT scan, SPECT, PET scan) for progression monitoring

Autoimmune or inflammatory (e.g., multiple sclerosis)

MULTIPLE SCLEROSIS

Signs and symptoms: variable depending on lesion location

> Spinal cord: sensory or motor dysfunction; Lhermitte sign (paresthesias radiating down the extremities or trunk with neck flexion); bowel, bladder or erectile dysfunction
>
> Brainstem: double vision; swallowing, speech difficulties; vertigo; pseudobulbar palsy
>
> Cerebrum: cognitive impairment; depression; upper motor neuron signs; unilateral motor or sensory deficits
>
> Cerebellum: problems with balance and coordination; vertigo
>
> Other symptoms: tonic spasms; fatigue; pain; exercise intolerance; temperature sensitivity; painful unilateral loss of visual acuity

Risk factors: younger than 50, female

Investigations: brain and spinal cord MRI, including advanced MRI techniques, with established occurrence of multiple episodes; CSF analysis

TRAUMA

Examples of trauma include head trauma and spinal trauma.

VASCULAR

Signs and symptoms: history of vascular conditions, such as stroke, cerebellar arterial dissection, vasculitis, hemorrhage (burst aneurysm, arteriovenous malformation), hypertension, repeat subarachnoid bleeding

OTHER (E.G., GENETIC)

Genetic condition

Signs and symptoms: family history of neuropathy such as Charcot-Marie-Tooth disease (common)

> Charcot-Marie-Tooth disease: symptom onset in adolescence or early adulthood, with gradual progression of symptoms; motor and sensory deficits; weakness in the foot and lower leg muscles (typical); foot deformities (high arch, hammer toes)

Keys to patient encounter

Key concerns

Distinguish muscular, nerve, and upper neurological disorders.

Characterize the distribution of the weakness, or localize the region of the weakness.

Determine the underlying cause.

History

HISTORY OF PRESENT ILLNESS

The key question is whether the patient has true weakness as opposed to fatigue. As a general rule, patients with true weakness describe specific symptoms of dysfunction.

Ask how quickly the weakness developed, how constant it is, how it has progressed, and what makes it better or worse.

Examples of characteristic features include:

Myasthenia gravis: weakness worse with sustained exertion

Infection: sudden-onset weakness

Degenerative disorders: progressive weakness

Patients who are malingering or have a conversion disorder may describe inconsistent histories, or weakness when performing some tasks but not others.

PAST MEDICAL HISTORY

Ask about HIV, Lyme disease, granulomatous disorders, malignancy, and underlying systemic illness (e.g., diabetes). Determine if the patient's immunizations are up to date.

FAMILY HISTORY

Ask about family members with similar symptoms. Ask about neuropathy, Huntington disease, and MD.

MEDICATIONS

Ask about neoplastic agents, steroids, and statins.

SOCIAL HISTORY

Ask about alcohol abuse. Ask about possible occupational or toxic exposures.

Physical exam

Physical examination is a key aspect of diagnosis.

Neurological: Perform a full exam, including sensation, strength, and reflexes, and assessment of the sphincter and cranial nerves.

Investigations

CBC

Fasting glucose or HbA_{1c}

Electrolytes (see *Notes on labs and assessments*)

CK

Creatinine

Calcium

Liver function (see *Notes on labs and assessments*)

OTHER SPECIFIC INVESTIGATIONS

Tensilon test in suspected myasthenia gravis (provides rapid diagnosis in some patients, but is rarely done clinically

LP to look for protein, cells, and oligoclonal bands in suspected Guillain-Barré syndrome or MS

MRI or CT scan in suspected myelopathy or stroke

Muscle biopsy in suspected myopathy

EMG in suspected Guillain-Barré syndrome, motor neuron disease, or myasthenia gravis

Genetic testing in suspected inherited disease

Management

Management depends on the specific entity identified. Immediately correct any electrolyte abnormalities. Optimally control any underlying disease. Discontinue any causative drugs. Refer the patient to a neurologist, physiotherapist, occupational therapist, or a stroke clinic as appropriate.

WEIGHT PRESENTATIONS

Weight gain, obesity

Differential diagnosis

INCREASED ENERGY INTAKE

Dietary cause (e.g., high fat/sugar diet, overeating)

HIGH FAT/SUGAR DIET

Signs and symptoms: history of high intake of foods with refined carbohydrates and fats (e.g., fast food, processed foods), and beverages containing sugar (soda, juice, alcohol)

OVEREATING

Signs and symptoms: polyphagia or hyperphagia (increased appetite or excessive hunger; no satiety from consuming food) due to diabetes, depression, stress (common causes)

Social and behavioral cause (e.g., socioeconomic cause, psychosocial cause)

SOCIOECONOMIC CAUSE

There is a higher incidence of obesity in children and adults living in poverty, perhaps due to lack of access to good nutrition because of expense or location.

PSYCHOSOCIAL CAUSE

Signs and symptoms: sleeping < 6 hours a night; chronic sleep disturbance; employed in shift work; depression or stress

Iatrogenic cause (e.g., drugs, hormones, hypothalamic surgery)

DRUGS

Drugs associated with weight gain include atypical antipsychotics (these are associated with marked weight gain), steroids, some SSRIs, amitriptyline, mood stabilizers (e.g., lithium, valproic acid, carbamazepine), and antiepileptics (e.g., valproate, gabapentin).

HORMONES

Signs and symptoms: history of hypothyroidism, polycystic ovary syndrome (common), or Cushing syndrome (rare)

DECREASED ENERGY EXPENDITURE (E.G., SEDENTARY LIFESTYLE, SMOKING CESSATION)

Signs and symptoms: history of recent change in exercise habits (e.g., new job that involves more sitting; loss of mobility from injury or illness), or recent smoking cessation

NEUROENDOCRINE CONDITION (E.G., HYPOTHYROIDISM, CUSHING SYNDROME, POLYCYSTIC OVARY SYNDROME)

Hypothyroidism

Signs and symptoms: history of hypothyroidism or symptoms of hypothyroidism (cold intolerance, decreased reflexes, dry skin, weight gain, impaired cognition)
Investigations: elevated thyrotropin (TSH)

Cushing syndrome

Signs and symptoms: history of glucocorticoid therapy; cushingoid features (round, red face; pronounced abdominal weight; hump on the upper back; thin arms and legs; hypertension; stretch marks; acne)

Investigations: high cortisol levels on either a 24-hour urine cortisol test or dexamethasone suppression test

Polycystic ovary syndrome

Signs and symptoms: symptom onset after puberty, with increased rate of hair growth and male-pattern hair growth; irregular menstruation; infertility; obesity; acne

Investigations: LH:FSH ratio (elevated: 2:1 or 3:1) (usual); elevated testosterone; US for ovarian cysts; normal prolactin levels; normal thyroid function

Genetic (e.g., Prader-Willi syndrome)

PRADER-WILLI SYNDROME

Survival past 50 years is low unless this condition is treated.

Signs and symptoms (adults and children in general): excess fat in the central body; small hands and feet; prominent nasal bridge; thin upper lip; downturned mouth; almond-shaped eyes; high narrow forehead; tapered fingers; soft, easily bruised skin; light skin and hair compared to family members; incomplete sexual development; frequent skin picking; delayed motor development

> Prenatal and neonate: reduced fetal movement; abnormal fetal position; excessive amniotic fluid; breech or cesarean birth; lethargy; hypotonia; poor sucking; hypogonadism
>
> Children: delayed intellectual development; excessive sleeping; strabismus; scoliosis; cryptorchidism; speech delay; poor physical coordination; hyperphagia; excessive weight gain; sleep disorders; delayed puberty; short stature; obesity; extreme flexibility
>
> Adults: infertility; hypogonadism; sparse pubic hair; obesity; hypotonia; learning and cognitive disabilities; diabetes (often)

Investigations: DNA-based methylation testing for Prader-Willi syndrome and Angelman syndrome

Epigenetic

Some causes are well understood, including Prader-Willi syndrome (this is usually paternally imprinted) and abnormalities of the *GNAS* locus.

There are likely other epigenetic causes that are poorly understood.

Investigations: genetic testing

Keys to patient encounter

Key concerns

Determine the degree and pattern of obesity.
Exclude primary treatable causes.
Assess the risk of associated morbidity and mortality.

History

HISTORY OF PRESENT ILLNESS

Ask how much weight the patient has gained and over what timeframe. Ask whether the weight gain is intentional or unintentional.

Ask about associated symptoms and listen for features consistent with undiagnosed hypothyroidism (e.g., cold intolerance, dry skin, impaired cognition), Cushing syndrome (e.g., hump on the upper back, stretch marks, acne), and polycystic ovary syndrome (e.g., male-pattern hair growth, irregular menstruation, infertility).

Ask about sleep disruption, depression, and stress.

RISK FACTORS FOR CARDIOVASCULAR DISEASE

Because obesity is a major risk factor for cardiovascular disease, ask about additional risk factors for cardiovascular disease including family history, diabetes, smoking, hypertension, dyslipidemia, and sleep apnea.

PAST MEDICAL HISTORY

Ask about hypothyroidism, Cushing syndrome, polycystic ovary syndrome, and Prader-Willi syndrome.

MEDICATIONS

Ask about changes in medications, and about atypical antipsychotics, steroids, SSRIs, amitriptyline, mood stabilizers, and antiepileptics.

SOCIAL HISTORY

Ask whether the patient has recently stopped smoking. Ask about diet and changes in exercise routines. Ask about social and psychosocial impacts the patient is experiencing because of their weight.

Physical exam

Vital signs: Look for bradycardia (this suggests hypothyroidism) and hypertension (this suggests Cushing syndrome).

General inspection: Note the distribution of fat (e.g., truncal with a hump on the upper back in Cushing syndrome).

Waist and hip measurements: Measure the waist circumference, or determine the waist-to-hip ratio, and calculate the patient's BMI (see *Notes on labs and assessments*).

Dermatological: Assess the patient for acanthosis nigricans (hyperpigmentation often found in the armpits, groin, and folds of the neck), which suggests insulin resistance.

Investigations

Thyrotropin (TSH)

Glucose

Lipids

Other specific tests in suspected Cushing syndrome or polycystic ovary syndrome (see the differential diagnosis)

Management

Counsel the patient regarding exercise, diet, and behavior modification. Discuss indications for—and risks and benefits of—antiobesity drugs and bariatric surgery.

POINTER

Achieving stable weight

Remember that for a stable weight, calories in equal calories out.

WEIGHT PRESENTATIONS

Weight loss, eating disorders, anorexia

Differential diagnosis

DECREASED NUTRITIONAL INTAKE

Psychiatric disease (e.g., anorexia nervosa, bulimia)

ANOREXIA NERVOSA[1(pp338–339)]

Signs and symptoms: significantly low body weight; intense fear of gaining weight or persistent behavior that interferes with gaining weight; excessive focus on body weight or shape in self-evaluation, or persistent lack of recognition of current low body weight

BULIMIA NERVOSA[1(p345)]

Signs and symptoms: recurrent binge eating, followed by behaviors to prevent weight gain (e.g., vomiting, abuse of laxatives, excessive exercise, fasting); binging and weight-loss behaviors that both occur ≥ 1 time per week for ≥ 3 months; excessive focus on body weight or shape in self-evaluation

Medical disease (e.g., chronic illness, esophageal cancer)

CHRONIC ILLNESS

Examples of chronic illness include kidney disease and adrenal insufficiency.

Signs and symptoms:

Kidney disease: bilateral lower limb swelling; shortness of breath; paroxysmal nocturnal dyspnea; orthopnea

Chronic primary adrenal insufficiency: abdominal pain; fatigue; hyperpigmentation; orthostatic light-headedness

ESOPHAGEAL CANCER

Signs and symptoms: none in early esophageal cancer (typical); difficulty swallowing; worsening indigestion or heartburn; chest pain; coughing; weight loss

Investigations: barium swallow imaging for esophageal assessment; endoscopy to examine the esophagus; biopsy; CT and PET scan to determine the stage of the cancer

Substance abuse or medications (e.g., alcohol, opiates, cocaine, amphetamines, anticancer drugs)

INCREASED ENERGY EXPENDITURE

Hormonal condition (e.g., hyperthyroidism)

HYPERTHYROIDISM

Signs and symptoms: history of hyperthyroidism or symptoms of hyperthyroidism (changes in menstrual patterns, enlarged thyroid, tachycardia, palpitations, diarrhea, muscle weakness, tremor, hyperactive reflexes, weight loss, sweating, thinning hair)

Investigations: decreased thyrotropin (TSH)

Chronic illness (e.g., chronic obstructive pulmonary disease, congestive heart failure)

CHRONIC OBSTRUCTIVE PULMONARY DISEASE

Signs and symptoms: wheezing; chest tightness; chronic productive cough; clubbing of fingers; cyanosis around the lips and in the extremities; decreased oxygen saturation; decreased capacity on pulmonary function testing

Risk factors: smoking; occupational exposure; intrinsic lung disease

Investigations: chest x-ray

CONGESTIVE HEART FAILURE

Signs and symptoms: history of heart disease (or risk factors for heart disease: diabetes, hypertension, hyperlipidemia, smoking) or hepatic vein thrombosis (Budd-Chiari syndrome); severe shortness of breath; elevated JVP; edema in the abdomen and legs; pink phlegm; heart murmurs and extra cardiac sounds

Investigations: chest x-ray to detect pulmonary edema; NT-proBNP; echocardiogram to distinguish forms of HF; cardiac stress testing, either with exercise or pharmacological agent

Malignancy

Signs and symptoms: weight loss, night sweats, fatigue, fever, organ-specific symptoms (e.g., bone pain)

Infection

Signs and symptoms: weight loss that develops over weeks or months (weight loss is clinically important if an adult loses > 5% of body weight or > 5 kg over 6 months)

If due to fungal infections: fever, night sweats, fatigue, cough, shortness of breath

If due to parasitic infections: fever, abdominal pain, bloating, diarrhea, eosinophilia, history of travel in developing countries

If due to viral infection (HIV): fever, shortness of breath, cough, lymphadenopathy, diarrhea, oral candidiasis (white oral plaques)

If due to TB: fever; night sweats; cough; hemoptysis; exposure to infected persons; poor, crowded living conditions

Investigations: stool test for ova and parasites; blood test to detect HIV; sputum culture to detect TB

Increased physical activity (e.g., runners)

CALORIC LOSS

Malabsorption (e.g., diarrhea)

CHOLESTASIS

This is slowed or blocked bile flow from the liver caused by acute hepatitis, alcoholic liver disease, primary biliary cirrhosis, pancreatitis, gallstones, and certain drugs.

Signs and symptoms: pale fatty stools; dark urine; itching; nausea; right upper quadrant abdominal pain; jaundice

CELIAC DISEASE

Signs and symptoms: family history of celiac disease, or signs and symptoms of celiac disease (chronic abdominal pain, rashes)

Investigations: positive serum anti-tTG (with IgA level); duodenal biopsy to detect villous blunting

INFLAMMATORY BOWEL DISEASE

Signs and symptoms: younger than 30 (usually); family history of inflammatory bowel disease; fluctuating symptoms with periods of exacerbation and remission; diarrhea (possibly with nocturnal waking); blood in the stool; abdominal pain; weight loss; fever; fatigue; right lower quadrant and periumbilical pain; extraintestinal manifestations (e.g., uveitis, arthritis)

Crohn disease: right lower quadrant mass, uveitis, arthritis

Investigations: elevated CRP (this suggests active inflammation); fecal calprotectin; colonoscopy with biopsy (this is a standard diagnostic procedure); CT scan or MRI (findings: diagnostic structural changes associated with inflammatory bowel disease)

Diabetes

Signs and symptoms: personal or family history of diabetes; history of diabetic complications and/or inadequate monitoring; polydipsia, polyuria, and/or weight loss

Investigations: fasting glucose or HbA_{1c}

Keys to patient encounter

Key concerns

Identify the primary mechanism of weight loss: decreased nutritional intake or increased expenditure.

Investigate for underlying medical conditions, where appropriate.

History

Ask how much weight the patient has lost and over what timeframe. Ask if the weight loss is intentional or unintentional.

Ask about associated symptoms. Examples of characteristic symptoms include:

COPD: shortness of breath, wheezing

Esophageal cancer: difficulty swallowing

Malabsorption: abdominal pain, diarrhea

Diabetes: polydipsia, polyuria

Ask about the symptoms of anorexia nervosa and bulimia (e.g., fear of gaining weight and lack of perspective on current weight in anorexia nervosa; binge eating followed by vomiting in bulimia).

SOCIAL HISTORY

Ask about the patient's usual exercise routines.

Physical exam

Vital signs

Height and weight: Calculate the patient's BMI (see *Notes on labs and assessments*).

Mouth: Patients with bulimia may show damage to tooth enamel from stomach acid.

Cardiovascular:

- Auscultate the heart for murmurs or extra sounds (CHF).
- Examine the legs for peripheral edema (CHF).

Respiratory: Auscultate the lungs for wheezing (COPD) and rales (CHF).

POINTER

Achieving stable weight

Remember that for a stable weight, calories in equal calories out.

Investigations

Serum glucose

Thyrotropin (TSH)

Serum albumin as indicated to further investigate nutritional status

Other specific tests as indicated by the history and physical exam (see the differential diagnosis)

Management

If you identify decreased nutritional intake, refer the patient to a dietitian or specialized treatment program. In cases of anorexia nervosa, refer the patient for counseling and to an eating disorders clinic.

If you identify increased energy expenditure, management depends on the specific diagnosis.

REFERENCE

1. American Psychiatric Association. Diagnostic and statistical manual of mental disorders. 5th ed. Arlington, VA: American Psychiatric Association; 2013. 991 p.

Notes on labs and assessments

Body mass index

In 2023, the American Medical Association (AMA) recommended using BMI in conjunction with other valid measures of body fat, such as:

- visceral fat
- body adiposity index
- body composition
- relative fat mass
- waist circumference
- genetic and/or metabolic factors

The AMA's decision arose from the limitations of BMI as a measure of body fat in clinical medicine. The AMA identified those limitations as the historical harm of BMI, its use to exclude people based on race, and its foundation in data from a narrow (white) segment of the population.

Electrolytes

Serum electrolytes

The usual electrolyte panel (also called "lytes") consists of sodium, potassium, chloride, and bicarbonate (HCO_3^-). Some labs report bicarbonate as CO_2; this essentially measures the same thing as the vast majority of CO_2 in the body occurs in the form of HCO_3^-.

Urine electrolytes

Like serum electrolytes, urine electrolytes include sodium, potassium, and chloride. However, urine electrolytes do not include bicarbonate or CO_2. CO_2 is removed from the body by the lungs, not in urine.

Lipids

Lipid tests (lipid profile, lipid panel, cholesterol test) consist of 4 measures:

- low-density lipoprotein cholesterol (LDL-c)
- high-density lipoprotein cholesterol (HDL-c)
- triglycerides (TG)
- total cholesterol (TC)

Additional measurements may be derived from these, including the ratio of total cholesterol to HDL and the ratio of LDL to HDL.

Other tests for cholesterol exist but are not as widely used, including:

- very low-density lipoprotein (VLDL)
- apolipoprotein-B100 (apoB)
- lipoprotein(a)

Of these less widely used lipid tests, apo(B) is sometimes used as an alternative to LDL-c testing.

Liver function

There is no universally accepted list of laboratory tests for assessing the liver. Moreover, common liver "function" tests include tests that look at liver inflammation rather than the actual function of the liver.

Tests that measure how well the liver is working

Albumin: This main protein in the blood is made in the liver and therefore low levels may indicate reduced liver function.

Total protein: Because most of the protein in the blood is albumin, total protein may be used as a proxy measure for serum albumin level.

Bilirubin (including total bilirubin, direct/conjugated bilirubin and indirect/unconjugated bilirubin): Bilirubin is created by the breakdown of RBCs. Initially, bilirubin is water insoluble and is called "indirect" or "unconjugated" bilirubin. Isolated indirect hyperbilirubinemia is commonly associated with hemolysis. Indirect bilirubin is carried to the liver where it is converted to a water soluble form of bilirubin known as "direct" or "conjugated bilirubin." Common causes of elevated direct hyperbilirubinemia include alcohol abuse, infectious hepatitis, drug reactions, autoimmune disorders, gallstones, pancreatitis, and malignancies. Total bilirubin is the sum of direct and indirect bilirubin levels. It should be noted that this explanation is somewhat simplified as "direct" and "indirect" refer to the laboratory method used and "conjugated" and "unconjugated" refer to the actual metabolites. However, these terms are generally used interchangeably.

INR/PTT: These tests measure the ability of the blood to clot. Since clotting factors are synthesized in the liver, an elevated INR may indicate reduced liver function.

ALP: Elevated levels are nonspecific but may be seen with bile duct obstruction.

5'-nucleotidase: This enzyme is specific to the liver and is elevated with bile duct obstruction.

Tests that measure liver inflammation

ALT: This enzyme is specific to the liver and is released into the blood in the setting of acute liver damage.

AST: This enzyme is also released into the blood in the setting of acute liver damage but is nonspecific and is found in a number of other organs as well as in red blood cells.

γ-glutamyl transferase: This enzyme is elevated in the setting of acute liver damage (especially with alcohol abuse) as well as with bile duct obstruction.

Common starting panel

While specific "liver function" panels differ by laboratory and by local practice, a common starting panel includes albumin, INR/PTT, bilirubin (total and direct), ALP, AST, ALT, and γ-glutamyl transferase.

Abbreviations

AAA	abdominal aortic aneurysm
ABG	arterial blood gas
ABI	ankle-brachial index
ACE	angiotensin-converting enzyme
ACL	anterior cruciate ligament
ACLS	advanced cardiac life support
ACS	acute coronary syndrome
ACTH	adrenocorticotropic hormone
ADH	antidiuretic hormone
ADHD	attention deficit hyperactivity disorder
ADL	activities of daily living
AF	atrial fibrillation
AFP	α1-fetoprotein
AHase	antihyaluronidase
ALP	alkaline phosphatase
ALS	amyotrophic lateral sclerosis
ALT	alanine transaminase
ANA	antinuclear antibodies
ANCA	antineutrophil cytoplasmic antibody
aPTT	activated partial thromboplastin time
ARB	angiotensin receptor blocker
ARDS	acute respiratory distress syndrome
ART	antiretroviral therapy
ASKase	antistreptokinase
ASO	antistreptolysin
AST	aspartate aminotransferase
AVM	arteriovenous malformation
β-HCG	chorionic gonadotropin
BMI	body mass index
BP	blood pressure
BPH	benign prostatic hyperplasia
BUN	blood urea nitrogen
CA 125	cancer antigen 125
CA 19-9	cancer antigen 19-9
CABG	coronary artery bypass graft
CAD	coronary artery disease
C. albicans	*Candida albicans*
CBC	complete blood count
CCB	calcium channel blocker

CD	clusters of differentiation (e.g., CD4)
C. difficile	*Clostridium difficile*
CEA	carcinoembryonic antigen
CF	cystic fibrosis
CHD	congenital heart disease
CHF	congestive heart failure
CK	creatine kinase
CKD	chronic kidney disease
CK-MB	creatine kinase MB
CMV	Cytomegalovirus
CNS	central nervous system
CO_2	carbon dioxide
COPD	chronic obstructive pulmonary disease
C. parapsilosis	*Candida parapsilosis*
CPR	cardiopulmonary resuscitation
CRP	C-reactive protein
C-section	cesarean section
CSF	cerebrospinal fluid
CT	computed tomography
CVA	cerebrovascular accident
CVD	cardiovascular disease
DAT	direct antiglobulin test
DHEA-S	dehydroepiandrosterone sulfate
DIC	disseminated intravascular coagulation
DNase	deoxyribonuclease
DRE	digital rectal exam
dsDNA	double-stranded DNA
DSM-5	*Diagnostic and Statistical Manual of Mental Disorders (Fifth Edition)*
DVT	deep vein thrombosis
EBV	Epstein-Barr virus
ECG	electrocardiogram
ECMO	extracorporeal membrane oxygenation
E. coli	*Escherichia coli*
ED	emergency department
EEG	electroencephalogram
EGF	epidermal growth factor
eGFR	estimated glomerular filtration rate
ELISA	enzyme-linked immunosorbent assay
EMG	electromyogram
ENT	ear, nose, throat
ERCP	endoscopic retrograde cholangiopancreatography
ESR	erythrocyte sedimentation rate
ESRD	end-stage renal disease
FEV	forced expiratory volume

FEV_1	forced expiratory volume in the first second of expiration
FFP	fresh frozen plasma
FISH	fluorescence in situ hybridization
FSH	follicle-stimulating hormone
G6PD	glucose-6-phosphate dehydrogenase
GBM	glomerular basement membrane
GCS	Glasgow Coma Scale
GERD	gastroesophageal reflux disease
GFR	glomerular filtration rate
GGT	ϒ-glutamyl transferase
GI	gastrointestinal
GU	genitourinary
HAART	highly active antiretroviral therapy
HAC	hepatitis A virus
HAV	hepatitis A virus
Hb	hemoglobin
HbA_{1c}	glycated hemoglobin
HBsAg	hepatitis B surface antigen
HBV	hepatitis B virus
HCO_3^-	bicarbonate
HCV	hepatitis C virus
HEV	hepatitis E virus
HF	heart failure
H. influenzae	*Haemophilus influenzae*
HIV	human immunodeficiency virus
HLA	human leukocyte antigen
HPF	high-power field
HPLC	high performance liquid chromatography
HPV	human papillomavirus
H. pylori	*Helicobacter pylori*
HRT	hormone replacement therapy
HSV	herpes simplex virus
HUS	hemolytic uremic syndrome
ICU	intensive care unit
IgA	immunoglobulin A
IgE	immunoglobulin E
IGF-1	insulinlike growth factor-1
IgG	immunoglobulin G
IgM	immunoglobulin M
INR	international normalized ratio
IUD	intrauterine device
IUGR	intrauterine growth retardation
IV	intravenous
JVP	jugular venous pressure
KOH	potassium hydroxide

KUB	kidneys, ureter, bladder
LDH	lactate dehydrogenase
LDL	low-density lipoprotein
LFT	liver function test
LH	luteinizing hormone
L. monocytogenes	*Listeria monocytogenes*
LMWH	low-molecular-weight heparin
LP	lumbar puncture
LSD	lysergic acid diethylamide
MAHA	microangiopathic hemolytic anemia
MAIO	monoamine oxidase inhibitors
MCHC	mean corpuscular hemoglobin concentration
MCV	mean corpuscular volume
MD	muscular dystrophy
MEK	mitogen-activated protein kinase kinase
MELAS	mitochondrial encephalomyopathy, lactic acidosis, and stroke-like episodes
MET	metabolic equivalent task
M. genitalium	*Mycoplasma genitalium*
MI	myocardial infarction
MMSE	Mini-Mental State Exam
MRA	magnetic resonance angiography
MRCP	magnetic resonance cholangiopancreatography
MRI	magnetic resonance imaging
MS	multiple sclerosis
MSE	mental status exam
NAAT	nucleic acid amplification test
NAD	nicotinamide adenine dinucleotide
NICU	neonatal intensive care unit
N. meningitidis	*Neisseria meningitidis*
NSAID	nonsteroidal antiinflammatory drug
NSTEMI	non–ST-segment elevation myocardial infarction
NT-proBNP	N-terminal pro–brain natriuretic peptide
OC	oral contraceptive
OCD	obsessive-compulsive disorder
OTC	over the counter
$PaCO_2$	partial pressure of carbon dioxide
PaO_2	partial pressure of oxygen
PCI	percutaneous coronary intervention
PCR	polymerase chain reaction
PE	pulmonary embolism
PET	positron emission tomography
PID	pelvic inflammatory disease
PPI	proton pump inhibitor
PSA	prostate-specific antigen
PT	prothrombin time

PTH	parathyroid hormone
PTSD	posttraumatic stress disorder
PTT	partial thromboplastin time
PUD	peptic ulcer disease
RA	rheumatoid arthritis
RBC	red blood cell
RDW	red blood cell distribution width
RNA	ribonucleic acid
RSV	respiratory syncytial virus
RT-PCR	reverse transcriptase–polymerase chain reaction
S. aureus	*Streptococcus aureus*
SDH	subdural hematoma
SIDS	sudden infant death syndrome
SLE	systemic lupus erythematosus
SNRI	serotonin and norepinephrine reuptake inhibitor
SPECT	single-photon emission computed tomography
S. pneumoniae	*Streptococcus pneumoniae*
SSRI	selective serotonin reuptake inhibitor
STEMI	ST-segment elevation myocardial infarction
STI	sexually transmitted infection
S. viridans	*Streptococcus viridans*
T_3	triiodothyronine
T_4	thyroxine
TB	tuberculosis
TBI	traumatic brain injury
TBSA	total body surface area
TCA	tricyclic antidepressant
TIA	transient ischemic attack
TIBC	total iron binding capacity
TMJ	temporomandibular joint
TORCH	**to**xoplasmosis, **r**ubella, CMV, HIV, HSV
T. pallidum	*Treponema pallidum*
TSH	thyroid-stimulating hormone (thyrotropin)
tTG	tissue transglutaminase
TTP	thrombotic thrombocytopenic purpura
ULN	upper limit of normal
URTI	upper respiratory tract infection
US	ultrasound
UTI	urinary tract infection
U. urealyticum	*Ureaplasma urealyticum*
UV	ultraviolet
VDRL	Venereal Disease Research Laboratory test
VF	ventricular fibrillation
V/Q scan	ventilation-perfusion scan
VT	ventricular tachycardia
VZV	varicella-zoster virus

W. bancrofti	*Wuchereria bancrofti*
WBC	white blood cell

Index

This index lists clinical presentations and the entities in the differential diagnoses of clinical presentations, in addition to topics in the "pointer" feature of this resource.

Clinical presentations are main entries with bold page numbers. See, for example, *abdominal distention.*

Entities are main entries followed by subentries. The subentries list the clinical presentations in which the entities appear, along with the starting page number of each clinical presentation. See, for example, *abdominal aortic aneurysm.*

When an index entry is both a clinical presentation and an entity in one or more differential diagnoses, it will include both a bolded page number (indicating where it appears as a clinical presentation) and subentries beginning with *and in* (indicating the clinical presentations in which the entry appears as an entity). See, for example, *abdominal mass.*

Pointers are labeled and listed by topic either as main index entries or as subentries under clinical presentations or entities. See, for example, *causes by location (pointer)* under *abdominal pain, acute.*

B

C

F

U

About the author

Dr. Christopher Naugler is a Diagnostic and Clinical Pathologist and Family Physician. He has held a number of senior medical leadership positions including Associate Dean of Undergraduate Medical Education at the Cumming School of Medicine, University of Calgary. Dr. Naugler is the author of 250 scientific publications and several books.

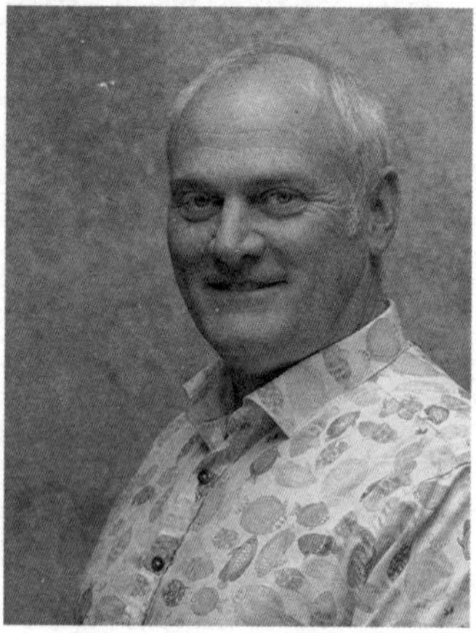